Emergency Psychiatry

Concepts, Methods, and Practices

CRITICAL ISSUES IN PSYCHIATRY
An Educational Series for Residents and Clinicians

Series Editor: Sherwyn M. Woods, M.D., Ph.D.
University of Southern California School of Medicine
Los Angeles, California

Recent volumes in the series:

LAW IN THE PRACTICE OF PSYCHIATRY
Seymour L. Halleck, M.D.

NEUROPSYCHIATRIC FEATURES OF MEDICAL DISORDERS
James W. Jefferson, M.D., and John R. Marshall, M.D.

ADULT DEVELOPMENT: A New Dimension in Psychodynamic Theory
and Practice
Calvin A. Colarusso, M.D., and Robert A. Nemiroff, M.D.

SCHIZOPHRENIA
John S. Strauss, M.D., and William T. Carpenter, Jr., M.D.

EXTRAORDINARY DISORDERS OF HUMAN BEHAVIOR
Edited by Claude T. H. Friedmann, M.D., and Robert A. Faguet, M.D.

MARITAL THERAPY: A Combined Psychodynamic–Behavioral Approach
R. Taylor Segraves, M.D., Ph.D.

TREATMENT INTERVENTIONS IN HUMAN SEXUALITY
Edited by Carol C. Nadelson, M.D., and David B. Marcotte, M.D.

CLINICAL PERSPECTIVES ON THE SUPERVISION OF
PSYCHOANALYSIS AND PSYCHOTHERAPY
Edited by Leopold Caligor, Ph.D., Philip M. Bromberg, Ph.D.,
and James D. Meltzer, Ph.D.

MOOD DISORDERS : Toward a New Psychobiology
Peter C. Whybrow, M.D., Hagop S. Akiskal, M.D., and
William T. McKinney, Jr., M.D.

EMERGENCY PSYCHIATRY: Concepts, Methods, and Practices
Edited by Ellen L. Bassuk, M.D., and Ann W. Birk, Ph.D.

DRUG AND ALCOHOL ABUSE: A Clinical Guide to Diagnosis
and Treatment, Second Edition
Marc A. Schuckit, M.D.

THE RACE AGAINST TIME: Psychotherapy and Psychoanalysis
in the Second Half of Life
Edited by Robert A. Nemiroff, M.D., and Calvin A. Colarusso, M.D.

A Continuation Order Plan is available for this series. A continuation order will bring
delivery of each new volume immediately upon publication. Volumes are billed only
upon actual shipment. For further information please contact the publisher.

Emergency Psychiatry
Concepts, Methods, and Practices

Edited by

Ellen L. Bassuk, M.D.
Harvard Medical School
Boston, Massachusetts

and

Ann W. Birk, Ph.D.
Learning Therapies, Inc.
Newton, Massachusetts

Plenum Press • New York and London

Library of Congress Cataloging in Publication Data

Main entry under title:

Emergency psychiatry.

(Critical issues in psychiatry)
Includes bibliographies and index.
1. Crisis intervention (Psychiatry) 2. Psychiatric emergencies. I. Bassuk, Ellen L.,
1945–   . II. Birk, Ann W., 1944–   . III. Series. [DNLM: 1. Crisis Intervention. 2. Emergencies. 3. Mental Disorders. 4. Mental Health Services. WM 401 E534]
RC480.6.E45   1984   616.89′025   84-11709
ISBN 0-306-41655-7

© 1984 Plenum Press, New York
A Division of Plenum Publishing Corporation
233 Spring Street, New York, N.Y. 10013

Printed in the United States of America

Contributors

Iris Lee Bagwell, M.Ed., Director, Adolescent Day Center, West-Ros-Park Mental Health Center, Roslindale, Massachusetts 02131

Arthur Barsky, III, M.D., Chief, Acute Psychiatry Service, Massachusetts General Hospital, Boston, Massachusetts 02114, and Assistant Professor of Psychiatry, Harvard Medical School, Boston, Massachusetts 02115

Ellen L. Bassuk, M.D., Associate Professor of Psychiatry, Harvard Medical School, Boston, Massachusetts 02115

Michael J. Bennett, M.D., Staff Psychiatrist, Harvard Community Health Plan, Boston, Massachusetts 02215, and formerly Chief of Mental Health Services, Kenmore Center, Harvard Community Health Plan, Boston, Massachusetts 02115

Henry A. Beyer, J.D., Interim Director, Center for Law and Health Sciences, Boston University School of Law, Boston, Massachusetts 02215

Ann W. Birk, Ph.D., Learning Therapies, Inc., Newton, Massachusetts 02163

Lee Birk, M.D., Associate Clinical Professor of Psychiatry, Harvard Medical School, Boston, Massachusetts 02115

W. R. Cote, R.N.C., C.A.C., Director of Outpatient and Emergency Services, Northeast Kingdom Mental Health Services, St. Johnsbury, Vermont 05819

James M. Donovan, Ph.D., Assistant Professor of Psychiatry, Harvard Medical School, Boston, Massachusetts 02115, and Staff Psychiatrist, Harvard Community Health Plan, Boston, Massachusetts 02215

Rosemary Evans, M.S.W., Social Work Consultant, New England Resource Center for Protective Services, Judge Baker Guidance Center, Boston, Massachusetts 02115

Ronnie Fuchs, M.D., Chief Resident in Psychiatry, Beth Israel Hospital, Boston, Massachusetts 02215, and Clinical Fellow in Psychiatry, Harvard Medical School, Boston, Massachusetts 02115

A. J. Gelenberg, M.D., Associate Professor of Psychiatry, Harvard Medical School, Boston, Massachusetts 02115

Barbara Schuler Gilmore, R.N., M.S.N., C.S., Coordinator of Outpatient Mental Health Service and The Crisis and Emergency Team, Newton-Wellesley Hospital, Newton Lower Falls, Massachusetts 02162

Roberta S. Isberg, M.D., Resident in Psychiatry, Beth Israel Hospital, Boston, Massachusetts 02215, and Clinical Fellow in Psychiatry, Harvard Medical School, Boston, Massachusetts 02115

James P. Jones, Ph.D., Psychologist, Emergency Service, West-Ros-Park Mental Health Center, Roslindale, Massachusetts 02131; present address: Department of Mental Health, Cape Ann Area Office, Beverley, Massachusetts 01919

Alvin Kahn, M.D., Clinical Instructor in Psychiatry, Harvard Medical School, Boston, Massachusetts 02115

Helene W. Kress, A.C.S.W., Director of Social Service, Framingham Hospital, Framingham, Massachusetts 01701

F. D. Lisnow, M.Ed., C.A.C., Director of Consultation Education and Community Care Programs, Northeast Kingdom Mental Health Services, St. Johnsbury, Vermont 05819

Sarah L. Minden, M.D., Instructor in Psychiatry, Harvard Medical School, and Associate Physician (Psychiatry), Brigham and Women's Hospital, Boston, Massachusetts 02115

Steven M. Mirin, M.D., Associate Clinical Professor of Psychiatry, Harvard Medical School, Boston, Massachusetts 02115, Medical Director, Westwood Lodge Hospital, Westwood, Massachusetts 02090, and Research Psychiatrist, Alcohol and Drug Abuse Research Center, McLean Hospital, Belmont, Massachusetts 02178

Peter J. Panzarino, Jr., M.D., Instructor of Psychiatry, Harvard Medical School, Boston, Massachusetts 02115, and Staff Psychiatrist, McLean Hospital, Belmont, Massachusetts 02178

Mark R. Proctor, M.D., Clinical Instructor in Psychiatry, Harvard Medical School, Boston, Massachusetts 02115, and Director, Stress Disorders Program, Department of Psychiatry, Beth Israel Hospital, Boston, Massachusetts 02215

Daniel W. Rosenn, M.D., Instructor in Psychiatry, Harvard Medical School, and Director of Ambulatory Services, Hall–Mercer Children's Center, McLean Hospital, Belmont, Massachusetts 02178

Ronnie F. Ryback, M.S.W., A.C.S.W., Senior Clinical Social Worker, Specialty Unit, Beth Israel Hospital, Boston, Massachusetts 02215

Steven E. Samuel, M.Ed., Formerly Assistant Director of Emergency Service, West-Ros-Park Mental Health Center, Roslindale, Massachusetts 02131; present address: Counseling Psychology Department, Temple University, Philadelphia, Pennsylvania 19122

Maria C. Sauzier, M.D., Assistant Clinical Professor in Psychiatry, Tufts University Medical School, Boston, Massachusetts 02111, and Clinical Instructor in Psychiatry, Harvard Medical School, Boston, Massachusetts 02115

S. C. Schoonover, M.D., Instructor of Psychiatry, Harvard Medical School, Boston, Massachusetts 02115

Andrew E. Skodol, M.D., Associate Professor of Psychiatry, College of Physicians and Surgeons of Columbia University, New York, New York 10032, and Research Psychiatrist, Biometrics Research Department, New York State Psychiatric Institute, New York, New York 10032

Florence Sullivan, M.S.W., Social Work Consultant, New England Resource Center for Protective Services, Judge Baker Guidance Center, Boston, Massachusetts 02115

Roger D. Weiss, M.D., Instructor in Psychiatry, Harvard Medical School, Boston, Massachusetts 02115, and Psychiatrist in Charge, Drug Dependence Treatment Unit, McLean Hospital, Belmont, Massachusetts 02178

Foreword

This eagerly awaited volume occupies an important place in the series Critical Issues in Psychiatry. Most mental health professionals are quite at home with ordinary day-to-day crises of clinical practice but relatively unprepared for the true psychiatric emergency. Such emergencies are too infrequent for most of us to experience a real sense of competence. On the other hand, emergency room psychiatrists as well as residents and other trainees have long wished for a truly comprehensive textbook that would cover the spectrum of emergency psychiatry. This book is just such a definitive and comprehensive volume for the specialist, while at the same time a clear, succinct, and comprehensive reference for the clinician.

The authors consistently present a systematic model of emergency care, emphasizing the interconnection between the process of emergency intervention and the specific features of clinical crisis. They are true to the principle that one's system of care should be built on priorities. It is immediately apparent that these are highly experienced clinicians as well as teachers.

It is difficult to imagine a clinical situation that is not addressed by this book. It includes chapters on triage, assessment, and treatment planning; emergencies associated with all the various psychopathologies; age groups from childhood to old age; the emergency management of violent and suicidal patients as well as rape and disaster victims; emergencies secondary to substance abuse and prescribed medications; psychotherapeutic and psychopharmacologic intervention; as well as the relevant legal, social, and community issues involved in emergency care.

This book belongs to that select few that I always keep within easy reach and which I find indispensable to clinical practice.

Sherwyn M. Woods

Preface

The hallmark of emergency psychiatry is, in some sense, its immediate availability. Unlike other forms of psychiatric treatment that rely for their structure on the scheduling of regular sessions, emergency care is literally on-line psychiatry. The physical setting, the staff and its expertise, the diagnostic instruments, and therapeutic aids constitute a self-sufficient unit whose collective function is the rapid containment of psychiatric crises.

The burden of on-line capability is twofold: There is, on the one hand, the practical necessity of treating a high, but irregularly spaced, volume of walk-in admissions, and there is, on the other hand, the technical correlate of any emergency care system, the demand that clinical omniscience unite in some form with limited intervention and rapid disposition. While the emergency clinician must be prepared to recognize and manage virtually any disturbance within the range and variation of potential psychiatric crises, his actual role is transient and tightly circumscribed. This irreducible gap between capability— the breadth and complexity of clinical skills required of front-line caretakers— and delivery—the actual scope of their interventions—constitutes the paradoxical core of emergency psychiatry.

This volume evolved from a wish to translate this essential clinical paradox into a systematic model for emergency care. The model was developed in two stages: Originally it grew out of the conceptual framework housing an experimental teaching curriculum for multidisciplinary emergency caretakers. With funding from the National Institute of Mental Health's Division of Manpower Research and Demonstration (NIMH #5 T24 MH15958), and with the collaboration of the Vermont Department of Mental Health and the 10 Vermont Community Mental Health Centers, this training program was developed and tested. The program emphasized the interconnection between the process of emergency intervention and the specific features of clinical crisis. This initial phase of the project involved many hours of training, testing, revising, and refining to the point where the training program could be presented in the form of a videotape instructional module focusing on assessment, mental status examination, organic mental disorders, psychosis, and depression.

For this part of the project we are very grateful to Stephen C. Schoonover, M.D., from the Beth Israel Hospital; Douglas Jacobs, M.D., from Cambridge Hospital; Helene Kress, A.C.S.W., from Framingham Union Hospital; and Sandra S. Fox, Ph.D., from Judge Baker Guidance Clinic, who helped to make the training program a success, and to Terry Primack, who devoted long hours to the development of the videotape materials. Without the cooperation, support, and feedback of our trainees and the emergency services personnel of Vermont, the training program would lack much of its present form and substance. Special thanks to Dorothy King, who coordinated the emergency personnel in Vermont, and to Richard Searle, John Pierce, and Andrea Blanch of the Vermont Department of Mental Health, and to Joe Rainville, William Cote, and Nancy DeVries for their ongoing involvement and support. Robert Apsler, Ph.D., from Cambridge Hospital, coordinated the research effort. We are very appreciative of his work.

The second stage in the development of a provisional model for emergency psychiatric care came into place as three separate pathways emerged. The first led through a decade of doing the real work of emergency psychiatry, and always wondering if there was a better way. The second pathway emerged as the training project neared an end, and it became evident that emergency psychiatric management could be taught—and grasped. The third route involved a decade of hard thinking about psychiatry's conceptual apparatus: its classification system, treatment paradigms, and theoretical biases. If psychiatry could be said to have a collection of shared or cohesive conceptual underpinnings, nowhere would they be thrown into greater relief than in the emergency setting, where symptoms possess an urgent clarity and treatment strategies are directly tested by a critical reality. In the process of sharing, then blending and refining our ideas, the format for this volume took shape.

The decision to invite a variety of authors to contribute chapters was made, in large measure, because of the particular expertise each brings to his subject. But beyond that, it is also a reflection of the fact that emergency psychiatry is a complex, wide-ranging field whose practitioners will (and should) display a diversity of styles and approaches, however, uniform we might like to make its theoretical constructs. We would like to thank the authors not only for their visible contributions to these volumes but for the invisible contributions as well: cooperation, support, and patience. Many of these chapters underwent extensive revision as the editors tried to grapple with shifts in their own thoughts about emergency care. It has not been easy to unify the chapters so that they form a cohesive whole. Our greatest concern was that in doing the difficult task of reweaving style and content to fit our vision of an integrated work, we not sacrifice or violate the richness and individuality of the different chapters.

Special thanks to Sam Silverstein, Ph.D., and Beatrice Shriver, Ph.D., from NIMH, who actively supported our efforts; to Betty James and Associates for typing wizardry; to Hilary Evans, our editor at Plenum, who remained enthusiastic about the project despite its changes in direction; and finally, to Sherwyn Woods, M.D., Ph.D. for his excellent suggestions and encouragement.

Note: Initially the text contained both male and female pronouns in sentences that did not have a specific referent. To improve clarity and flow, however, we made an editorial decision to include only masculine pronouns.

Ellen L. Bassuk

Boston, Massachusetts

Ann W. Birk

Newton, Massachusetts

The Organizational Framework

The organization of this book is based on two principles: (1) that emergency psychiatry is a blend of process (see Parts I, II, and VIII) and content issues (see Parts III–VII describing Patients and Clinical Syndromes), and (2) that it is a system of care built on priorities.

Following the first organizational criterion, we arranged the chapters in this book according to whether they dealt more with the general process of care or more with the patients and clinical syndromes. That format, however, partially violated our second organizational principle: namely, that medical or psychiatric urgency should dictate the order of topics.

Our solution involves a compromise. The book itself has been arranged to preserve the distinction between what the clinician needs to know in advance and what the patient presents. The generic chapters on legal, psychopharmacological, and psychological management appear first—before the chapters concerning the patients and clinical syndromes. Although Part VIII also discusses process issues, we included it at the end because it refers to specific circumstances and approaches unique to certain settings.

The organizational framework contains a map of the book arranged according to technical stages, beginning with triage and followed by assessment, management, and treatment planning (see Figure 1 for a map of the process of emergency care). Under each, we refer to relevant chapters in the text. The first references in any particular group are to chapters discussing the most

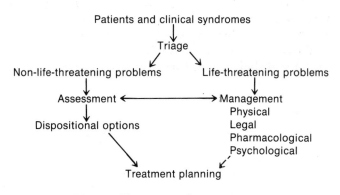

Figure 1. The process of emergency care.

Table 1. The Organizational Framework

Triage
  1. The First Few Minutes (Chapter 2)
  2. Alcohol Use and Abuse (Chapter 8)
  3. Drug Use and Abuse (Chapter 9)
  4. Emergency Management of Potentially Violent Patients (Chapter 6)
  5. Emergency Care of Suicidal Patients (Chapter 7)
  6. Part VII, Chapters 18 and 19; discusses children and elderly patients
  7. Part V; discusses organic etiologies of behavioral, cognitive, and affective disturbances
  8. All other clinical chapters
Assessment
  1. The Concept of Emergency Care (Chapter 1)
  2. Parts III–VII, inclusive; discuss the assessment of specific kinds of emergency patients and clinical syndromes
Management issues and options
  1. The Concept of Emergency Care (Chapter 1)
  2. The First Few Minutes; contains a discussion of all forms of management, including physical, required during the initial contact with the patient (Chapter 2)
  3. Part II—Chapters 3–5; discusses legal, pharmacological, and psychological management issues
  4. Part VIII—Chapters 20–25; discusses management issues and options in specific settings and under special circumstances
  5. Parts III–VII, inclusive; discuss the management of specific groups of emergency patients and clinical syndromes
Treatment planning
  1. The Concept of Emergency Care (Chapter 1)
  2. Parts III–VII, inclusive; discuss the treatment planning of specific groups of emergency patients and clinical syndromes
  3. Part VIII—Chapters 20–25; discusses treatment planning under special circumstances and in specific settings

general treatment of a topic, the latter references are to the most specific. (See Table 1 for a list of the chapters.)

For example, to learn more about general management issues, a reader might begin with the overview chapter, "The Concept of Emergency Care." For management specific to a psychotic patient who might lose control, the reader is next referred to "The First Few Minutes," to the chapter on violence, and later to the relevant sections of the legal and psychopharmacological chapters. Where violence is a feature of other clinical syndromes, the reader is finally referred to appropriate sections of the chapters in Part V. Patients and Clinical Syndromes 3: Behavioral, Cognitive, and Affective Disturbances.

Contents

I. Emergency Care: An Overview

1. The Concept of Emergency Care 3

Ann W. Birk, Ph.D., and Ellen L. Bassuk, M.D.

1. Introduction 3
2. Emergency Psychiatry: A Systematic Approach 4
3. Emergency Psychiatry: The Process 8
4. Special Clinical Applications 14
5. Conclusion 17
   References 17

II. The Process of Emergency Care

2. The First Few Minutes: Identifying and Managing Life-Threatening Emergencies 21

Ellen L. Bassuk, M.D., and Andrew E. Skodol, M.D.

1. Introduction 21
2. Initial Assessment and Psychological Management 21
3. Determination of the Problem 23
4. Physical Management 25
5. Pharmacologic Management 29
6. Medical Management 31
7. Conclusion 35
   References 35

3. Legal Issues in a Psychiatric Emergency Setting 37

Henry A. Beyer, J.D.

1. Introduction 37
2. Autonomy, Privacy, and Informed Consent 37

  3. Informed Consent 38
  4. Substitute Consent 40
  5. Written versus Oral Consent 41
  6. Emergencies 42
  7. Confidentiality 44
  8. Special Mental Health Laws 46
  9. Dangerousness 47
 10. The Management of Dangerousness 48
 11. Least Restrictive Alternative 49
 12. Right to Treatment 49
 13. Right to Refuse Treatment 50
 14. Legal Liability 53
 15. Standards of Care 53
 16. Suicide 54
 17. The Hardest Part 56
     Notes 58

**4. General Principles of Pharmacologic Management in the Emergency
   Setting** 61

*Ellen L. Bassuk, M.D., Peter J. Panzarino, Jr., M.D.,
and Stephen C. Schoonover, M.D.*

  1. Introduction 61
  2. Evaluating the Patient and Choosing Medication 61
  3. Applying General Principles of Drug Use to the Emergency Setting. . 69
  4. Forming a Relationship with the Patient 71
  5. Conclusion 72
     References 73

5. The Therapeutic Stance 75

Alvin Kahn, M.D.

III. Patients and Clinical Syndromes 1: Potentially Life-Threatening

6. Emergency Management of Potentially Violent Patients 83

Andrew E. Skodol, M.D.

  1. Introduction 83
  2. General Assessment Issues 83
  3. Assessing and Managing the Potentially Violent Patient 85
  4. Treatment Options 91

5. Disposition 91
6. Conclusion 95
   References 95

7. Emergency Care of Suicidal Patients 97

Ellen L. Bassuk, M.D.

1. Introduction 97
2. Clinical Checklist for Assessment 99
3. Management 106
4. Treatment Planning 107
5. Conclusion 110
   Appendix: The Rating Scales 111
   References 124

IV. Patients and Clinical Syndromes 2: Medication-Related/Toxic Origins

8. Alcohol Use and Abuse 129

W. R. Cote, R.N.C., C.A.C., and F. D. Lisnow, M.Ed., C.A.C.

1. Introduction 129
2. Definitions 129
3. Pharmacology 130
4. Acute Intoxication 131
5. Sequelae of Chronic Intoxication 131
6. Alcohol Withdrawal 133
7. General Approach to Treatment Planning 137
8. Conclusion 138
   Bibliography 138

9. Drug Use and Abuse 141

Steven M. Mirin, M.D., and Roger D. Weiss, M.D.

1. Abuse of Opiate Drugs 141
2. Abuse of Central Nervous System (CNS) Depressants 147
3. Abuse of CNS Stimulants/Amphetamines 154
4. Abuse of CNS Stimulants/Cocaine 158
5. Abuse of Hallucinogens 160
6. Phencyclidine (PCP) Abuse 165
7. Marijuana Use and Abuse 168
8. Inhalant Abuse 173

9. Summary 174
Bibliography 175

10. *Emergency Presentations Related to Psychiatric Medication* 181
Stephen C. Schoonover, M.D., and Alan J. Gelenberg, M.D.

1. Introduction 181
2. Lithium Toxicity 181
3. Extrapyramidal Effects 183
4. Anticholinergic Syndromes 189
5. Conclusion 191
References 191

V. Patients and Clinical Syndromes 3: Behavioral, Cognitive, and Affective Disturbances

11. *Acute Psychoses* 195
Arthur Barsky, III, M.D.

1. Overview 195
2. Triage 196
3. Assessment 196
4. Differential Diagnosis 203
5. Management 209
6. Patient–Evaluator Interaction 213
7. Treatment Planning 214
References 217

12. *Presentation of Depression in an Emergency Setting* 219
Ronnie Fuchs, M.D.

1. Introduction 219
2. Assessment 220
3. Management and Disposition 222
4. Clinical Applications 224
5. Summary 231
Selected Reading 231

13. *Emergency Care of Anxious Patients* 233
Roberta S. Isberg, M.D.

1. Introduction 233
2. Assessment 234

3. Treatment 245
4. Conclusion 250
   Appendix 250
   References 259

VI. Patients and Clinical Syndromes 4: Victims of Situational Crises

14. Psychological Management of Disaster Victims 263

   Mark R. Proctor, M.D.

1. Introduction 263
2. Psychological Reactions to Disasters 263
3. Assessment 266
4. Management 267
5. Conclusion 270
   References 270

15. Emergency Care of Rape Victims 271

   Maria C. Sauzier, M.D.

1. Introduction 271
2. Definitions 271
3. Popular Myths versus the Facts 272
4. The Rape Crisis 273
5. Management 276
6. Conclusion 282
   References 282

16. Emergency Care of Battered Women 285

   Ronnie F. Ryback, M.S.W., A.C.S.W.

1. Introduction 285
2. Definitions 285
3. Background 285
4. The Victims, Their Families, and the Abusers 286
5. The Emergency Presentation 287
6. Assessment and Management of Identified Victims 289
7. Conclusion 291
   References 292

17. Child Abuse and Neglect 293

   Florence Sullivan, M.S.W., and Rosemary Evans, M.S.W.

   1. Introduction 293
   2. Dynamics of Child Abuse and Neglect 293
   3. Legal Issues 295
   4. Evaluation and Intervention 296
   5. Follow-Up 299
   6. Summary 299
        Bibliography 300

VII. Patients and Clinical Syndromes 5: Special Populations

18. Psychiatric Emergencies in Children and Adolescents 303

   Daniel W. Rosenn, M.D.

    1. Introduction 303
    2. Description of Childhood Psychiatric Emergencies 304
    3. General Considerations 304
    4. The Emergency Intervention 306
    5. Classification of Psychiatric Emergencies in Childhood and
         Adolescence 310
    6. The Specific Syndromes 313
    7. Suicidal Behaviors in Children and Adolescents 314
    8. Homicidal Behaviors in Children and Adolescents 325
    9. Firesetting 332
   10. Runaway Children and Adolescents 337
   11. School Refusal 340
   12. Other Problems 346
   13. Conclusion 346
         References 346

19. Elderly Psychiatric Emergency Patients 351

   Sarah L. Minden, M.D.

   1. Introduction 351
   2. Overview 351
   3. Working with the Geriatric Patient 352
   4. Assessment, Management, and Treatment 354
   5. Clinical Presentations 363
   6. Conclusion 367
        References 367

VIII. Special Settings, Circumstances, and Approaches

20. **Managing Emergencies in the Practice of Psychotherapy** 373

    Lee Birk, M.D., and Ann W. Birk, Ph.D.

1. Introduction 373
2. Types of Genuine Emergencies 374
3. Pseudoemergencies 376
4. Management 377
5. Conclusion 382
   Postscript 382

21. **General Hospital Psychiatric Emergency Services** 383

    Ellen L. Bassuk, M.D.

1. Introduction 383
2. Organization of Services 384
3. Staffing Patterns 389
4. Conclusion 390
   References 391

22. **Psychiatric Emergency Care in Resource-Poor Areas** 393

    W. R. Cote, R.M.C., C.A.C.

1. Introduction 393
2. The Intervention 394
3. Conclusion 398
   Bibliography 399

23. **Psychiatric Home Visiting Services** 401

    Steven E. Samuel, M.Ed., Iris Lee Bagwell, M.Ed.,
    and James P. Jones, Ph.D.

1. Introduction 401
2. Function, Composition, and Structure 401
3. Intervention Techniques 402
4. Conclusion 405
   Bibliography 405

24. **The Telephone in Psychiatric Emergencies** 407

    Barbara Schuler Gilmore, R.N., M.S.N., C.S.

1. Introduction 407
2. Hotlines 407

3. Crisis Centers and Other Emergency Facilities 408
4. Personnel 408
5. The Emergency Call 409
6. Conclusion 414
   References 414

25. *Role of Family and Networks in Emergency Psychotherapy* 417

   Helene W. Kress, A.C.S.W.

1. Introduction 417
2. Who Are the Significant Others? 417
3. Assessment 418
4. Management 420
5. Conclusion 422
   References 423

26. *Crisis Groups* 425

   Michael J. Bennett, M.D., and James M. Donovan, Ph.D.

1. Introduction 425
2. Why a Group? 426
3. Review of the Literature 426
4. Patient Evaluation and Selection 428
5. The Open Group in General 429
6. Technical Aspects 430
7. Treatment Outcome 433
8. Summary 435
   References 435

Index 437

I

Emergency Care
An Overview

The Concept of Emergency Care

Ann W. Birk, Ph.D., and Ellen L. Bassuk, M.D.

1. Introduction

Although it is generally assumed that emergency services provide care for persons with urgent, predominantly life-threatening problems, most emergencies are self-determined, if not actually elective.[1] When a person decides to call the local crisis center or go to the emergency department for help, his decision is based on a number of considerations. These include (1) the presence of an urgent situation defying his usual standards for affect, conduct, or experience; (2) the failure of his psychosocial network to circumscribe or to ameliorate the crisis; and (3) the convenience and immediate accessibility of the emergency service.

Psychiatric emergencies are not merely the immediate by-product of unbearable internal distress or psychobiological disturbance, however. They are the culmination of a complicated interplay of past and present events, biochemical and psychological processes, and individual, interpersonal, and systems dynamics. Erupting violence or heightened suicidal despair are discrete, highly visible points along a temporal continuum whose segments are otherwise only occasionally observed and seldom reliably documented. Strictly speaking, genuine psychiatric emergencies, such as these, indicate a serious problem requiring professional intervention. They occur when "general functioning has been severely impaired and the individual rendered incompetent or unable to assume responsibility"[2] (p. 547). However, these define one type of "crisis situation" calling for rapid symptom containment. Many others may require less intensive "emergency" interventions and include anticipated life transitions, traumatic experiences, maturational/developmental stages, psychopathological decompensation, existential despair, and even routine problems in daily living. While these and other situations define occasions for seeking help, they do not necessarily represent the reasons. To identify these, the clinician must understand the interplay of three factors: (1) the larger sociopolitical context in which care is provided, (2) the characteristics of the patients, and (3) the unique attributes of the emergency setting.

Twenty years ago (1963), the Community Mental Health Centers Act mandated emergency care an essential service. Since that time, deinstitutionali-

Ann W. Birk, Ph.D. • Learning Therapies, Inc., Newton Massachusetts 02163.   *Ellen L. Bassuk, M.D.* • Harvard Medical School, Boston, Massachusetts 02115.

zation, increasing medical specialization, and the proliferation of brief treatment modalities have contributed to the rapid growth of emergency facilities.[1,3] However, these services have barely kept pace with rapidly increasing demand. Groups of persons previously unconnected to psychiatry were brought under the protective cover of an expanded mental health network; these included the "worried well" and persons whose age, socioeconomic status, and general level of adaptive functioning interfered with the formation of more traditional alliances within the health care establishment. Moreover, the emergency setting's ready accessibility, convenience, anonymity, and liberal third-party reimbursement policies attracted young, unemployed, poor, and other disenfranchised persons. These complex trends contributed to gradual transformation of the emergency ward into a drop-in center whose emphasis concurrently shifted from rapid assessment and prompt disposition to immediate and sometimes definitive management. Within this context the traditional model of emergency care—evaluation and referral—has been gradually supplanted by services offering comprehensive and immediate treatment.

Although patients who use the emergency setting have common demographic and sociological characteristics, their symptoms, complaints, and needs conform to no single psychiatric profile.[4] Acute symptoms reflect the entire diagnostic spectrum. They are sometimes psychosocial in origin and may be complicated by underlying medical or psychiatric disturbances; at other times there are no discrete pathological conditions save a palpable deficiency in the patient's quality of life. Whether these persons present with "true" emergencies or with other needs, all require individualized care.

Conceptual paradigms emphasize the importance of grounding treatment decisions in solid etiologic foundations, but expediency has forced emergency interventions to begin at once and proceed quickly— most often with only a minimum of historical and clinical data and an alliance with the patient that is, at best, quite tenuous. The patient's urgency and the constraints of the setting conspire to collapse the process of emergency care into its densest form where exhaustive data collection, complicated psychodynamic hypotheses, and verifiable diagnostic assignments have no place. Frequently, a single intervention must embody complex therapeutic aims. Furthermore, appropriate dispositional alternatives are often unavailable, or the patient may not follow through on referral recommendations. The economics and exigencies of emergency care delivery nonetheless demand rapid processing of a large volume of patients.

The fact that hundreds of patients are evaluated and treated in emergency settings means that some part of this enormously complex work gets done. Studies have shown that what gets done depends in large measure on practical necessity balanced by normative general standards for assessment and treatment. What is needed, however, is a systematic approach to, or model for, crisis psychiatry that takes into account the unique characteristics of the patients, clinical process, and emergency setting.

2. Emergency Psychiatry: A Systematic Approach

The growth of brief treatment modalities has stemmed from the long overdue recognition that certain patients, for reasons of social class, capacity for insight, motivation, or financial status, could not be treated by long-term re-constructive psychoanalytic psychotherapy. Changing commitments within the professional community called for the development of immediate, effective, and economically feasible treatment alternatives for these patients. Although the incorporation of brief psychotherapies within the professional armamentarium was viewed by some as an ignominious surrender to the demands of expediency, it nonetheless infused contemporary psychiatry with a spirit of eclecticism, innovation, and pragmatism. The result, in practical terms, has been a proliferation of therapeutic modalities. These include short-term individual psychotherapy as well as systems approaches that are committed to the time-limited treatment of a central problem or target symptom. The result, in social terms, has been a professional division between those who regard the brief therapies as second-class, superficial, and only temporarily effective (if at all), and those who see them as effective, sufficient, and even necessary for certain patients.

The controversy about the efficacy of short-term treatment centers on the question of depth—depth of therapeutic focus and of change. The critics contend that depth of change can be no greater than depth of therapeutic focus, the latter correlating with duration of treatment. The change that occurs, they argue, has to do with symptom relief, possibly also with enhanced adaptive function, but not with psychodynamic restructuring. Assuming that symptoms will recur so long as the pathogenetic intrapsychic organization remains, the brief therapies are, *a priori*, of limited efficacy.

The defenders argue that depth of therapeutic focus need not be tied to treatment duration, and that depth of change need not correlate with depth of therapeutic focus. Assuming that symptom relief or superficial environmental manipulation may promote a shift in ego function that in turn catalyzes spontaneous dynamic reorganization, the time-limited psychotherapies can, *a priori*, engender permanent change in some patients.

Without begging the question of whether a single or brief intervention achieves symptom relief or dynamic change, it should be emphasized that the depth and locus of therapeutic agency in any type of psychiatric treatment are highly variable. They depend on the patient, the nature of the presenting symptoms, the quality of the therapeutic relationship, the particular nexus of psychobiological and psychosocial forces, and the tractability of key pathogenetic factors. Until psychiatric theory successfully substantiates the mechanisms of psychopathology with empirical evidence, hypotheses about therapeutic agency and efficacy will continue to stand strictly outside the limits of "proof." It cannot be argued too strongly, however, that no single treatment format can be applied with equal effectiveness to all psychiatric patients, nor can any eclectic commitment to rapid, immediate, and effective treatment options afford to ignore the subtle understanding of intrapsychic dynamics distilled from traditional long-term methodology.[5] The ultimate question should not be whether psychoanalytic psychotherapy is better than time-limited modalities, but how the assets of each can be combined to create a uniform methodology sufficiently effective, flexible, and brief to treat the volume, complexity, and variety of emergency patients.

The process of emergency psychotherapy involves an interplay of complicated factors. There is first and foremost the patient: individualized in personality, history, and fact, but sharing with others diagnostic labels and psychodynamic patterns. The patient is neither wholly unique nor a statistical figure; as a consequence, he requires an integrated approach that is both tailored and general. Under the best of circumstances, he must briefly describe his situation and clarify his concerns or requests. He must balance his expectations against his help-seeking stance, negotiate the oddly intimate interaction with a professional helper, and leave with the presenting distress relieved. Under the most typical circumstances, the patient has difficulty identifying the problem, presenting his history, and labeling his key personal and interpersonal assets and liabilities.

There is secondarily the clinician: a blend of personal history, professional training, experience, and theoretical orientation. Within a highly pressured time frame he must evaluate the patient for high-risk conditions and identify medically or psychiatrically urgent symptoms. He must organize his impressions of the crisis and try to understand why the patient chose the emergency setting rather than some other avenue. He must determine the precipitating events or stresses and establish the patient's baseline level of functioning from which to estimate the severity of pathology and its capacity to disrupt normal behavior. He must get a sense of the patient's interpersonal network, why it failed to contain the current crisis, and whether it will help to promote the patient's return to baseline, or obstruct it. He must manage the current crisis by appropriate, time-limited means. Finally, he must forecast both immediate and long-term outcome and balance this knowledge against the availability of actual dispositional alternatives. And during all of this, he must establish and maintain a working relationship with the patient and with the persons who accompanied him. He should offer reassurance, instruction, and clarification, and finally effect a successful transition to the next stage of treatment whether it is hospitalization, outpatient treatment, family therapy, or long-term monitoring of psychoactive medication—assuming, of course, that the patient can accept, use, pay for, and be supported by the treatment in question.

There is thirdly the setting: hectic, impersonal, and pressured by the need to stretch limited personnel and resources over a broader and broader base. Increasing use of emergency settings and serious gaps in the immediately available community network further stress the emergency clinician's capacity to arrange creative and individualized treatment programs.

And finally, there is the theoretical treatment structure, uniquely formed by the clinician's individual interpretation but based on a solid foundation of conceptual premises, methods, and technical principles. The cornerstone of emergency psychotherapy is its active, focused, goal-directed therapeutic stance. The duration of the intervention is severely limited, the scope of the therapeutic objective is correspondingly circumscribed, and the focus of the interview necessarily restricted. The resultant clinical process therefore combines traditional assessment and therapeutic approaches to produce a directed, mutually interactive effort. The central goal is to define and treat a focal problem, usually the conflictual area "nearest the surface." The choice of focus is central to the delineation of treatment objectives and disposition, but it may not be obvious. Indeed, defining an appropriate focus may be the dominant clinical task during the initial stage of the intervention.

The focus of any short-term strategy is partially determined by the internal organization of the problem to be addressed; emergency interventions are no different. Defining how a particular crisis is organized, however, is not easy, but the task can be simplified considerably by imposing a model on the specific situation and sorting relevant factors by category. In its simplest form, a psychiatric crisis is composed of two types of events, some operating as causes, agents, predisposing factors, precipitating events, or pathogenetic mechanisms and others as reactions, symptoms, effects, or consequences. It goes without saying that in actual fact, causes and effects tend to overlap, but the distinction is still not without heuristic value.

Under this model, psychiatric emergencies could in theory form three groups: (1) Cause and effect are clear and identified: that is, symptoms result from a specifiable cause; (2) effects or symptoms are known, but the etiology is either unknown or indeterminate; and (3) only a clearly identified predisposing condition or agent is present; effects or long-term sequelae are, as yet, undetermined. Examples of each include extreme agitation following ingestion of a toxic substance; mood disturbance with no clear-cut precipitant; and trauma, such as rape or death of a loved one, with a typical pattern of short-term symptomatology but no long-term effects yet evident.

The initial clinical tasks conforming to this classification involve (1) screening for identifiable precipitants, particularly treatable organic or medical etiologies; (2) formulating a treatment plan to alter or remove the identified causal conditions by the most effective short-term technique, such as medication, or referral for long-term treatment; and (3) using strategic forecasting to manage the short-term symptomatology and obviate the possibility of longer-range traumatic consequences.

The goal in each of these three general categories is to formulate a simple working hypothesis of causal relations that led to the current crisis. The hypothesis should use a minimum of inferential leaps and be based on the available evidence. It may be difficult to establish such a hypothesis, however, either because the relevant information is lacking or because some psychiatric effects have as yet no identified causes. Once a causal relationship is posited, the clinician must then determine the patient's current and past level of functioning, and the quality of his psychosocial network. On the basis of an assessment of the interplay among these factors, he must begin to plan an approach to treatment. When causal factors are unclear, the focus of therapeutic intent is not the distal end of the causal chain but the symptom cluster, where alleviating target symptoms may be the most ambitious aim of treatment. In other cases where the precipitants of psychiatric crisis are clearly defined, the treatment objective is to modify or remove these antecedent conditions by any effective technique—medication, environmental manipulation, crisis support, systems intervention, hospitalization, or insight.

In skeletal form, the emergency intervention is structured to address the most immediately visible and malleable pathogenetic factors at the deepest possible level of influence. In practical form, the emergency intervention is a complex, highly variable clinical process.

3. Emergency Psychiatry: The Process

The process of emergency care involves four phases: triage, assessment, management, and disposition. In actuality these phases overlap or occur in combination; it is useful, however, to divide the process into discrete phases for illustrative purposes.

3.1. Triage

According to the principles of triage, the clinician must first determine if the patient has a life-threatening problem, such as an acute medical illness, and is in good behavioral control. The safety of the patient, his family, other emergency patients, and the staff is the first priority. Once any life-threatening problems are identified and contained, the assessment proper can begin.

3.2. Assessment

During the assessment phase, emergency patients should be evaluated with respect to general psychological and medical status, interpersonal adjustment, functional disability, nature of support network, etiologic and diagnostic considerations, when relevant, and capacity to use available treatment resources. Of these, diagnostic classification has traditionally been assigned the greatest weight in treatment planning and disposition. There are two key factors, however, one abstract and the other practical, that militate against basing treatment decisions on diagnostic labels.

Earlier classification schemes assumed that diagnoses reflected homogeneous psychopathological groups. In contrast, contemporary nosology is based on symptoms, syndromes, and clusters that are phenomenologically similar, but heterogeneous with respect to etiology, course, and outcome. Diagnosis by symptom-criteria or pathognomonic signs is a useful and necessary element of the clinical hypothesis, but in itself neither reliably predicts clinical outcome nor is a sufficient foundation for treatment planning. A more specific determination of the underlying precipitants, patient's current and past levels of functioning, and available psychosocial supports is required for that.

Moreover, because most emergency facilities are open 24 hours a day and offer walk-in treatment, patients who use this service have other characteristics in common: They generally have difficulty negotiating the complexities of established systems, they belong to poorer socioeconomic groups, are less well educated and insight-oriented than other demographic groups, and they are less capable of defining their problems or providing accurate and relevant psychiatric and personal histories. They typically lack a social system that routinely buffers life's stresses or provides information, material aid, and emotional support after crisis erupts.[4] The emergency situation itself limits data collection to a single point-in-time perspective, thus loading the information matrix heavily on the side of self-report data and two-dimensional clinical impressions. Subtle diagnostic distinctions are difficult to make under these conditions.

Even if it were possible to translate these data into an accurate diagnosis, their usefulness as the major determinant of management and dispositional decisions is open to question. There is no demonstrated connection between therapeutic alternatives with reliable outcomes and diagnostic classifications. In fact, therapeutic outcome may have more to do with such variables as the patient's general psychological and medical status, the severity and chronicity of symptoms, the quality of his interpersonal network, and the congruence of treatment options with patient's resources, motivation, and general emotional/cognitive style than with the actual nature or type of psychopathology.

The assessment phase of the emergency intervention should, therefore, focus on variables that affect management and dispositional decisions, such as (1) the immediate crisis, (2) the longer-range clinical forecast, and (3) the available treatment options.

The current crisis or the ostensible reason for the patient's emergency visit is composed of the presenting complaint and its etiology. The clinician's first task is to evaluate the immediate severity of the crisis and its capacity to threaten the long-range welfare of the patient or others. Symptoms, including medical/toxic conditions or behavior patterns that threaten or potentially threaten the well-being of the patient or others take precedence over all other aspects of the presentation—including even the expressed wishes of patient or family if those run counter to safety considerations. Screening for life-threatening medical conditions or overtly dangerous behaviors, impulses, or wishes should begin with the initial contact and continue throughout the intervention. This is followed by formulation of a clinical hypothesis.

The clinical hypothesis is a working formulation of the case designating some aspect of the current crisis and associated symptomatology as the therapeutic focus. It must meet several criteria: It must be clearly circumscribed, relevant to the production of the current crisis or the experience of it, congruent with the patient's understanding of his problem, and malleable. Choice of focus will in some sense determine the therapeutic goal; if excessive reactive affect or acute aggressive behavior is designated the focus of treatment, then resolution need only involve symptom relief. If chronic domestic violence is the focus, resolution requires a deeper level of systems-restructuring. Thus, the clinician's primary task during the assessment phase is to dissect the present crisis from its remote determinants: that is, to focus on the level of causation nearest the surface and identify those precipitants, if any, that are readily treatable. Medical or organic etiology should be ruled out first; the problem might abate or disappear if treated appropriately (see Part IV). Where no apparent organic cause is found, the determinants may be either functional and internal to the patient (see Parts V, VII) or situational and therefore external to the patient (see Part VI). In any case, it should be possible to specify target variables: aspects of the patient's personality, cognitive style, or interpersonal environment that are either causing, maintaining, or influencing the symptomatic clinical picture. Choice of therapeutic focus depends on isolating one or more of these target variables for strategic manipulation.

Developing a clinical hypothesis that is simple, useful, and accurate involves complicated information-processing. All information about a patient is, in some sense, relevant; even the hierarchical relationship that historical data have to some current problem can only be determined after the fact. There is no *a priori* methodology for assessment, but there are a few general guidelines:

- Focus on the presenting complaint or symptomatology.
- Work backwards through time to substantiate the clinical picture and to suggest or verify the operation of particular pathogenic factors.
- Use the mental status examination to verify areas and levels of disruption in current functioning. In combination with the presenting clinical picture, the examination might also suggest areas for further medical/organic screening.
- Compare current level of functioning to premorbid level.
- Maintain a high index of suspicion about the presence of organicity. Symptoms and signs include:
  ○ fluctuating levels of consciousness with some lucid intervals.
  ○ disorientation and short-term memory loss.
  ○ perceptual distortions and predominantly visual hallucinations.
  ○ sudden, acute onset of symptoms—to be ascertained by history, not by direct observation.
  ○ abnormal vital signs.
  ○ any physical complaints and abnormal physical findings.
- Use the psychiatric history specifically to provide evidence about prior symptomatic episodes or patterns of crisis with particular modes of resolution and adaptation.
- Use the psychodynamic history to identify and define pivotal events. These highlight the quality and perspective of the patient's general emotional orientation, roles, relationships, and ability to use the support network.
- Use the quality of the therapeutic relationship to clarify relative degrees of interpersonal reactiveness, independence, need for distance, empathy, and insight.

As the assessment phase nears completion, it should be possible to formulate the clinical hypothesis. This, in combination with the forecast and inventory of the available treatment options, forms the basis for management and dispositional decisions. The clinical hypothesis defines an appropriate focus for the emergency intervention, and a reasonable, but limited treatment objective. The forecast combines statistical measures (e.g., demographic factors related to increased risk of suicide) generally applicable to discrete patient populations with personalized historical data and suggests a probable course and outcome for the current crisis, both with and without treatment.

In the emergency setting the liabilities of more traditional modes of evaluation take on added significance as certain dispositions, such as hospitalization and long-term psychotherapy, becoming increasingly less popular and more difficult to provide. In addition, the current gaps in the implementation of a comprehensive community system have led to a further narrowing of available long-range treatment options. At the same time, however, short-term options have expanded. The accordionlike trend in dispositional alternatives should be reflected in a complementary shift in the assessment process. That is, an inventory of the patient's and community's resources should receive equal weight with the clinical presentation and forecast.

The decision to use a particular treatment strategy, whether on a short- or long-term basis, is related to *both* the nature of the clinical crisis and the availability of treatment resources. It is not, and should not be regarded as a unidirectional decision. The ideal treatment plan is rendered least effective if the chosen treatment is unavailable, involves long waiting periods, is too far away, or is prohibitively expensive. As a rule of thumb, it may be necessary to rework the clinical hypothesis several times—first from the perspective of the clinical presentation itself, exclusive of practical considerations like insurance coverage and availability of treatment resources, and second from the perspective of all available dispositional options. These include short-term solutions within the family system—supervision, confinement, or support—to longer-range outpatient or community programs. When dispositional options are limited by practical constraints, the therapeutic goal should also shift.

3.3. Management

The third phase of emergency intervention has traditionally involved management of the patient. This phase has become increasingly more important in this setting, particularly with the recent shifts in the mental health care delivery system.[6] Again, it should be emphasized that it is artificial to separate what is really a continuous and intertwined process into three phases except to highlight abstract structural differences relating to distinct clinical goals: i.e., acquiring sufficient data versus using them for crisis resolution. In fact, the initial stages of the interview can be viewed as early steps in an ongoing problem-solving process that overlaps with the intervention itself. The tasks as defined by the earliest goals of the evaluation process shift subtly from the collection of information and establishment of rapport with the patient to active, collaborative problem-solving. While deliberately focusing on the current situation, the therapist and the patient together collect and begin to integrate material in a structured, step-by-step process. The problem is defined in terms of its risks and consequences to the patient and others, its emotional impact and meaning, and its origins so far as they can be grasped. The common theme throughout is the problem at hand; the primary goal a working definition of the problem and a practical rationale for its resolution.

A secondary, but essential, objective of most emergency interventions is to build a therapeutic relationship from which to effect successful crisis resolution and to begin the process of engaging the patient in ongoing treatment. Establishing and maintaining rapport during the entire interview may make the critical difference between successful treatment and follow-up, and dropping-out. Although the patient may develop an automatic positive transference to the institution affiliated with the emergency service, he has not yet formed a genuine therapeutic alliance with the clinician.

The initial process of engagement may require patience, persistence, and outreach. One of the most challenging aspects of this work is to monitor and try to influence the patient's involvement in treatment. The evolution of the relationship during the emergency intervention provides information crucial to the choice of disposition. A patient who responds to an empathic interaction by becoming calmer and more communicative can be managed differently from a person who withdraws and remains unresponsive to the therapist. Patients who experience the interaction as threatening or risky and cannot sustain a consistent level of contact with the interviewer may benefit less from a therapeutic modality that relies heavily on the formation of a relatively steady alliance.

The emergency clinician should actively promote problem-solving activities and establish rapport, by using and combining various technical strategies. These include:

- operant shaping either to reinforce positive, adaptive responses or interrupt problematic, counterproductive, resistant responses.
- acknowledging and labeling the patient's feelings.
- empathic listening.
- reality testing, instruction, and reshaping cognitive misconceptions.
- offering reassurance, support, and, in appropriate cases, direct advice.
- labeling the need for, and helping the mastery of, new types of skills—asking for help, communicating, perceiving self and others more accurately.
- clarifying and, when appropriate, interpreting the meaning of the crisis.

It goes without saying that in every patient where the underlying precipitant is treatable by medication, medical techniques, restraint, isolation, or hospitalization, those measures take immediate precedence over psychotherapeutic strategies.

3.4. Treatment Planning

The final phase of the treatment process is to resolve the crisis and develop realistic, long-range dispositional options. While there is an increasing demand for immediate, definitive crisis management approaches within the emergency setting, there are some patient groups that will not benefit immediately by treatment, and various types of crisis and emergency facilities that cannot provide definitive care. Under these conditions, referral is the critical function of the emergency service.

Disposition or referral requires that the patient's needs be matched with available treatment modalities, support services, and resources. Successful implementation depends on accurately identifying the patient's current needs and concerns, closing the gap between the patient's wishes and what he can realistically expect, and facilitating his acceptance of the proposed disposition. Understanding the patient's requests is essential to this process.[7] Often these are only indirectly expressed by the patient; the therapist may have to elicit them actively. Furthermore, however sound the rationale for a specific disposition, the patient is unlikely to accept it if it departs too far from his expectations.

Once the patient's needs and requests are defined, the clinician can begin to determine the available treatment resources in his community. Generally, the least restrictive disposition that still meets the patient's therapeutic needs should be chosen: that is, fulfilling the "objective of maintaining the greatest degree of freedom, self-determination, autonomy, dignity, and integrity of body, mind, and spirit for the individual while he participates in treatment or receives services"[8] (p. 44). The concept of restriction is difficult to interpret, for it involves a poorly defined set of variables, such as location, expense, milieu philosophy, or staffing patterns, and requires comparing incomparables like medication and residential treatment.[9]

Because of limited resource availability and shifting treatment philosophies (e.g., deinstitutionalization), usual and customary dispositional alternatives may be either scarce or unpopular. It may be necessary to arrange a suboptimal treatment plan, depending on, for example, the creative mobilization of members of the patient's family or community network. Whatever the actual or philosophical limitation of services, the emergency clinician should know of, or have access to information about the complete range of resources in his community, and should understand the practical, personal, and interpersonal liabilities his patient brings to the long-range treatment forecast.

Once the dispositional plan has been formulated, it should be discussed with the patient and those close to him. So far, the patient has collaborated in the crisis management; the groundwork has presumably been laid for the rationale behind the referral. The starting point in negotiating a mutually acceptable treatment plan is the patient's requests, expectations, and wishes. Once defined, the gap between those wishes and the clinician's assessment should be systematically reduced by a series of negotiated steps: The clinician should explain the plan in a simple, straightforward manner, and the patient should discuss his reactions, concerns and questions.[10] Ultimately, of course, the patient has the right to accept or reject the proposed course of action. If he accepts, his continued motivation and compliance are significantly reinforced if the clinician specifically plans the transition to the next stage of treatment before ending the emergency interview. Arrangements should be made directly by the emergency clinician, appointments set up, procedural details and policies openly discussed. The emergency clinician should continue to follow the patient until he has been assigned to an interim caretaker or has actually started the next treatment phase.

4. Special Clinical Applications

Although emergency care often implies a single visit (with follow-up) and a therapeutic focus distinct from the patient's involvement with the therapist himself or with an outside therapist, it is not uncommon for some patients to use the emergency setting habitually and repeatedly, bring a crisis in ongoing psychotherapy into the emergency setting, or respond to the emergency clinician with such intensity that the transference reaction itself becomes the dominant theme. With each of these patient groups, the emergency clinician must understand their unique patterns of seeking help and their special needs.

4.1. Repeaters

Although the pattern of repetitive or habitual use may seem antithetical to the goals of emergency management, a consistent subgroup of patients will nonetheless use the emergency ward repeatedly. These patients, referred to as repeaters, require a treatment approach that is supportive and tailored specifically to their needs. Various authors estimate that these patients account for from 7 to 17.9% of the total psychiatric emergency population.[11]

Repeaters represent a discrete clinical group characterized by a common symptom profile, a similar treatment history, and a typical style of interacting with therapists.[11] These three dimensions are interrelated, synergistically reinforcing each other and resulting in a self-defeating clinical pattern. To put it simply, help is ambivalently sought and then, with equal ambivalence, rejected. Although these chronic crisis patients follow a similar symptomatic treatment pattern, they are demographically and diagnostically heterogeneous. Their receiving similar diagnostic labels, such as "borderline," and therefore appearing to conform to a specific psychiatric designation may be an accident of institutional bias.

Beginning with symptoms, these patients complain of urgent needs that are accentuated by unrealistic expectations and entitled wishes for immediate relief. They relate in a generally negativistic manner and are regarded as demanding and manipulative. The patient's desires and demands are usually quite different from the real clinical possibilities, opening the door to intense frustration and angry ambivalence on both sides.

These repeater patients have a paucity of supportive interpersonal networks. They tend to interact with their social environments in much the same manner as they do in the emergency setting, leaving those resources exhausted and depleted. Over a period of time, the patient's social supports gradually recede and weaken, a factor that is bound to reinforce reliance on anonymous caretakers.

Managing these patients is not an easy task in itself, but the difficulty is inevitably compounded by the therapist's own response. Trained to help and nurturant by temperament, the therapist may find himself using therapeutic strategies or opting for dispositional alternatives that reflect his internal discomfort more than his clinical judgment. For example, repeaters tend to be hospitalized more than nonrepeaters.

To obviate this intervention pattern, the therapist needs to have a conceptual framework into which to fit his work with repeaters. The engagement and containment of these patients in the emergency setting should be viewed as a protracted process characterized by frequent flights from the helper. Cycles of intense engagement followed by equally intense disengagement are a predictable part of their behavior. Repeaters are not easily able to tolerate the limits of a relationship; they may experience distance as abandonment and closeness as entrapment. The space within a relationship represents a fine line that is easily violated.

Managing these patients requires a flexible approach. The patient's autonomy should be supported, but each emergency visit should be viewed as an opportunity to encourage the patient's engagement and participation in treatment. Some of these patients will ultimately form a positive transference to the emergency setting that will help them maintain a relatively consistent level of functioning. Although such an approach runs the risk of diluting the transference and sacrificing the possibility of working through aspects of the patient's problems with close relationships, it does keep the patient under the protective mantle of a single health care facility. For some of these patients, group therapy in an outpatient setting is an effective, relatively stabilizing disposition.

Perhaps the most difficult aspect in managing any patient whose expectations and interpersonal stance defy satisfaction is the therapist's own discomfort. Because these patients are consistently manipulative, uncooperative, and ambivalently help-rejecting, the therapist must remind himself that the patient's style reflects early developmental problems. Such an understanding should help the therapist resist being drawn into the transference struggle and instead should help him to respond empathically despite provocation. In addition, a supportive approach combined with operant shaping strategies that reinforce the patient's appropriate behavior, cooperativeness, and efforts at self-analysis while ignoring or setting limits on demanding or inappropriate behavior can be effective when interacting with repeaters.

4.2. Patients in Ongoing Treatment

Although many patients are currently in treatment elsewhere, they still choose to use the psychiatric emergency department.[12,13] It has been estimated that at least one-third of emergency patients are in concurrent treatment. Whatever the presenting complaint, the emergency evaluator should always investigate why these patients didn't return to their primary caretaker for help. Some patients deny that this is an issue; however, it most often reflects a crisis in psychotherapy that is generally related to "(1) clinical difficulties; (2) consumer dissatisfaction; (3) empathic distance; and (4) interactional issues, either transference or countertransference or both"[13] (p. 95). Common immediate precipitants to the emergency visit include missed sessions (therapist's vacations), altered length of sessions, medication issues, contact outside the therapy session, other changes in the therapeutic process, or a combination of these events. The emergency evaluator should view his role as that of consultant to the primary treatment; he should attempt to identify therapy factors that interfere with a more effective working alliance. His role is not to judge the effectiveness of the therapy but to facilitate more open communication between patient and therapist. Although occasionally more extensive consultation may be indicated, most patients can either be referred back to their primary therapist or referred elsewhere (e.g., hospitalization) after discussion among the various caretakers and the patient.

Many patients with outside therapists who repeatedly visit the emergency ward carry a diagnosis of borderline. They present with concerns and complaints about their treatment. For these patients, repeated use of the emergency facility may be an inevitable part of the process of psychotherapy. Often the patient cannot tolerate ambivalent feelings about the therapist and may use the defense of splitting. The patient may view the therapist as the bad, devalued object and the emergency clinician as the good, overidealized object, or vice versa. The emergency evaluator should recognize this defensive operation and attempt to define the precipitant of the visit, always focusing on the therapeutic relationship. He should discuss and reality-test some of the patient's distortions about the therapist, and encourage the patient to return and talk with the therapist about his feelings. After getting permission from the patient, the evaluator should contact the therapist, and together they should develop an integrated approach to care. If the emergency visits are frequent, the patient, therapist, and emergency clinician should work out an acceptable plan for managing these visits.

4.3. Specific Transference Issues

Managing the transference in the therapist–patient relationship is a central feature of most therapies, including the single and brief interventions (see Chapter 5). Since the task-oriented focus of crisis intervention and other short-term modalities tends to suppress the spontaneous expression of transference material, however, this aspect of treatment has been underemphasized; the problem-solving task or content of short-term treatments may be weighted more heavily than the patient's relationship with the therapist or process of treatment. The interaction between patient and therapist is nonetheless central to the success of treatment. The therapist should actively promote the formation of a carefully controlled positive transference that will help to gain the patient's cooperation and facilitate his involvement with treatment. In shorter-term therapies, the therapist–patient relationship is more a treatment catalyst than the central focus of treatment as in the analytic formats.

Various emergency patients rapidly form intense and binding attachments to professional helpers, including emergency personnel. In these persons a transference relationship may replace the real or fantasized loss that generated the crisis. Continuity in the therapeutic relationship, the implicit promise of a lasting attachment, and the active confrontation of crisis issues may be sufficient to contain further regression while allowing the patient to mobilize ego skills and environmental resources. Other patients may endow the emergency clinician with omnipotent and magical properties and cannot effectively function without persistent contact with the therapist. Referral for longer-term psychotherapy may precipitate a secondary termination crisis. Shorter-term strategies to contain the symptoms may be the only dispositional option available to the emergency clinician.

The difficulties in the management of transference emphasize the general complexity of emergency care. The importance of matching the therapist's stance and intervention with the patient's needs is clear. While therapist stance and intervention may be relatively set in theory, they are flexible and individualized in practice. Patients' needs, however, are inherently bimodal, distributed at one end of the spectrum according to the clinician's perspective, and defined at the other end by the patient's loftiest wishes.

5. Conclusion

The process of emergency psychiatry as discussed in this volume is a distillate of theory, logic, and experience—the hard core of psychiatric science. But so long as clinical psychiatry involves the intersection of two individuals who happen to be doctor and patient for that moment in time, there will be a soft core as well. It is this ineffable human element that infuses knowledge and technical skill, allowing them to touch, and alter human misery.

References

1. Bassuk EL, Gerson S: Into the breach: Emergency psychiatry in the general hospital. *Gen Hosp Psychiatry* 1:31–45, 1979.
2. Baldwin B: A paradigm for the classification of emotional crises: Implications for crisis intervention. *Am J Orthopsychiatry* 48:538–551, 1978.
3. Bassuk EL, Gerson S: Deinstitutionalization and mental health services. *Sci Am* 238:46–53, 1978.
4. Gerson S, Bassuk EL: Psychiatric emergencies: An overview. *Am J Psychiatry* 137:1–11, 1980.
5. Auerbach S., Kilman P: Crisis intervention: A review of outcome research. *Psychol Bull* 84:1189–1217, 1977.
6. Bassuk EL, Schoonover S: The private general hospital emergency service in a decade of transition. *Hosp Comm Psychiatry* 32:181–185, 1981.
7. Lazare A, Eisenthal S, Wasserman L, et al: Patient requests in a walk-in clinic. *Compr Psychiatry* 16:467–477, 1975.
8. Report to the President from the President's Commission of Mental Health, vol 1. Washington, D.C., 1978, p 44.

9. Bachrach L: Is the least restrictive alternative always the best? Sociological and semantic implications. *Hosp Comm Psychiatry* 31:97–103, 1980.
10. Lazare A, Eisenthal S, Wasserman L: The customer approach to parenthood. *Arch Gen Psychiatry* 32:553, 1976.
11. Bassuk EL, Gerson S: Chronic crisis patients: A discrete clinical group. *Am J Psychiatry* 137:1513–1517, 1980.
12. Kass F, Karasu T, Walsh T: Emergency room patients in concurrent therapy: A neglected clinical phenomenon. *Am J Psychiatry* 136:91–92, 1979.
13. Skodol A, Kass F, Charles, E: Crisis in psychotherapy: Principles of emergency consultation and intervention. *Am J Orthopsychiatry* 49:585–597, 1979.

II

The Process of Emergency Care

The First Few Minutes

Identifying and Managing Life-Threatening Emergencies

Ellen L. Bassuk, M.D., and Andrew E. Skodol, M.D.

1. Introduction

A small percentage of patients using emergency settings present with problems requiring immediate containment and treatment. Within the first few minutes of meeting any patient, the clinician must complete a focused assessment and, in a few cases, rapidly translate his observations and impressions into action. Although the patient may be uncommunicative, resistant, and difficult to contain, even a very brief examination provides important clues about the nature of the disorder (e.g., organic versus functional) and forms a basis for developing a rational and safe management plan.

The most important goal of any emergency evaluation is to identify and treat life-threatening or potentially life-threatening problems. These include (1) agitated, menacing, self-destructive, and out-of-control behaviors; (2) serious and chronic self-neglect; and (3) serious medical problems either coexisting with or causing psychiatric symptoms. This chapter describes the initial assessment and immediate psychological, physical, pharmacological, or medical management of patients presenting with truly urgent conditions. Although screening for true emergencies should continue throughout the clinical intervention, the initial encounter often sets the tone for the entire session and may affect the patient's ability to stay in control.

2. Initial Assessment and Psychological Management

Evaluating an emergency patient begins with the earliest interaction and is interlaced with immediate management considerations. For the particularly agitated or bizarre patient, the clinician should try to recognize potentially reversible problems in reality testing, judgment, and impulse control (e.g., or-

Ellen L. Bassuk, M.D. • Harvard Medical School, Boston, Massachusetts 02115. *Andrew E. Skodol, M.D.* • College of Physicians and Surgeons of Columbia University, New York, New York 10032, and Biometrics Research Department, New York State Psychiatric Institute, New York, New York 10032.

ganic and functional psychosis) and provide reconstitutive treatment while simultaneously attending to the premonitory signs of violence: Any subtle or abrupt changes in mood, behavior, or speech may indicate that the patient is about to lose control.

The interviewer should be guided by his observations and impressions of the patient. He should listen to the patient's associations, shifts in conversation, and discrepancies between verbal reports and nonverbal behaviors. He should direct his participation in the interaction to soothing potentially explosive anxiety. A confrontive, direct approach with a paranoid individual, for example, may increase the patient's defensiveness and hostility while a supportive intervention may calm him.

In spite of the anxiety-provoking context, the clinician should try to remain calm and decisive. The agitated patient should be removed from the stimulating atmosphere of the waiting room to the quietest area available. Separating the patient from family members is generally appropriate, unless their presence has an obviously calming influence. Avoiding the agitated patient or deferring action will only aggravate the situation, contribute to a more dangerous patient later, or alienate other personnel.

If the agitated patient is in reasonable control, the interview may continue. The clinician should sit at a comfortable distance from the patient. The patient should be permitted to sit closer to the door, affording an easy escape route should violent impulses or panic develop. Most emergency interviewing rooms have a buzzer that can be unobtrusively sounded if violence erupts, or are equipped with Plexiglas wall panels so that the interview can be monitored by staff or security personnel. If the patient is less well controlled, the clinician may elect to have additional staff, security personnel, or police stationed in the interviewing room. If the patient appears to be losing control, the clinician should state emphatically that control will be reinstituted if necessary.

No matter how hostile or provocative patient behavior becomes, it should be remembered that it is a manifestation of illness. The clinician should firmly structure expectations and set limits, without anger, challenge, or confrontation. For example, he might say to a psychotic patient who is responding to voices and believes that the staff is part of a CIA conspiracy: "I know you are frightened. You are safe here. No one is trying to hurt you. If you are unable to stay in control, we will help you." Acknowledging and labeling feelings ("I know you are frightened"), correcting cognitive distortions ("I'm the doctor and not part of the CIA or any conspiracy"), and providing realistic reassurance ("You are safe here") are important supportive interviewing techniques.[1] Exception to these recommendations is made for patients using phencyclidine (PCP) since supportive interviewing can exacerbate their agitation. Once diagnosed they should be isolated immediately in a "quiet" room (see Chapter 9). They cannot be "talked down."

In these, as in all other emergency encounters, the clinician should gather essential information by asking critical historical questions and administering indicated parts of the mental status examination and physical examination. The difference between the truly urgent condition and other "emergencies" is the moment-by-moment monitoring required. The course of the intervention may be dramatically altered at any time by the need for physical restraint, medical intervention, or forcible medication. Occasionally, physical restraint may be necessary to ensure an adequate examination.

2.1. History

Whenever a relatively controlled situation permits, the clinician should obtain information about the nature, duration, and course of the present illness; history of medication use and drug abuse; and current and past major medical and psychiatric illnesses and treatments. These questions help to differentiate between organic and functional disorders. While it is useful for persons accompanying the patient to the ER to provide supplementary information, most psychiatric patients are unaccompanied and therefore are responsible for their own histories.

2.2. Mental Status Examination (MSE)

The MSE enables the physician to elicit relatively objective data about the patient's behavioral, psychological, and intellectual functioning (see Tables 1 and 2). It consists of initial impressions, systematic observations, and standardized questions that generally can be gathered informally. Neurological and mental functioning can be assessed from the patient's level of consciousness, size and reactivity of pupils, extraocular movements, skin color and turgor, gait, speech, thought flow and content, perceptions, judgment, and insight. To differentiate an organic from a functional problem, specific questions must be asked to probe the extent of disorientation, memory loss, impaired concentration, or decreased intellectual functioning. Severely impaired cognitive capacity suggests an organic etiology.[4–7] An agitated patient, however, may be unable to answer specific questions, thus limiting the usefulness of the MSE.

2.3. Vital Signs and Physical Examination

The evaluator should obtain vital signs (i.e., pulse, blood pressure, respiration, and temperature). They may point to the presence of medical or toxic problems and, at the least, provide a baseline that can be used to monitor the patient over time.

Without compromising the patient's stability, a physical examination, even a brief one, should be administered. If it is necessary to restrain or medicate a patient to complete the examination or obtain essential laboratory tests (e.g., blood sugar), it should be done promptly. Normal findings, however, do not necessarily rule out organic etiology.

3. Determination of the Problem

Using observations and clinical impressions, history, and findings from the MSE and physical examination, the clinician should attempt to determine

Table 1. The Mental Status Examination[a]

1. Appearance	How does the patient look?
	Neat and clean or dirty and unkempt
	Bizarre or inappropriate
	Pupils—round, regular and equal
	Extraocular movements
	Skin color and turgor
and	
Behavior	How does the patient act?
	Strange, threatening, or violent
	Unusual motor activity such as grimacing or tremors
	Impaired gait
	Psychomotor retardation, agitation
2. Speech	How does the patient talk?
	Rate, tone, quantity
3. Thought content	What's on the patient's mind?
	Delusions, suicide, bodily concerns, thought broadcasting and withdrawal
and	
Thought flow	How are thoughts connected?
	Randomly, logically
4. Mood	How does the patient feel?
	Sad, down, blue, high
and	
Affect	What emotions are being expressed?
	Anger, fear, grief
5. Perceptions	What does the patient see, hear, etc.?
	Illusions, hallucinations
6. Cognitive capacity	What does the patient know?
	Orientation, attention span, memory, intellectual functioning, insight, and judgment; special tests of localized cerebral function

[a] Adapted from Bassuk et al.[2]

if the agitated behavior reflects an organic or functional disorder (see Table 2). This distinction has a marked influence on his subsequent course of action (see Chapter 4). Identifying an organic etiology points to the treatment of a specific disease or toxic process; functional etiology does not. The latter term implies only that the disorder has no identifiable organic causes and may or may not be medicable. In general, a patient is more likely to have an organic mental disorder, as opposed to a functional disorder, if he is older than 40 years, the onset is acute, and the symptoms are intermittent and fluctuating. Other indicators include impaired level of consciousness (e.g., the "clouded consciousness" of delirium) and diminished cognitive function. Important exceptions are acute amphetamine toxicity and alcoholic hallucinosis, in which the patient has a clear sensorium and intact cognitive capacity.[8] Clinical manifestations, diagnostic considerations, and treatment of several substance-induced organic mental disorders are described and contrasted to functional disorders in Table 3.

Table 2. Mental Status Findings That Help in the Differential Diagnosis between Organic Brain Syndrome and Functional Psychiatric Disorder[a]

Mental Status	Organic brain syndrome	Functional psychiatric disorder
Level of consciousness	Stuporous, lethargic, or sleepy, sometimes hyperalert	Stuporous or hyperalert; rarely lethargic or sleepy
Facial expression	Often empty	Rarely empty
Muscle tone	Often decreased (increased with phencyclidine)	Seldom decreased
Respiration	Often slow or irregular	Normal to rapid and regular
Speech	Often slurred	Not slurred
Voice	Often weak	Normal strength or loud
Concentration span	Decreased	Decreased or normal
Retention or recall	Decreased	Normal
Memory	Decreased	Normal
Orientation	Decreased	Normal
Hallucinations	Visual or auditory	Rarely visual; if auditory, source generally not located
Motor signs	Coarse tremor, nystagmus, ataxia	None or fine regular tremor

[a] Adapted from Glickman.[3]

Distinguishing between organic and functional disorders, however, is often extremely difficult. If a patient is severely anxious, depressed, or preoccupied he may have difficulty concentrating, which obscures the interpretation of the MSE. Similarly, various psychiatric syndromes can mimic organic disease (e.g., "pseudodementia" in elderly depressed patients and severely disorganized psychotic patients). Other illnesses, such as temporal lobe elipesy (TLE), may have both medical and psychiatric components.[10]

Agitated behavior may be a manifestation of a wide range of nonorganic psychiatric disorders, including various psychotic disorders (e.g., schizophrenia, bipolar disorder), borderline personality disorder, or antisocial personality disorder (see Chapter 6). Out-of-control behavior is more likely in syndromes marked by disturbed reality testing, poor impulse control, and impaired judgment. In contrast, severely agitated patients with major depressive illness are unlikely to lose control; these patients may appear extremely restless, pacing continuously and wringing their hands, but they generally are not threatening. Haloperidol may effectively decrease the acute distress of these individuals (see Chapter 12).

4. Physical Management

Forceful managing of the violent, acutely agitated, or threatening individual in the volatile atmosphere of the ER is frightening even for the most skilled clinician, but it may be necessary. Whether no action is taken or active measures applied, physical injury looms as a real possibility.[11-13] A major goal is

Table 3. Substance-Induced Organic Mental Disorders versus Functional Disorders in Patients Presenting with Agitated Behavior[a]

Physical examination	Probable cause	Treatment
Agitation with blank stare,[b] anxiety, stupor, aggression, panic, bizarre behavior → Elevated blood pressure and heart rate, vertical and horizontal nystagmus, analgesia to pinprick, muscular rigidity, salivation, vomiting	→ Phencyclidine (PCP) →	Minimal intervention (no talking down) Sensory deprivation with observation at a distance Diazepam for intoxication Haloperidol for psychosis No phenothiazines Diazepam for seizures Alpha-blockers or diazoxide for severe hypertension
Agitation with persecutory delusions or euphoria with irritability → Sympathetic signs: blood pressure elevation, tachycardia, tachypnea, mydriasis, diaphoresis, motor restlessness, tremor	→ Amphetamine and/or cocaine or other sympathomimetics →	Controlled environment Acidify urine Control hyperpyrexia, seizures (diazepam), behavior (haloperidol) No sedatives
No sympathetic signs →	Consider schizophrenia, schizophreniform disorder, paranoid disorder, bipolar disorder, brief reactive psychosis, atypical psychosis	

Sensory distortion, hypersensitivity of all senses, euphoria, hallucinations, pseudohallucinations

→ Sympathetic excess → Epinephrine-type hallucinogens; STP, mescaline, nutmeg → Controlled environment, support and reassurance (talking down); haloperidol for behavior control

→ Minimal changes → Indole-type hallucinogens; LSD, psilocybin →

Undistinguishable acute delirium

→ Muscarinic blockade: dilated and sluggishly reactive pupils, blurred vision, flushed face, paralytic ileus, constipation, urinary retention, fever, and hyperreflexia → Pilocarpine, or methacholine → Physostigmine

→ Muscarinic blockade not present → Reclassify patient by physical examination; if the findings are not clear, consider mixed or unusual presentation; consider polydrug ingestion when psychological and physical presentations are contradictory or confusing → Conservative—with observation and protection as needed

[a] Adapted from DiSclafani et al.[9]

[b] The patient with moderate dose or high dose PCP ingestion may present with stupor or coma and later exhibit low dose signs and symptoms.

Table 4. Physical Management[a]

---

1. Develop specific protocols describing methods of restraint.
2. Determine composition of team (optimally six persons, though five is usually safe).
    a. One person directs restraint procedure, controls patient's head.
    b. One person restrains each limb.
    c. One person administers medication.
3. Review the specific plan for restraint, including assignment of roles.
4. Have necessary equipment and medication available.
5. Inform the patient about treatment options.
6. Ask the patient to lie down to apply restraints.
7. Apply restraints and, perhaps, medicate.
8. Continue to talk with patient about his feelings and procedural issues.
9. Never leave the patient alone.
10. Convene a meeting of caretakers to discuss continuing patient observation and subsequent plans, including removal of restraints, medication, disposition.
11. Remove restraints—one limb at a time.

---

[a] From Bassuk.[1]

to ensure the safety of staff, patient, and other persons. The clinician should approach the patient with both caution and confidence, acknowledging the danger, but not allowing fear to dominate.[14,15] He should attempt to establish rapport by appealing to the patient's strengths, structuring expectations, encouraging impulse control, and explaining alternative treatment choices. From the outset, the clinician should assert that maintaining control is a top priority and prerequisite to effective treatment. If the patient still is unable to cooperate, the clinician should not bargain or argue. He should combine physical restraint and/or medication, describe the plan in a straightforward and direct manner, and implement it quickly.

4.1. Physical Restraint

Physical restraint can be an effective therapeutic technique. Understanding restraint techniques, their combination with psychological and pharmacological treatments, the staff's reactions, and relevant legal issues is essential for optimal physical management (see Chapter 3). Each emergency unit should develop realistic protocols and practice procedures for restraint.[1]

General guidelines for physically restraining a patient are useful but must be tailored to each clinical circumstance (see Table 4). Whenever possible, a physician should give the order, but the on-line staff should also have the authority to call for restraint. No matter who gives the order, police and/or security should be notified. Before the patient is confronted, the requisite number of personnel—at least four, preferably five or six—and proper equipment should be on hand. Leather restraints with padded bracelets for wrists and ankles are preferable to nylon and Velcro restraints, which may not hold a large person. Members of the restraint team should be certain of their respective roles, *in advance.*

Initially, the clinician should request that the patient submit to restraint voluntarily. He might say: "We would like you to lie down on the stretcher so we can restrain you for your own protection." If the patient does not respond, do not further cajole him. Instead, the team should take physical control of the patient and bring him to a horizontal position on the stretcher. To avoid aspiration and possible airway obstruction, do not restrain a patient in a supine "spread-eagle" position. The amount of physical force should always be the least necessary to restrain the patient safely. Each person should grasp a limb and one person should hold the patient's head to limit movement. Starting with the arms, each limb should be placed in a leather bracelet. A staff member should remain with the patient, reassuring him and encouraging him to talk. The remainder of the team should convene for discussion of their observations and formulation of subsequent plans, including use of medication, criteria for removing restraints, and disposition.[1] Patients who continue to fight restraint may suffer soft-tissue damage. If so, efforts should be made to soothe the patient, using medication if necessary. For some extremely agitated patients, physical restraint may be contraindicated because of the risk of physical injury.

If the patient is brought to the ER in restraints, the clinician should carefully assess the current clinical status before removing them. Because of the soft-tissue damage frequently caused by handcuffs on struggling patients, clinicians sometimes make the mistake of releasing them too quickly—with disastrous consequences.

4.2. Weapons

Occasionally, a clinician is threatened with a weapon. Experienced emergency workers have recommended a wide range of responses. Often, such maneuvers cannot be planned, and their effectiveness depends on their spontaneity. Few rules are available to guide a response to a threatening situation, with one exception: Under no circumstances should the clinician forcefully attempt to disarm the individual. He should either attempt to leave the room or insist that the patient put the weapon on the floor.

5. Pharmacologic Management

The initial decision to medicate a patient depends on the clinical presentation and his responses to the emergency intervention. Is the patient assaultive, violent, and out of control or is he intermittently violent but currently in control? Generally, the patient who is at the limits of control or actively violent should receive high-potency antipsychotic medications, such as the piperazine phenothiazines, haloperidol (Haldol), or thiothixene (Navane).[16] Although these drugs cause a high incidence of acute dystonic reactions, they have fewer adverse cardiovascular effects such as arrhythmias and postural hypotension (see Chapter 4).

Table 5. Rapid Neuroleptization[a]

1. Use only after treatment with less intrusive measures.
2. Carefully weigh risks and benefits.
3. Administer intramuscular haloperidol (Haldol).
4. Dosage
   a. 2.5 mg to 10 mg haloperidol IM given every 30 to 60 minutes.
   b. Varies from 1 to 10 mg per dose.
   c. Patients typically require one to four injections.
   d. Total daily doses = 100 to 120 mg/day.
5. Response is evident within minutes.
6. Common adverse effects
   Hypotension
   Sedation
   Extrapyramidal effects (e.g., acute dystonia)
7. After acute treatment, patients generally require oral antipsychotic medication.

[a] From Bassuk et al.,[8] and Donlon et al.[17]

The use of medications is always combined with psychological interventions and sometimes with physical restraint. If the MSE and PE, for example, suggest that the patient has an organic mental disorder (see Table 2), the clinician must weigh the risks and benefits of medication against those of physical restraint. Since high-potency antipsychotics, such as haloperidol, may potentiate other CNS depressants, depress CNS function, or produce adverse extrapyramidal effects such as acute dystonias, they may complicate the ongoing evaluation of suspected organic brain syndrome. In these cases, the lowest possible effective dose should be administered and the clinical status carefully monitored (e.g., particularly level of consciousness). Generally, the initial dose is somewhat lower than for patients with functional disorders (e.g., haloperidol 0.5–2.0 mg). Antipsychotic agents are contraindicated for agitated patients with an anticholinergic syndrome. While not absolutely contraindicated, antipsychotic medication may be unnecessary for the previously violent patient who is calming down but remains restrained. However, if the patient's agitation escalates or he continues to manifest excited behavior, combined pharmacological and physical treatment may be required. Occasionally, an excited patient may continue to fight restraints, risking the danger of fractures, soft-tissue injury, and, rarely, rhabdomyolysis (in patients taking high doses of phencyclidine); in these individuals chemical restraints may be preferred.[16] Although safety dictates action in these cases, the clinician must not ignore the patient's legal rights (see Chapter 3).

Some excited patients with functional disorders may require frequently repeated doses of high-potency antipsychotic agents—an approach known as *rapid neuroleptization*[8,17] (see Table 5). Although clinicians generally try to avoid physical restraint, its risks and benefits should be carefully weighed against those of high-dose medication. In a rare patient, rapid neuroleptization may be potentially dangerous—resulting in laryngospasm (treated with diazepam 5 to 10 mg IV) and even sudden death. Containment of symptoms (i.e.,

Table 6. Level of Consciousness[a]

Alert wakefulness—The patient "responds immediately, fully and appropriately to visual, auditory or tactile stimulation."

Lethargy—The patient appears drowsy and inactive; his responses are delayed or incomplete.

Obtundation—The patient seems indifferent; he "maintains wakefulness, but little more."

Stupor—The patient "can only be aroused by vigorous and continuous external stimulation."

Coma—The patient's "responses to stimulation are either completely lost (deep coma) or reduced to only rudimentary reflex motor responses (moderately deep coma)."

---

[a] From Plum and Posner.[18]

behavioral control) results from the drug's neuroleptic and sedative properties and not from the abatement of psychotic symptoms. In practice, haloperidol (Haldol) is the most common drug used for rapid neuroleptization, although the other high-potency antipsychotic drugs may be used in a similar manner.

The dose of haloperidol should be individualized, but the effective dose generally ranges from 2.5 to 10 mg IM (range of 1 to 10 mg) and can be administered every 30 to 60 minutes. Patients typically require one to four injections. The drug should be mixed and drawn into the syringe immediately before use and should not be stored after mixing. The total dose should not exceed 100 to 120 mg per day. Once contained, patients who have been treated by rapid neuroleptization for out-of-control behavior usually require continued treatment with antipsychotic medication.[8,17] They should be monitored continuously.

6. Medical Management

Patients with medical problems requiring immediate treatment may present with behavioral symptoms that coexist with and/or mask their medical origin. Clues to the medical etiology of the disorder may include the patient's level of consciousness, appearance, and behavior, other findings on the MSE, and the results of the physical examination (see Tables 1, 2, and 6). The clinician should try to differentiate between a medical and a functional disorder by testing cognitive capacity (e.g., orientation, memory, ability to concentrate) and extending the physical examination to include simple neurological or cardiopulmonary tests.

Most often, the emergency medical physician has primary responsibility for the care of medically urgent conditions. It is not impossible, however, for the mental health clinician to be the only caretaker available or to see psychiatric emergencies with life-threatening medical sequelae, e.g., suicide attempts, cardiac arrests, and self-mutilation. Therefore, he should have some facility with general life support measures, such as cardiopulmonary resuscitation, and should be familiar with those behavioral disorders that commonly present with medical signs and symptoms.

The subsequent section describes the management of two common psychiatric emergencies with immediately life-threatening medical implications:

Table 7. Toxic Drugs Frequently Used in Suicide Attempts[a,b]

Key: 1000 milligrams (mg) = 15 grains (gr) = 1 gram (g)
MLD = minimum lethal dose
Notes: 1. Special adjustments for scoring are found at the end of the chart.
    2. If tab strength is recorded, make sure the common dosage in column 4 corresponds with the strength ingested.
    3. Fifth column rates toxicity. Mild = 0–33% of MLD (patient not expected to die); Moderate = 34–66% of MLD (a patient with a moderate rating could die); and Severe = 67% of MLD (this patient might well die).
    4. Class—Use only with a mixed drug overdose (see #2 at end of this chart for instructions about its use).

Drug	Est. MLD	Commonly available doses	Est. MLD number of tabs at most common dosage	Toxicity (at most common dosage)			Class
				Mild	Moderate	Severe	
Aspirin, Bufferin, Anacin, Excedrin (acetylsalicylics)	30 g	5 gr (3 gr)	90/5 gr	1–30	31–60	61+	3
Amytal (amobarbital)	1.5 g	15, 30, 50, 100 mg	30/50 mg	1–10	11–20	21+	2
Benadryl (diphenhydramine hydrochloride)	3 g	25 50 mg	60/50 mg	1–20	21–40	41+	3
Butisol (sodium butabarbital)	1 g	15, 30, 50, 100 mg	30/30 mg	1–10	11–20	21+	2
Carbrital (sodium pentobarbital)	1 g	75, 100 mg	10/100 mg	1–3	4–7	8+	2
Darvon (propoxyphene hydrochloride)	2 g	30, 65 mg	30/65 mg	1–10	11–20	21+	3
Demerol (meperidine hydrochloride)	1.2 g	50, 100 mg	24/50 mg	1–8	9–16	17+	3
Dilantin (phenytoin sodium)	3 g	30, 100 mg	30/100 mg	1–10	11–20	21+	5
Doriden (glutethimide)	8 g	250, 500 mg	16/500 mg	1–5	6–10	11+	1
Dramamine (dimenhydrinate)	5 g	50 mg	100/50 mg	1–33	34–66	67+	3
Elavil (amitriptyline hydrochloride)	3 g	10, 25, 50 mg	120/25 mg	1–40	41–80	81+	7
Equanil, Miltown (meprobamate)	15 g	200, 400 mg	38/400 mg	1–12	13–24	25+	5
Librium (chlordiazepoxide hydrochloride)	5 g	5, 10, 25 mg	500/10 mg	1–166	167–332	333+	5

Drug							
Luminal (phenobarbital)	1.5 g	15, 30, 100 mg	45/30 mg	1–15	16–30	31+	2
Mellaril (thioridazine)	3 g	10, 25, 50, 100, 150, 200 mg	100/25 mg	1–33	34–66	67+	4
Nembutal (sodium pentobarbital)	1 g	30, 50, 100 mg	10/100 mg	1–3	4–7	8+	2
Noludar (methyprylon)	5 g	50, 200, 300 mg	17/300 mg	1–6	7–12	13+	5
Nytol, Sominex (methapyrilene +)	3.5 g	25, 50 mg	140/25 mg	1–46	47–92	93+	3
Percodan (oxycodone hydrochloride)	0.5 g	4.5 mg	124/4.5 mg	1–42	43–84	85+	3
Placidyl (ethchlorvynol)	15 g	100, 200, 500 mg	30/500 mg	1–10	11–20	21+	5
Seconal (secobarbital sodium)	1.5 g	30, 50, 100 mg	15/100 mg	1–5	6–10	11+	2
Serax (oxazepam)	10 g	10, 15, 30 mg	333/30 mg	1–111	112–223	224+	5
Stelazine (trifluoperazine hydrochloride)	2.5 g	1, 2, 5, 10 mg	500/5 mg	1–166	167–332	333+	4
Thorazine (chlorpromazine)	2.2 g	10, 25, 30, 50, 75, 200 mg	44/50 mg	1–15	16–30	31+	4
Tofranil (imipramine hydrochloride)	2.5 g	10, 25, 50 mg	100/25 mg	1–33	34–66	67+	7
Tuinal (amobarbital sodium and secobarbital sodium)	1.5 g	50, 100, 200 mg	15/100 mg	1–5	6–10	11+	2
Valium (diazepam)	8 g	2, 5, 10 mg	1600/5 mg	1–553	534–1066	1067+	5
Valmid (ethinamate)	15 g	500 mg	30/500 mg	1–10	11–20	21+	5

a Special adjustment for scoring:

1. When any ingestion is accompanied by ETOH, increase tab/strength count by 50% before scoring toxicity.
2. Mixed drug ingestion—class division
   When 80% of the mixed drugs are within the same numerical class (column 6), take the single drug with the lowest MLD (columns 2 and 4) and compute all ingested tabs as being the single drug.
   When 80% of the mixed drugs are not within the same numerical class, compute the most lethal drug within the lowest ingested numerical class and raise one category.
3. If it is established that a person is a regular drug user, then reduce the number of ingested miligrams by ⅓ before using the chart for calculations. This procedure should correct for tolerance levels.
4. Ingestion with another agent (i.e., slashing)—rate most lethal agent.

b This table is a guide to toxicity. It should *not* be used as the only source for determining treatment. Adapted from Sterling-Smith.[22]

(1) coma and (2) overdose. These conditions are most often related to substance abuse. The clinician should carefully examine the patient, determine the level of consciousness (see Table 6), and provide appropriate treatment.

General guidelines for treating comatose patients with drug-related problems[19,20] include:

1. *Establish adequate respiration* by administering oxygen by mask, inserting an airway, or intubating the patient with a cuffed endotracheal tube. Draw arterial blood gases.
2. *Maintain perfusion pressure and circulation* by inserting an intravenous line and administering vasopressors as necessary.
3. *Administer various drugs to determine diagnoses.*

   a. Give two 50-cc ampules of 50% glucose in water after drawing blood for a glucose level.

   b. If the patient remains comatose, administer the opiate antagonist naloxone (Narcan). (See Chapter 9, pp. 143–144 for dosage schedule.)

   c. If the patient still does not respond and it is known that an anticholinergic agent was taken such as a heterocyclic antidepressant, administer physostigmine salicylate (Antilirium). (See Chapter 10.)

   d. Additional measures include treating seizures and cerebral edema and controlling body temperature. Obtain baseline bloods and other necessary diagnostic studies (e.g., arterial blood gases).

Individuals who have overdosed either accidentally or intentionally (e.g., suicide attempt) constitute another large group of emergency patients often requiring medical care. General guidelines for immediate treatment of these persons[21] include:

1. Ensure that the airway is open. If the patient slips into coma he should be intubated with a cuffed endotracheal tube. Support respiration as necessary.
2. Administer oxygen if indicated.
3. Induce vomiting with syrup of ipecac orally (30 ml in an adult or 15 ml in a child) *except* if the patient:

   a. is stuporous or comatose.

   b. has seizures.

   c. is pregnant.

   d. has overdosed on phenothiazines (e.g., chlorpromazine [Thorazine and others]) because they are antiemetics.

   e. has a possible acute myocardial infarction.

   f. has ingested a corrosive material (i.e., strong acids or alkalis or petroleum product such as kerosene, lighter fluid, gasoline, or furniture polish).
4. Give the patient large amounts of water after the ipecac and encourage him to move about.
5. Start an intravenous line with D5W.
6. Monitor the cardiac rhythm.

Table 7 describes those drugs commonly used in suicide attempts. It provides general guidelines for estimating the lethality of an overdose. Clinicians should use it only in combination with a careful history, MSE, and physical examination; it is not a substitute for specific information about the patient. For description of the clinical manifestations and management of specific overdoses see the chapters in Part IV.

7. Conclusion

One of the most challenging aspects of emergency work is the process of screening and care during the first few minutes. That small, pressured block of time encapsulates the toughest work of emergency psychiatry: identifying the dangerously violent patient and the medically urgent condition. Immediate action is required with virtually no data—action that continually reminds the emergency physician that he is briefly, but very profoundly, responsible for the welfare and, occasionally, life of his patients.

References

1. Bassuk EL: Management of the acutely ill psychiatric patient, in Noble J (ed): *Textbook of General Medicine and Primary Care*. Boston, Little, Brown and Co, 1984.
2. Bassuk EL, Fox S, Prendergast K: *Behavioral Emergencies: A Field Guide for EMTs and Paramedics*. Boston, Little, Brown and Co, 1983.
3. Glickman L: *Psychiatric Consultation in the General Hospital*. New York, Marcel Dekker, Inc, 1980, p 70.
4. Taylor M: *The Neuropsychiatric Mental Status Examination*. New York, Spectrum, 1981.
5. Folstein M, Folstein S, McHugh P: Mini mental state, *J Psychiatr Res* 12:189–198, 1975.
6. Jacobs J, Bernard M, Delgado A, et al: Screening for organic mental syndromes in the medically ill. *Ann Intern Med* 86:40–46, 1977.
7. Kaufman D, Weinberger M, Strain J, et al: Detection of cognitive defects by a brief mental status examination. *Gen Hosp Psychiatry* 1:247–255, 1979.
8. Bassuk EL, Schoonover SC, Gelenberg AJ (eds): *The Practitioner's Guide to Psychoactive Drugs,* ed 2. New York, Plenum Publishing Corp, 1983.
9. DiSclafani A II, Hall RC, Gardner ER: Drug-induced psychosis: Emergency diagnosis and management. *Psychosomatics* 22, October 1981.
10. Benson FD, Blumer D: *Psychiatric Aspects of Neurologic Disease*. New York, Grune and Stratton, 1975.
11. Tardiff K, Sweilamm A: Assault, suicide and mental illness, *Arch Gen Psychiatry* 37:164–169, 1980.
12. Madden DJ, Lion JR, Penna NW: Assaults on psychiatrists by patients. *Am J Psychiatry* 133:422–425, 1976.
13. Fortell E: A study of violent behavior among patients in psychiatric hospitals. *Br J Psychiatry* 136:216–221, 1980.
14. Lion JR, Pasternak SA: Countertransference reactions to violent patients. *Am J Psychiatry* 130:207–210, 1973.
15. DiBella CA: Educating staff to manage threatening paranoid patients. *Am J Psychiatry* 136:333–335, 1979.
16. Gelenberg AJ: Psychiatric emergencies: The psychotic patient. *Drug Ther* May 1981, pp 25–36.

17. Donlon P, Hopkin J, Tupin J: Overview: Efficacy and safety of the rapid neuroleptization method with injectable haloperidol. *Am J Psychiatry* 136:273–279, 1979.
18. Plum F, Posner M: *Diagnosis of Stupor and Coma*. Philadelphia, FA Davis Co, 1966, p 2.
19. Goldfrank L, Bresnitz E: Opioids. *Hosp Physician* October 1978, pp 26–37.
20. Costrini NV, Thomson W (eds): *Manual of Medical Therapeutics*, ed 22. Boston, Little, Brown and Co, 1977.
21. Caroline N: *Emergency Care in the Streets*. Boston, Little, Brown and Co, 1979, pp 350, 355.
22. Sterling-Smith, RS: A medical toxicology index: An evaluation of commonly used suicidal drugs, in Beck, AT, Resnik, HLP, Lettieri, DJ (eds): *The Prediction of Suicide*. Bowie, Md., The Charles Press Publishers, 1974, pp 216–218.

Legal Issues in a Psychiatric Emergency Setting

Henry A. Beyer, J.D.

1. Introduction

One might ask why there should be special legal rules applicable to the provision of psychiatric emergency services and not other emergency medical services. Aren't the legal principles the same, regardless of the type of services rendered? Although the same basic legal doctrines apply to both situations, certain important aspects of those doctrines are so pronounced in the case of a mentally disturbed patient that special discussion is warranted. For example, a psychiatric patient may be unable to give a legally valid competent consent to treatment or may pose a greater than average threat of losing control and causing serious physical harm. These characteristics have caused courts and legislatures to accord special treatment to the psychiatric emergency patient. Therefore, in this chapter, we will first describe the law relevant to all medical emergencies and then discuss in detail specific features applicable to psychiatric emergencies.

2. Autonomy, Privacy, and Informed Consent

American society and law place a very high, and still growing, value on the concept of personal autonomy. This concept is accorded legal recognition in many ways but, most generally, under the doctrine of the right of privacy. It has been a common law right (that is, a right recognized by English and American courts) for centuries and was defined succinctly in the 1880s as "the right to be let alone." In more recent years, the United States Supreme Court has given the privacy right a constitutional basis by holding that it is founded in the Fourteenth Amendment's concept of personal liberty and that it gives a woman the right to exercise significant control over her own body.[1] In the words of the Massachusetts Supreme Judicial Court, "the constitutional right to privacy . . . is an expression of the sanctity of individual free choice and self determination as fundamental constituents of life."[2]

Henry A. Beyer, J.D. • Center for Law and Health Sciences, Boston University School of Law, Boston, Massachusetts 02215.

3. Informed Consent

In the medical field, the autonomy and privacy principles are expressed in the doctrine of informed consent. This doctrine stipulates that a physician may not treat a patient until he has explained to the patient the possible risks and expected benefits of the proposed treatment, has outlined alternative courses of action, and has received from the patient a consent that is "informed," "voluntary," and "competent." Treatment without such consent may constitute negligence or a legal "battery."

Courts have differed from time to time and from state to state in deciding under what conditions a consenting patient has been adequately informed: that is, precisely how much must the patient be told? The trend in recent years has been decidedly toward requiring the provision of more information. In general, it can be said that patients must be given all the material facts to enable them to exercise self-determination in deciding about the proposed treatment. With regard to medication, for example, the patient should be told the expected benefits of the proposed drug and the probability that such benefits will actually be obtained; the possible neurologic and other adverse effects of the recommended drug and their probability of occurrence; what alternative drugs might be prescribed and their advantages and disadvantages; what alternative treatment modalities might be employed, along with their pros and cons; the risks of not accepting treatment; and any other facts that a reasonable person might find relevant to making the decision of whether to accept the treatment. Courts have made clear that this explanation should be given, not in a "lengthy polysyllabic discourse," but in terms understandable to the layperson.

Although the general rule is that all material facts must be presented, courts have on occasion found that doctors have the right to withhold certain information from particular patients. The California Supreme Court has held that "a disclosure need not be made beyond that required within the medical community when a doctor can prove . . . that he relied on facts that would demonstrate to a reasonable man the disclosure would so seriously upset the patient that the patient would not have been able to dispassionately weigh the risks of refusing to undergo the recommended treatment."[3] This exception to the general rule is a very narrow one, however. In one case, the court held that the doctor should have informed the patient that shock therapy involves some small risk of bones being fractured even though at the time of consent the patient was depressed, upset, agitated, crying, had marital problems, and had been drinking.[4]

In order for a patient's consent to treatment to be valid, it must be given "voluntarily." A "consent" that is forced from a patient is no consent at all. But there are, of course, varying degrees of pressure ranging from mild persuasion to overt physical force, and it is not always clear at what point permissible persuasion becomes coercion sufficient to invalidate a consent. Verbal suggestions or recommendations are certainly permissible, provided that they are accompanied by the provision of sufficient information, as discussed above. On the other hand, a threat (for example, that medication must be taken orally or it will be forcibly administered by injection) exceeds the bounds of permissible persuasion. A patient who takes medication as a result of such a threat cannot be said to have given legal consent.

One of the most common problems of voluntariness within the psychiatric context involves admission to a psychiatric facility. Although most persons who now enter psychiatric facilities do so "voluntarily," it is also true that many of those persons would not do so were it not for coercive factors. For example, persons may be told that if they do not sign a voluntary admission form, they will be involuntarily committed. Such admissions have generally been deemed "voluntary" in practically all states. At least one court, however, has rejected this fiction. In 1978, the Appellate Court of Illinois, noting that false imprisonment may occur as a result of words alone, held that a jury should determine the reasonableness of a patient's apprehension that if she did not rescind her request for discharge from a general hospital's psychiatric unit, her psychiatrist would have her committed to a state hospital.[5] It remains to be seen whether courts in other states will adopt this more stringent test of voluntariness.

The third element of informed consent—competence—must be considered from two aspects: legal competence and actual competence. In order for a person's consent to be valid, he must be both legally competent and competent in fact. Legal competence is the more easily determined. A person who has reached the age of majority (18 years of age in almost all states) is considered legally competent unless judged by a court of law to be incompetent. Involuntary civil commitment to a mental health facility notwithstanding, a person is still legally competent unless explicitly declared otherwise by a court of law.

Actual competence, on the other hand, is determined by a psychiatric or psychological judgment about the person's mental state. Does he have the cognitive and emotional capacity to understand and decide the matter for which his consent is sought? If not, his consent is not competent in fact and is therefore not valid.

Applying these legal principles within the hospital context is sometimes not easy.

> Consider, for example, the case of Mr. R., a 53-year-old male, brought to the emergency room complaining of crushing chest pain of one hour's duration. He is fully evaluated by the emergency physician; the findings are consistent with a severe myocardial infarction (heart attack) and admission is strongly recommended. The patient is panicky, refuses further treatment, and asks for his clothes so that he can leave. His wife and children are called, but they are unable to reason with him. As a last resort, the psychiatrist is called to evaluate him. Mr. R. seems overwhelmed with anxiety and tells the psychiatrist that his 50-year-old brother died three weeks ago of a heart attack and that his father died at the age of 53 of the same illness. He has worried his entire life about being like his father. The major findings on mental status examination are consistent with extreme anxiety, but the patient has no evidence of a thought disorder or suicidal ideation. Despite

the psychiatrist's attempts to help him with his fears, Mr. R. remains panicky and adamantly refuses to stay.

In this case the clinician's strong desire to meet the patient's physiologic need is pitted against his duty to respect Mr. R.'s legal right of privacy. Since Mr. R. is legally and actually competent, and has been fully informed of the risks of leaving the hospital, he has the legal right to leave. Attempts may be made to persuade him to stay, but he may not be retained by force. As difficult as it may be for the clinician, Mr. R.'s right to control his own fate must be respected.

Mr. R.'s situation differs only in degree from that of Robert H. Jackson, an associate justice of the United States Supreme Court from 1941 until 1954. In his last year on the Court, Justice Jackson suffered a severe heart attack. His doctors described to him the options—years of comparative inactivity or a continuation of his normal activity with the risk of death at any time. He chose the latter and suffered a fatal heart attack shortly thereafter.[6] No one interfered with Justice Jackson's elected course, nor would they have been legally able to do so if they had tried.

4. Substitute Consent

Both Mr. R. and Justice Jackson were considered mentally and legally competent to give or withhold consent to treatment. It is clear, however, that many persons in serious need of treatment are not capable of giving a valid, informed consent. The law therefore recognizes a number of ways in which others can supply a "substitute" consent for such persons.

Parents have general authority to give legally valid consent for the treatment of their minor children. Although this parental power is not without limit (parental consent is not legally sufficient, for example, for the sexual sterilization of a minor), it does extend, in most states, to the admission of such children to mental health facilities and to their treatment there. In some states, including Massachusetts, there is some question concerning parents' right to provide substitute consent in the psychiatric context for 16- and 17-year-olds. This question arises from statutes that grant to persons 16 or over the right to apply for voluntary admission to a mental hospital.[7] A Connecticut court,[8] the Massachusetts Department of Mental Health regulations,[9] and others have concluded that a right to admit oneself implies a corresponding right to release oneself. Thus, if parents provide substitute consent to the admission of their 16- or 17-year-old child, could that child not immediately retract such consent? In a state with such a statutory provision, therefore, it is advisable to obtain the consent of both the child in this two-year age group and his parents.

Legal guardians have traditionally had roughly the same authority with respect to their wards as parents have with respect to their children. Guardians are appointed by a probate or family court to guard, protect, and make decisions for persons deemed incompetent to care for themselves. Traditionally, guardianships are "plenary," that is, full or total. The guardian is authorized to decide and speak for his ward in practically all situations.

In recent years, however, guardians' powers have become more limited in several respects. First, many guardianships are no longer plenary. Some courts are appointing "limited" guardians with authority to decide and speak for their wards only on specific matters in which the wards are judged incapable of deciding for themselves. To determine whether or not a limited guardian's authority extends to decisions concerning mental health services, the court's guardianship order must be examined.

Second, in some states, the powers of even plenary guardians have recently been restricted in various contexts, some of which involve mental health. In Massachusetts, for example, a 1977 statute provides that a plenary guardian can no longer admit his ward to a mental health facility as a voluntary patient without the explicit authorization of the court that created the guardianship.[10] The Massachusetts Supreme Judicial Court has, in recent years, restricted a guardian's powers even further. In a 1981 case entitled *In re Richard Roe III*, the court ruled that the legal guardian (the father) of a nonhospitalized young adult male, diagnosed as suffering from paranoid schizophrenia, could not validly consent to the administration of antipsychotic medication to his ward (son).[11] "In order to accord proper respect to [the] basic right of all individuals [to refuse such treatment, the court held] that if an incompetent individual refuses antipsychotic drugs, those charged with his protection must seek a judicial determination of substituted judgment."[12] In a 1983 opinion, *Rogers vs. Commissioner*, the same court extended this right to involuntary patients in state mental hospitals.[13] "[A] committed mental patient is competent and has the right to make treatment decisions until the patient is adjudicated incompetent by a judge. If a patient is adjudicated incompetent, a judge, using a substituted judgment standard, shall decide whether the patient [if competent] would have consented to the administration of antipsychotic drugs."[14] If the judge's substituted judgment decision is for use of the drugs, the "burden shifts to the incompetent patient's guardian to seek modification of the order, should such modification be needed before the time for periodic review."[15]

The *Roe III* court also indicated that although there "is no bright line dividing those decisions which are (and ought to be) made by a guardian from those for which a judicial determination is necessary," the requirement for judicial rather than guardian decision-making applies as well to psychosurgery and electroconvulsive therapy.[16]

5. Written versus Oral Consent

Except in a few specific cases, the law does not require that consent to treatment be given in writing; oral consent can be equally valid and binding. The problem with oral consent, however, is documentation. What did the patient actually say? Was full consent given or was it qualified in some way? Exactly how much information was provided to the patient before he consented? Unfortunately, patients and health care providers may remember differently the precise parameters of the consent, particularly in the traumatic conetxt of a psychiatric emergency. Therefore, a signed consent form, although not legally necessary, is advisable. The form should be written in layperson's language and should contain as much information as possible relevant to the treatment procedure in question. If written consent is not possible, it is advisable to have the consent witnessed so that the extent of the information provided and the fact of the patient's consent are in some sense documented.

6. Emergencies

One other long-recognized exception to the requirement for informed consent applies in emergency situations. If the delay involved in obtaining informed consent before beginning treatment would result in serious harm, or if the patient requiring treatment is unconscious, incompetent, a minor, or unable for some other reason to provide a valid consent, courts have developed the concept of "implied" consent. Thus, doctors have been found to have acted properly in administering emergency treatment without waiting to obtain an informed consent. In recent years, many states have codified this common law exception in statutes dealing with emergency treatment.[17]

In the mental health context, "emergency" has been defined as "circumstances in which a failure to [forcibly medicate] would bring about a substantial likelihood of physical harm to the patient or others."[18] The United States Court of Appeals for the First Circuit, in reviewing *Rogers vs. Okin*, a case that arose in Massachusetts, has suggested that this definition should be extended to include "situations in which the immediate administration of drugs is reasonably believed to be necessary to prevent further deterioration in the patient's mental health."[19] The court held that "[w]hile judicial determinations are certainly preferable in general, room must be left for responsible state officials to respond to exigencies that render totally impractical recourse to traditional forms of judicial process."[20]

In the 1981 *Roe III* case, however, the Massachusetts Supreme Judicial Court, while taking note of the court of appeals decision, laid stress on the fact that an emergency situation is one in which " 'immediate action' is required."[21] "[T]he relevant time period to be examined begins when the claimed emergency arises and ends when the individual who seeks to act in the emergency could, with reasonable diligence, obtain judicial review of his proposed actions. This time period will, of course, be brief. . . . We recognize that 'the interests of the patient himself would [not] be furthered by requiring responsible [parties] to stand by and watch him slip into possibly chronic illness while awaiting an adjudication.' . . . However, . . . unless the course of a disease is measured by hours, there need never be such a case in the courts of this Commonwealth."[22]

Most recently, the Massachusetts high court, in the *Rogers* case, agreed that "[a] patient may be treated with antipsychotic drugs against his will and without prior court approval to prevent the 'immediate, substantial and irreversible deterioration of a serious mental illness.' "[23] But if someone is medicated under such circumstances, "and the doctors expect to continue to treat the patient with antipsychotic medication over the patient's objection, the doctors must seek adjudication of incompetency, and, if the patient is adjudicated incompetent, the court must formulate a substituted judgment treatment plan."[24] In response to the hospital's argument that if doctors are unable to medicate, great disruption of the hospital environment will result and the safety of patients and staff will be threatened, the court concluded that "only if a patient poses an imminent threat of harm to himself or others, and only if there is no less intrusive alternative to antipsychotic drugs, may the Commonwealth invoke its police powers without prior court approval to treat the patient by forcible injection of antipsychotic drugs over the patient's objection."[25] And it went on to note: "The defendants suggest that certain patients, as a symptom of their illness, will periodically threaten violence. Predictable crises are not within the definition of emergency. . . . Therefore, in those cases, the consent of the patient for medication with antipsychotic drugs must be obtained in advance, while the patient is competent and calm. If the patient has been declared incompetent, the periodic episodes of violence should be considered in formulating the substituted judgment treatment plan."[26]

Because of the *Roe III* and *Rogers* cases, the rules concerning emergency medication are now much more clearly defined in Massachusetts than in most other states. Moreover, because these cases were decided on the basis of state law rather than the federal Constitution, they may or may not be followed in other states. Meanwhile, however, emergency room clinicians throughout the nation must regularly face the difficult task of applying the emergency and substitute consent rules. Consider the following case:

> A 34-year-old male, well known to the staff, is brought into the emergency department by the police. He has been acting "strange" and is unable to tell them where he lives. The patient has been diagnosed as "a chronic schizophrenic" who can be maintained successfully in the community so long as he takes his medications. He has stopped them, however, and now refuses to resume. The man is not under guardianship, and past experience has indicated that he is not committable.

"Strange" actions and an inability to provide one's address do not constitute a danger to self or others. Unless it can be shown that a few hours' delay in commencement of treatment will result in the immediate, substantial, and irreversible deterioration in the man's condition, the circumstances do not constitute an "emergency" in jurisdictions following the *Roe III* and *Rogers* rules. If the emergency room staff and any family members who can be reached are unable to persuade the patient to resume taking his medication, they should turn to the probate or family court for authority to medicate. The hospital counsel should be familiar with this process. The court will conduct an incompetency hearing and, if convinced of the man's incompetence to make treatment decisions, will appoint a guardian (in some states called a "committee") for the patient. The role of permanent guardian is ordinarily filled by a relative or friend of the patient; a temporary guardian, whose involvement with the patient is expected to end with the current crisis, may be a lawyer or other stranger not otherwise involved in the treatment decision.

In many jurisdictions, the guardian will possess the inherent power to consent to the patient's medication. In others, following *Roe III* and *Rogers*, the court itself will make the treatment decision. The standard to be applied in making this decision also differs with the jurisdiction. In some, the decision is to be based on the patient's "best interests." In others, the standard is one of "substituted judgment"—what decision would the patient himself make if he were competent to do so? Some of the factors to be considered when making a substituted judgment are (1) the patient's expressed preferences regarding treatment, (2) his religious beliefs, (3) the impact of the decision upon the patient's family, insofar as this impact would be likely to affect the patient's decision, (4) the probability of adverse effects, (5) the consequences if treatment is refused, and (6) the prognosis with treatment.[27] If it is believed that the patient would, if competent, make an unwise or foolish decision, the substitute decision-maker should make the same unwise or foolish decision, and the court must respect that decision as long as it would accept the same decision if made by a competent individual in the same circumstances.[28]

An objection has been raised that requiring clinicians and patients' families to turn to the judicial system for authority to medicate in cases like this will be impossibly time-consuming. In response, the Massachusetts Supreme Judicial Court asserts that "every judge recognizes that in any case where there is a possibility of immediate, substantial, and irreversible deterioration of serious mental illness, even the smallest of avoidable delays would be intolerable."[29] Only experience will determine whether the court's faith in the judicial system's ability to respond quickly in such situations is justified.

7. Confidentiality

All patients have a right to confidentiality with respect to medical matters and what is said between patient and doctor. Because free and open communication is essential to psychotherapy, and because much of our society attaches a damaging stigma to psychiatric problems, the confidentiality right is especially important in the mental health context. In general, confidentiality in this field means that the health care provider may not disclose information received from the patient or information concerning the patient's case to anyone not involved in the patient's care and treatment.

There are, however, exceptions to the general confidentiality rule that vary from state to state. Many state statutes and their implementing regulations permit disclosure of some identifiable patient information to the Department of Mental Health, some other state agencies such as Welfare and Education Departments, state and federal law enforcement agencies, courts, and insurers. Some statutes authorize the Department of Mental Health or a court to grant responsible access to psychiatric, legal, or social science researchers. Many states do, and should, explicitly permit disclosure to anyone (including the patient) upon the express consent of a competent patient.

One major exception to the medical confidentiality rule is a long-standing common law privilege of physicians to warn individuals whose life or health might be threatened by their patient's condition. Thus, doctors may violate confidentiality to warn others of their patient's contagious disease. The California Supreme Court, in a 1976 opinion, *Tarasoff vs. Regents of the University of California*, transformed this privilege into a legal duty within the mental health context by holding that "when a psychotherapist determines, or pursuant to the standards of his profession should determine, that his patient presents a serious danger of violence to another, he incurs an obligation to use reasonable care to protect the intended victim against such danger."[30] Although courts in Georgia, Kansas, Nebraska, and New Jersey have adopted similar rules,[31] a Maryland appellate court decided in 1980 that no duty to warn third parties exists in that state.[32] The question has not yet been decided in most states.

Related to, and sometimes confused with, a patient's general confidentiality right is the doctor–patient *testimonial privilege*. This term refers to a rule of evidence created by statute applying only in judicial proceedings. The privilege exists in most, but not all, states. Where it exists, it simply states that a doctor (or, in some states, a psychiatrist) may not disclose information he has learned in confidence from a patient without the patient's permission. There are, however, exceptions to the doctor–patient rule that vary from state to state. These include civil commitment proceedings and actions in which the patient brings into question his mental condition (e.g., the insanity defense). A very common exception relates to the reporting of public health and welfare problems. Perhaps all states have statutes similar to the following:

> [A]ny physician, medical intern, medical examiner, dentist, nurse, public or private school teacher, educational administrator, guidance or family counselor, probation officer, social worker or policeman who, in his professional capacity shall have reasonable cause to believe that a child under the age of eighteen years is suffering serious physical or emotional injury resulting from abuse inflicted upon him including sexual abuse, or from neglect, including malnutrition, or who is determined to be physically dependent upon an addictive drug at birth, shall immediately report such condition to the department [of Public Health] . . . provided, however, that whenever such person so required to report is a member of the staff of a medical or other public or private institution, school or facility, he shall immediately either notify the department or notify the person in charge of such institution, school or facility, or that person's designated agent, whereupon such person in charge or his said agent shall then become responsible to make the report. . . .[33]

In many states other statutes require the reporting of such items as gunshot and stab wounds, cases of acute poisoning caused by controlled substances, motor vehicle accidents, and venereal disease. These statutes vary widely from state to state and from context to context, some requiring a report of the event but not of the identity of the person(s) involved, others requiring complete details.

8. *Special Mental Health Laws*

Because of the special circumstances of the psychiatric context, all state legislatures have enacted special mental health statutes. These statutes vary considerably from state to state, and many have been substantially revised recently. A few years ago, most mental health statutes stated their applicability to all persons who were "in need of," or "suitable for" care and treatment. The recent trend has been to narrow the target group to mentally ill persons who present a danger to themselves or others, while still recognizing such persons' rights to autonomy and privacy.

Typically, these statutes provide for three types of entry into the mental health system: voluntary admission to psychiatric care facilities, involuntary commitment by a court, and emergency admission. A voluntary admission is one in which a competent person, after being fully informed of the options available, voluntarily enters a mental health facility. If the person has not reached the age of majority or the state's statutory age for voluntary admission (age 16 in a number of states), the child's parent or guardian may provide substitute consent. In many states, a legal guardian may similarly provide such substitute consent to admission for his ward. In some jurisdictions such as Massachusetts, however, this requires the explicit approval of the court that created the guardianship.

Voluntary admission to a mental hospital differs from voluntary admission to a general hospital in that the mental patient is usually not free to leave at any time. Instead, the patient may be required to give several days' notice of his intent to leave. This delay in release allows the hospital time to petition a court for the patient's involuntary commitment, if it is thought that the person's mental illness poses a serious danger to the patient or others. Admissions that require such notice before release are sometimes called "conditional voluntary." Many states also provide for admissions in which no predischarge notice is required. These are sometimes called "straight voluntary."

Involuntary civil commitment to a mental hospital may be ordered by a court, usually in response to petition by the hospital or a member of the patient's family. At a court hearing to determine whether commitment is required, it usually must be shown that the proposed patient is mentally ill and that there is a likelihood of serious harm because of that illness. In some states, civil commitments are for specific periods, such as six months or a year, after which time either the person must be discharged or a recommitment hearing must be conducted. In other states, civil commitment is for an indefinite period—that is, until the hospital superintendent or designated staff member finds that the patient is no longer mentally ill or dangerous. In these latter states, however, some courts are now requiring that there be periodic reviews (e.g., once per year) to determine whether continuing commitment is required.

Every state's statutes make some provision for the emergency detention and treatment of mentally ill persons. These emergency admission statutes permit persons who seem dangerous as a result of mental illness to be held involuntarily at designated mental health facilities for a short time (usually between two days and two weeks) after proceedings much less formal than a civil commitment hearing. Typically, an emergency admission requires only that one (or sometimes two) physicians (or, in some states, a police officer or a qualified psychologist) and the hospital admitting person decide that failure to admit the person could result in serious harm by reason of mental illness. During the person's emergency stay, the hospital staff may perform diagnostic tests, administer treatment (but see Section 13 below), decide whether to petition for involuntary civil commitment, and perhaps encourage the patient to sign voluntary admission forms.

9. Dangerousness

The element of "dangerousness" or "likelihood of serious harm," found in the standards for both civil commitment and emergency admissions, is generally of three types: dangerousness to self, dangerousness to others, or inability to protect oneself in the community. Dangerousness to self is usually manifested in attempts or threats of suicide but may sometimes consist of serious self-mutilation. Dangerousness to others is typically evidenced by attempts or threats to do serious physical harm to others combined with an apparent ability to inflict such harm. Inability to protect oneself in the community is manifested in such actions as failure to eat, to protect oneself from the elements, or to seek or accept needed medical attention to such an extent that one's life is endangered. It may also be evidenced by instances of wandering heedlessly into busy streets or other life-threatening situations. In some states' statutes, this element of the commitment standard is stated in more general terms as an inability to care for one's physical needs or as being "in need of care and treatment." Statutory enactments as well as court decisions during the past decade, however, indicate a clear trend toward restricting involuntary civil commitment to mentally ill persons who are dangerous and toward increasing the severity of harm required to support a finding of dangerousness.

Although all states permit civil commitment only upon proof of "mental illness" (or "mental disorder"), most statutes fail to define the term *mental illness*, or they define it only vaguely or circularly as a condition that impairs mental health or that requires hospitalization. Similarly, most statutes fail to state the magnitude of harm, its probability of occurrence, or the degree of immediacy that is required to satisfy their commitment standards. Although most laws give little guidance as to the type of proof needed to establish these elements, a few states now require evidence of a recent, overt dangerous act or credible threat. The Pennsylvania Mental Health Procedures Act, for example, provides that "clear and present danger to others shall be shown by establishing that within the past 30 days the person has inflicted or attempted to inflict serious bodily harm on another and that there is a reasonable probability that such conduct will be repeated."[34]

Although the United States Supreme Court has not ruled on the constitutionality of the various civil commitment standards or the type of evidence required to establish them, it has decided what level of proof is constitutionally required. In its 1979 opinion in *Addington vs. Texas*, the Court held that the commitment standard must be satisfied by at least "clear and convincing" proof.[35] This "clear and convincing" standard of proof falls between the "beyond a reasonable doubt" standard employed in criminal trials and the "preponderance of the evidence" standard used in other civil litigation. A number of states, however, have gone beyond *Addington* and require, on the basis of a statute or the state constitution, proof beyond a reasonable doubt.[36]

10. The Management of Dangerousness

The provision of services to dangerous mentally ill persons sometimes violates certain rights of those persons. Civil commitment and emergency admission involve limitations of rights. Other situations requiring rights-abridgments may occur at any point in the course of a patient's care and treatment. Among the treatment techniques that limit a patient's liberty rights are time-out, seclusion, and physical, mechanical, or chemical restraints.

The first point to be ascertained before interfering with another person's liberty or other legal rights is the authority to do so. In the psychiatric care context, there are two major sources for such authority: contract or statute. In the context of private practice or a private psychiatric facility, the person seeking mental health services may waive certain rights in the admission application or other contract granting consent to care and treatment. The validity of such contractual waivers, however, is frequently beset with uncertainties. The essential elements of informed consent, as discussed above, are applicable to such a contract. The specific type of rights-interference authorized must be stated in detail; courts are increasingly unwilling to uphold the legality of "blanket" consent provisions. The competence of a mentally ill person to enter into such an agreement may also be a contestable matter. Finally, courts are beginning to question the voluntariness of an agreement that is entered under the explicit or implicit threat of civil commitment.[37]

The other source of authority for restricting a patient's rights is statutory. As noted above, some state statutes authorize physicians or certain others to restrain persons whom they believe to be mentally ill during the course of an emergency admission. Mental health care providers employed by the state or by certain facilities or programs licensed by the state to care for involuntary patients may have additional statutory authority to restrict a patient's rights during the course of care and treatment. These providers are acting as agents of the state and, as such, are exercising the state's police power to protect society, and its *parens patriae* (paternalistic power) to care for those who are incapable of caring for themselves. The authority of mental health care providers acting as agents of the state differs greatly from state to state and is usually detailed in regulations of the Department of Mental Health or the comparable state agency. Regulations typically specify which members of the treatment team may authorize mechanical restraints or other various restrictions, under what circumstances, for what time periods, and with what documentation.

11. Least Restrictive Alternative

Regardless of the source of authority for limiting a patient's rights, it is essential that any such actions be taken in good faith—that is, for the benefit of the patient rather than staff or others—and that they be the least restrictive, least drastic, least intrusive means of handling the situation. The legal principle of "least restrictive alternative" mandates that when government has a legitimate societal goal to serve, it should act through means that curtail individual freedom no more than is necessary to secure that goal. Under this principle, electroconvulsive therapy should not be administered if talking therapy can achieve the same results; a patient should not be confined in a state hospital if weekly visits to a clinic will suffice; four hours' seclusion is not permissible if five minutes of physical holding will settle a crisis situation.

The question arises whether the use of psychotropic medications as chemical restraint is more or less restrictive than civil commitment, seclusion, or various types of mechanical restraints. Few courts have even addressed this question in the general case. Most seem inclined to focus on the particular facts of the case before them—the specific intended effects and adverse side effects of the particular drug, the degree and duration of liberty restrictions imposed by the mechanical restraints, and the degree of discomfort inherent in alternative approaches. In its *Roe III* decision, however, the Massachusetts Supreme Judicial Court ruled that "[i]n order to satisfy the least intrusive means test, the incompetent is entitled to choose, by way of substituted judgment, between involuntary commitment and involuntary medication."[38] The court indicated that, in Massachusetts at least, the authority to make such a substituted judgment lies with the court.

12. Right to Treatment

Once a patient has been admitted to a facility or program for psychiatric treatment, he has a right to receive treatment. For voluntary patients at private facilities, this right is based upon their contractual relationship with the facility. For patients in state hospitals and some other state-licensed, certified, or supported facilities or programs, treatment is frequently a statutory right. For involuntary patients (probably including persons on emergency admission and conditional voluntary status), it is widely believed that the right to treatment has a constitutional basis.

The United States Supreme Court has not ruled directly on this issue. In the 1975 case, *O'Connor vs. Donaldson*, the Court held only that "a state cannot constitutionally confine without more a nondangerous individual who is capable of surviving safely in freedom by himself or with the help of willing and responsible family members or friends."[39] Although the phrase "without more" has been generally interpreted to mean "without treatment," the Court noted explicitly in *Donaldson* that "there is no reason now to decide whether mentally ill persons dangerous to themselves or others have a right to treatment upon compulsory confinement by the State, or whether the State may compulsorily confine a nondangerous, mentally ill individual for the purpose of treatment."[40] In a June 1982 opinion the high Court ruled that a mentally retarded man involuntarily confined to a state facility for mentally retarded persons had a constitutional right to safe conditions, freedom from unreasonable restraint, and "minimally adequate" training to enable him to better control his aggressive behavior so that he could be allowed more freedom of movement.[41] Once again, however, the Court sidestepped the more general question. It explicitly refused to decide whether an institutionalized mentally retarded person "has some general constitutional right to training per se."[42]

Despite the Supreme Court's reluctance to decide the issue, lower federal courts and some state courts have held that all involuntarily confined patients have a constitutional right to receive such treatment as will give them a realistic opportunity to be cured or to improve their mental condition.[43] They point out that provision of treatment is the stated purpose of civil commitment, and confinement in a mental hospital without treatment would be equivalent to imprisonment, but imprisonment imposed without the due process safeguards of a criminal trial.

Courts have faced greater difficulty, however, in deciding what constitutes adequate or appropriate treatment. A few extreme or experimental behavior modification techniques, such as the use of the emetic apomorphine on nonconsenting residents of a state secure medical facility, have been found to constitute cruel and unusual punishment.[44] And psychosurgery for involuntarily detained mental patients has been judicially banned in at least one jurisdiction.[45] In general, however, the courts and legislatures have been reluctant to interfere in mental health professionals' determinations of appropriate treatment. In decisions upholding the right to treatment, courts have stated that, although they may not have the expertise to judge between different types of therapies, they *are* capable of determining when *no* treatment is being given. They have indicated, for example, that mere warehousing does not constitute milieu therapy. Beyond that, however, the right to treatment issue has essentially involved requiring improved institutional conditions and facilities, better staff–patient ratios, and individualized treatment plans.[46]

13. Right to Refuse Treatment

Courts have long recognized a person's general right to refuse treatment for physical illness. This right is a natural corollary of the informed consent to treatment requirement discussed above. Only in very recent years, however, has this right been held to apply to mental patients. The traditional approach had been to presume that psychiatric patients are not competent to make decisions regarding their treatment, and therefore to entrust mental health care providers with this responsibility. Since 1979, however, federal and state courts in several states have held that mental patients should be permitted to make the decisions concerning their own treatment unless they are in emergency situations or have been judged legally incompetent. Most courts hold that even a civil commitment does not, by itself, deprive a patient of the right to make decisions concerning his own treatment.

In the recent *Rogers vs. Commissioner* opinion, discussed above, the Massachusetts Supreme Judicial Court ruled that "a committed mental patient is competent and has the right to make treatment decisions until the patient is adjudicated incompetent by a judge. If a patient is adjudicated incompetent, a judge, using a substituted judgment standard, shall decide whether the patient [if competent] would have consented to the administration of antipsychotic drugs. . . . No State interest justifies the use of antipsychotic drugs in a non-emergency situation without the patient's consent. Antipsychotic drugs which are used to prevent violence to third persons, to prevent suicide, or to preserve security, are being used as chemical restraints and must follow the strictures of [a state statute and regulations governing the use of restraints]. A patient may be treated with antipsychotic drugs against his will and without prior court approval to prevent the 'immediate, substantial, and irreversible deterioration of a serious mental illness.' [But i]f a patient is medicated [in such circumstances], and the doctors expect to continue to treat the patient with antipsychotic medication over the patient's objection, the doctors . . . must seek adjudication of incompetency, and, if the patient is adjudicated incompetent, the court must formulate a substituted judgment treatment plan."[47]

The court rejected the defendants' argument that doctors "should be responsible for making treatment decisions for involuntarily committed patients, whether competent or not. . . . 'Every competent adult has a right to forego treatment, or even cure, if it entails what for him are intolerable consequences or risks however unwise his sense of values may be in the eyes of the medical profession.'"[48] The court noted that "[b]ecause a person is competent until adjudicated incompetent, . . . a patient's acceptance of antipsychotic drugs ordinarily does not require judicial proceedings. . . . [H]owever, . . . because incompetent persons cannot meaningfully consent to medical treatment, a substituted judgment by a judge should be undertaken for the incompetent patient even if the patient accepts medical treatment."[49]

In most states, however, courts have not yet squarely addressed this question. And those that have have arrived at different results.[50] In California, for example, mental patients and the Department of Mental Health have recently entered into a Consent Decree, approved by the federal court, which permits the administration of antipsychotic medication without informed consent under certain specified circumstances, upon the approval, not of a judge, but of an "independent reviewer" employed by the department.[51] Because of the variations among states' laws, as well as the uncertainties inherent in such situations, it is evident that a patient's right to refuse treatment can pose difficult legal and ethical issues to an emergency room staff. Consider, for example, the following case:

> A disheveled 23-year-old male comes into a general hospital emergency ward talking loudly, incoherently, and at times aggressively. The psychiatrist is called to evaluate him. He concludes that the patient is acutely psychotic, only marginally in control, and needs medication. The patient refuses treatment and threatens the physician. He is medicated forcibly and, after several hours, seems to be calmer. His thought disorder is improved. Arrangements for evaluation at the local state hospital are made, but the patient does not have insurance. A commitment paper requesting admission is signed by the emergency ward psychiatrist. When the patient arrives at the state hospital he is somewhat improved and in good control. They find out that he lives with his father, has been out of work for six months, has become increasingly seclusive, and had a similar episode three years ago. He is currently not in treatment. The state hospital is overbedded and feels that he can be evaluated for partial hospitalization and aftercare. He is discharged with an appointment scheduled for the next day. Twelve hours later he is brought in by the police after seriously assaulting a neighbor in his apartment building.

What are the legal issues in this all-too-common scenario? One is, of course, the forcible administration of medication. As discussed above in Section 4, the overriding of a patient's refusal is legally permissible in an emergency. The question is, however, was this an emergency situation? Was the young man's threat of assault a serious one? And was the danger so immediate that no judicial review could have been obtained before serious harm occurred?

If the patient actually presented a substantial likelihood of immediate physical harm to the psychiatrist or others (and the later neighborhood assault supports a claim that it did), some action is clearly justified. But what action? Was there a "less restrictive alternative"? That is, did there exist other means of countering his aggressive potential that would have been less intrusive than a mind-altering drug? Could he, for example, have been physically held until he was admitted to the state hospital, a judicial incompetency hearing was conducted (see discussion above in Section 6), or his aggressive tendencies subsided? Might mechanical restraints have been more or less restrictive than medication? In addressing a closely analogous question in *Roe III*, the Massachusetts Supreme Judicial Court said:

> We are unwilling to establish a universal rule as to which is less intrusive—involuntary commitment or involuntary medication with mind-altering drugs. Since we feel that such a determination must be individually made, we conclude that the less intrusive means is the means of restraint which would be chosen by the ward if he were competent to choose.[52]

As mentioned above, in Section 10, state regulations usually govern the use of mechanical restraints. One other consideration in the case at hand (admittedly, most apparent in retrospect) is that, if mechanical restraints had been used rather than medication, the patient's verbal threats might have continued and admission to the state hospital would thus have been more likely.

14. Legal Liability

Like all persons, mental health care providers can be held legally liable for their actions. Although liability can be for breach of contract or for a criminal act, most legal liability actions are civil suits charging malpractice or negligence, a civil wrong or "tort."

To prevail in a negligence suit, the patient must prove four things: (1) that the provider had a duty of care, (2) that the duty was breached, (3) that the patient was injured, and (4) that the patient's injury was caused by the provider's breach of duty. Elements (2), (3), and (4) present factual questions requiring the presentation of testimony and/or physical evidence concerning the patient's particular situation. Element (1), on the other hand, presents both factual and legal questions: Did the particular provider owe a duty of care to this individual, and, if so, what is the standard of care against which that duty should be measured?

15. Standards of Care

Violation of a statute, ordinance, or regulation is evidence of negligence with respect to all consequences the rule was intended to prevent. Whenever, as in many psychiatric care situations, there is no controlling statute, ordinance, or regulation, the test of whether a person has acted negligently is whether the person has acted as a "reasonable" person would have acted under the same or similar circumstances. If the so-designated actor belongs to a profession possessing specialized knowledge or skill superior to that of the ordinary person, the law demands that his actions be consistent with that special knowledge or skill. Where the actor is a physician, the test that courts in many states apply is to ask whether the doctor acted as a reasonably prudent practitioner from the same school of medicine, in the same or similar community, would have acted under the same or similar circumstances. In many states, however, courts have abandoned the "locality" aspect of the rule.

Standards for physicians with medical specialities, such as psychiatry, also differ from state to state but generally take into account the greater skill resulting from their specialization. In Massachusetts, for example, "[o]ne holding himself out as a specialist should be held to the standard of care and skill of the average member of the profession practising [sic] the specialty, taking into account the advances in the profession. And, as in the case of the general practitioner, it is permissible to consider the medical resources available to him."[53]

As mentioned above, standards of care for different professional and paraprofessional providers may also be set or modified by state statutes that apply in various contexts. Many states have "Good Samaritan" statutes, which absolve licensed professionals and some other persons from civil liability for negligence in rendering aid in good faith at the scene of an emergency. In 1973 Massachusetts added to its law a new chapter relating to emergency medical care. It includes a provision that no registered doctor or nurse shall be liable in a suit for damages that result from advice, consultation, or orders given in good faith to qualified ambulance operators and attendants by radio, telephone, or other remote means of communication under emergency conditions; nor shall the ambulance operator or attendant be liable as a result of acts or omissions based upon such advice, consultation, or orders.[54] Another section provides that no certified emergency medical technician, who in the performance of his duties and in good faith renders emergency first aid or transportation to an injured or incapacitated person, shall be personally liable as a result.[55] Although such statutes and regulations vary widely from state to state in the context to which they apply as well as in their specific provisions, a common requirement is that the actions were taken "in good faith": that is, for the intended benefit of the patient.

16. Suicide

Suicide presents such an extreme and irreversible attack upon normal societal standards that it merits special attention in both medical and legal literature.[56] Some persons argue that it is every individual's right to end his life given sufficient reason, and several organizations have been established to defend and advance that view.[57] But Anglo-American law has traditionally prohibited suicide (or, at least, attempts at suicide), and many states have had specific statutes to that effect.

Although the criminal penalities formerly associated with suicide have been almost totally repealed in recent years, states are still grappling with methods of preventing the act.[58]

> A compromise approach would be to impose a "cooling off period," a relatively short period of time . . . during which the would-be suicide could be involuntarily detained in order to give him time in which to regain perspective lost because of depression or other mental disability.[59]

California has adopted a qualified version of this approach in its Lanterman-Petris-Short Mental Health Act. Under its provisions, "Suicidal patients must be released on demand after thirty-one days of involuntary commitment unless a judicial determination is made that the [person] is 'gravely disabled' in which case a conservator would be appointed who might continue the confinement on that basis."[60]

If a recent, serious suicide attempt results from mental illness, that action clearly satisfies one of the criteria for civil commitment—that a person presents a danger to himself.[61] Since the taking of one's own life represents the paramount example of harm to self and also, in many cases, seriously disrupts the social order, law has traditionally recognized the state's right to prevent suicide under both its *parens patriae* and police powers. The staff of a state-licensed psychiatric emergency unit, as agents of the state, share in that authority. In addition, if the suicidal person is a patient entrusted to their care, they have a duty to attempt to prevent his self-destruction.

One major legal issue in this area concerns the determination of the likelihood of suicide. How probable must it be that a person will attempt to take his life in order for that person to be judged a danger to self and thus subject to civil commitment or other abridgments of his liberty rights? And how apparent must this danger be in order for mental health staff to be held liable for failing to recognize it? A related question concerns the degree and type of measures that mental health staff members are legally required to take in order to prevent a suicide, once the danger is recognized.

The legal standards for determining committability and liability based on assessed dangerousness to self vary from state to state, are constantly changing, and are generally unclear even in a given state. One attorney's 1975 observation remains valid today:

> Generally the cases from New York give an understanding of problems involved in determining "the law" in this area of hospital liability. Starting from a lack of foreseeability of suicide in 1891, the New York courts developed a rigid standard of care by the hospital through the 1920s and 1930s. In the 1940s the courts seemed to swing away from close supervision in response to medical pleas for more freedom for mental patients. Cases in the late 1950s and through the 1960s do not reflect a predominant theme. Going into the 1970s, the field of hospital liability for patient suicide and self-injury seems wide open for the imaginative advocate.[62]

In determining liability, all courts appear to apply some test of "reasonable forseeability." In a suit concerning the suicide of a Connecticut VA hospital patient, a United States Court of Appeals noted that "unlike blood pressure or pulse rates, emotional states cannot be calibrated with precision."[63] But if the patient's suicide was "reasonably foreseeable on the basis of [his] past history," then the hospital staff was negligent in not providing close supervision. Courts vary considerably, however, in their opinions of what circumstances make a suicide reasonably foreseeable. Factors that are frequently considered include the patient's history of suicide attempts, their seriousness, and their recentness. Less important, but frequently also relevant, are threats of suicide, particularly if they are recent, perceived as serious by a "reliable" observer, and documented in the patient's record.

The qualifications of the person making the risk determination are also important. In *Cohen vs State of New York*, the state was held liable for the death of a patient who committed suicide on the day of his release from a state hospital psychiatric ward.[64] The court found that the patient had been treated and released by a physician in his first year of residency—"a doctor not qualified in an unsupervised status to make a judgment [concerning release]." The fault, said the court, lay not with the treating physician and superior resident and attending doctor as individuals, "but rather with the lack of policies requiring more direct management of a patient's treatment by a qualified psychiatrist."

In view of such decisions, and the generally unclear and unsettled status of the law, it would appear prudent for hospitals to formalize at least the following elements: Any staff member who observes a patient exhibiting suicidal tendencies, through statements or behavior, shall report this immediately to a member of the medical staff. A qualified member of the medical staff shall then, at the earliest opportunity, write an order stating that the patient does or does not require constant supervision and, if not, whether other precautions should be followed. Until such time as this order is written, the patient shall not be left unattended. Facilities should ensure, of course, that any such policies that are adopted are actually implemented and followed. Many courts have held that a hospital's failure to follow its own rules is evidence of negligence.

Protective measures (other than constant supervision) which might be taken with patients considered suicidal include removal of dangerous articles (clothing, necklaces, razors, lighters, eating utensils, drugs, etc.), confinement in "safe," non-hazardous rooms or areas, use of psychotropic medication or mechanical restraints, or civil commitment.[65] This, however,

> is not to suggest that every potential suicide must be locked in a padded cell. The law and modern psychiatry have now both come to the belated conclusion that an overly restrictive environment can be as destructive as an overly permissive one. But while we must accept some calculated risks in order to insure the patient's legal rights and provide him with the most effective therapy, we must also admit that errors in judgment do occur and that when they do, medical authorities must assume their rightful share of the responsibility.[66]

17. The Hardest Part

Perhaps the hardest part of a psychiatric emergency professional's job is acknowledging that not all patients' problems can be solved psychiatrically or legally. Even though the staff may feel certain of what a patient needs or should do, it is sometimes not possible to bring about that result without the use of force. And force may not be legally permitted because of the value our society places on the patient's right to privacy and autonomy even when that patient makes faulty judgments.

Consider the case of Mary:

> Mary is a 19-year-old female who is brought into the emergency ward by her father after a serious Tylenol overdose. After 24 hours of treatment and observation on the ER, her Tylenol level has decreased to therapeutic levels and she is more alert. This is her third major overdose in the past month. On each occasion, outpatient treatment was recommended, but Mary did not follow through. She now denies any suicidal intent and shows no evidence of psychosis. She denies that the current ingestion was related to her feelings but insists instead that she took the pills to treat her low back pain. Mary says that her only problem was that she was not allowed to go outside of her home unless accompanied by her parents. She had no friends, nor any social activity. She had been looking for secretarial work, and her mother insisted on going to interviews with her. For a brief moment she

was able to acknowledge how trapped and desperate she was, but then she quickly denied these feelings and went on to rationalize her mother's position. In the middle of the interview the parents arrive, threatening litigation if Mary is not allowed to leave immediately. Her father appears intoxicated and her mother and grandmother paranoid and threatening. The psychiatrist tries to discuss Mary's behavior with them, particularly the seriousness of all three overdoses and the meaning of the escalating suicidal behavior. No one in the family system will acknowledge that the ingestion was an overdose or that the patient was troubled in any way. What are the dispositional alternatives?

At 19, Mary is legally an adult in practically all states. As such, she has the right to speak for herself. It is she, not her parents, who has the legal right to accept or refuse treatment. Although there may be a danger, a "likelihood of serious harm," Mary exhibits no psychosis. If it cannot be shown that the danger results from mental illness, it is probably not possible to have her civilly committed. And after her Tylenol level has been reduced, the situation is not an "emergency" by either the *Rogers vs. Okin* or *Roe III* definition.

Just how "paranoid" are Mary's mother and grandmother? Could it be argued that they constitute a danger to others (namely Mary) by reason of their own "mental illness" and should therefore be committed? Again, because civil commitment statutes are being more narrowly construed in all states, it is quite doubtful that this could be done. Also, it is questionable whether commitment of her mother and grandmother would have the desired effect of freeing Mary from their overbearing control. Would the situation be at all improved by even raising the possibility of civil commitment of Mary or others? It might well have the opposite effect of bringing the family together to resist a perceived attack from without.

Although attempted suicide may no longer be classified as a crime, strong societal disapproval persists. And persons who aid or abet a suicide attempt are considered criminals in many states.[67] Although it would undoubtedly be impossible to have Mary's family charged with this crime (the requisite intent being absent), it may be worth considering what the effect might be on the family of a suggestion that such a prosecution might be possible. Could the family be persuaded that outpatient treatment is the best way of forestalling such an eventuality? Although there might be some risk of uniting the family in their resistance to what is perceived as outside attack, the ER staff might persuade them that the staff's allegiance is to the family and their aim is to avoid any such prosecution (which would be brought by the prosecutor's office rather than the staff).

When all is said and done, however, the ER staff may not be able to persuade Mary or her family to follow their advice. She may insist upon leaving, thus beginning the next and possibly final act in what the staff feels is an avoidable tragedy. Although understandably frustrated and depressed by their inability to prevent this, the staff may profit from recalling the case of Justice Jackson and remembering that, in order for society to preserve personal autonomy, people must have a right to be wrong.[68]

Notes

1. *Roe vs Wade*, 410 US 113 (1973).
2. *Superintendent of Belchertown State School vs Saikewicz*, 370 NE 2nd 417, at 426 (Mass, 1977).
3. *Cobbs vs Grant*, 502 P2d 1 (Cal, 1972).
4. *Mitchell vs Robinson*, 334 SW2d 11 (Mo, 1960).
5. *Marcus vs Liebman*, 375 NE2d 486 (Ill App Ct, 1978).
6. Dershowitz, A: Psychiatry in the legal process: A knife that cuts both ways, in Brooks A (ed): *Law, Psychiatry and the Mental Health System*. Boston, Little Brown and Co, 1974, pp 609, 615.
7. See, e.g., Mass Gen Laws, ch 123, sec 10.
8. *Melville vs Sabbatino*, 30 Conn Sup 320, 313 A2d 886 (1973).
9. Mass 104 CMR 3.04(7) and 104 CMR 3.14(5).
10. Mass Gen Laws, ch 201, secs 6, 6A, and 14.
11. 421 NE 2d 40 (1981).
12. Ibid., at 51.
13. *Rogers vs Commissioner*, 390 Mass 489 (1983).
14. Ibid., at 491.
15. Ibid., at 507.
16. 421 NE 2d at 52.
17. See, e.g., W Va Code, ch 16, sec 4C-11.
18. *Rogers vs Okin*, 634 F 2d 650 (1st Cir, 1980), at 659; vacated and remanded *sub nom Mills vs Rogers*, 457 US 291 (1982).
19. Ibid., at 634 F 2d 659–660.
20. Ibid., at 660.
21. *In re Richard Roe III*, note 11, above, at 54.
22. Ibid., at 55.
23. 390 Mass at 491.
24. Ibid. (footnote omitted).
25. Ibid., at 510–511.
26. Ibid., at 511, n 26.
27. Each of these factors is discussed in *In re Richard Roe III*, note 11, above, at 56–59.
28. Ibid., at 59, n 20.
29. Ibid., at 55.
30. *Tarasoff vs Regents of the University of California*, 551 P 2d 334 (Cal, 1976).
31. *Bradley Center vs Wessner*, 51 USLW 2275 (Ga Super Ct, 1982); *Durflinger vs Artiles*, 52 USLW 2361 (Kans Super Ct, 1983); *Lipari vs Sears Roebuck*, 497 F. Supp 185 (D Neb 1980); *McIntosh vs Milane*, 168 NJ Super 466 (1979).
32. *Shaw vs Glickman*, 415 A2d 625 (Md App 1980).
33. Mass Gen Laws, ch 119, sec 51A.
34. Pa Act of July 9, 1976, PL 817, No 143, sec 301(b), interpreted and applied in *Comm ex rel Gibson vs DiGiacinto*, 395 A2d 938 (Pa Super Ct, 1978).
35. 99 S Ct 1804 (1979).
36. See, e.g., *Superintendent of Worcester State Hospital vs Hagburg*, 374 Mass 271, 372 NE2d 242 (1978).
37. See *Marcus vs Liebman*, note 5, above.
38. *In re Richard Roe III*, note 11, above, at 61.
39. *O'Connor vs Donaldson*, 422 US 563 (1975).
40. Ibid., at 573.
41. *Romeo vs Youngberg*, 644 F2d 147 (3rd Cir, 1980); remanded 102 S Ct 2452 (1982).
42. Ibid., at 102 S Ct 2459.
43. See, e.g., *Wyatt vs Stickney*, 325 F Supp 781, 334 F Supp 1341, 344 F Supp 373 (MD Ala, 1971–72); generally affirmed *sub nom Wyatt vs Aderholt*, 503 F2d, 1305 (5th Cir, 1974).

44. *Knecht vs Gillman*, 488 F2d 1136 (8th Cir, 1973).
45. *Kaimowitz vs Michigan Department of Mental Health*, CA No 73–19434–AW (Cir Ct, Wayne County, Mich, July 10, 1973), summarized at 42 USLW 2063 (July 31, 1973).
46. See, generally, *Wyatt vs Stickney*, note 43 above.
47. *Rogers vs Commissioner*, note 13 above, at 491.
48. Ibid., at 497–498.
49. Ibid., at 500, n 14.
50. See, e.g., *Rennie vs Klein*, 476 F Supp 1294 (D NJ, 1979), affirmed in part, 653 F2d 836 (3rd Cir, 1981); *Davis vs Hubbard*, 506 F Supp 915 (ND Ohio, 1980); *In re K.K.B.*, 609 P.2d 747 (Okla, 1980); *A.E. and R.R. vs Mitchell*, C 78–466 (USDC, D Utah, June 12, 1980). (Under Utah's statute, the requisite findings for involuntary commitment include, in effect, a finding that the person being committed is incompetent to consent to treatment.)
51. *Jamison vs Farabee*, No C 780445 WHO (USDC, ND Cal, Consent Decree, 4/26/83), reported at 7 Ment Disabil L Rep 436 (1983).
52. *In re Richard Roe III*, note 11, above, at 61, n 24.
53. *Brune vs Belinkoff*, 354 Mass 102 (1968), at 109.
54. Mass Gen Laws, ch 111C, sec 13.
55. Mass Gen Laws, ch 111C, sec 14.
56. See, e.g., Ruben LH: Managing suicidal behavior. *JAMA* 241(3): 282–284, 1979; Doctor and the law: On expert guidance and the suicide risk. *Medical World News,* March 1, 1974, Vol 15, p 46E; Cooper TR: Medical treatment facility liable for patient suicide and other self-injury. *J Legal Med* 3:20–29, 1975; Seiden RH: Suicide among the young: A review of the literature, 1900–1967. Joint Commission on Mental Health of Children, 1969 (A supplement to the bulletin of suicidology). See also Morgan HG: *Death Wishes: The Understanding and Management of Deliberate Self-Harm.* New York, John Wiley and Sons, 1979. In this book, suicide, "fatal self-harm," is distinguished from other, nonfatal "acute deliberate self-harm."
57. "Hemlock: A Society Supporting Active Voluntary Euthanasia for the Terminally Ill"; "The Society for the Right to Die"; and "Exit," a British group, which, in March 1980, announced plans to publish a manual entitled *A Guide to Self-Deliverance*, outlining "nonviolent" methods of committing suicide. *Science*, 1980, 209:1096–1097. Cf. "The American Association of Suicidology," a "multidisciplinary organization of professionals and non-professionals who share a conviction that the advancement of suicidology will contribute to our knowledge how best to reduce human self-destruction," and which sponsors a quarterly journal, *Suicide and Life-Threatening Behavior*.
58. For an exposition of the arguments that led to this repeal, see *The punishment of suicide—A need for change. Villanova Law Rev.* 14:463, 1969.
59. Brooks AD: *Law, Psychiatry and the Mental Health System.* Boston, Little, Brown and Co, 1974, p 701.
60. Ibid., at 701.
61. A California Court of Appeals has held that "[i]f a person is insane, he cannot form the intent to take his own life." Thus, "[i]nsane persons cannot commit suicide." *Searle vs Allstate Life Insurance Company*, as reported by the *New York Times*, September 4, 1979. This view, although critical to the interpretation of various provisions of insurance policies, is of only semantic interest to this discussion.
62. Cooper TR: Medical treatment facility liability for patient suicide and other self-injury. *J Legal Med* 2:20–29, 1975 (quote, 29; footnotes omitted).
63. *Dinnerstein vs United States*, 486 F2d 34 (2nd Cir, 1973).
64. 382 NYS2nd 128 (New York Superior Court, Appeals Division, 1976).
65. But see discussions above in sections 11 and 13.
66. *Dinnerstein,* note 63, above, at 38 (footnotes omitted).
67. See, e.g., Okla Stat Ann, Title 21, sec 818.
68. Text, above, at note 6.

General Principles of Pharmacologic Management in the Emergency Setting

Ellen L. Bassuk, M.D., Peter J. Panzarino, Jr., M.D., and Stephen C. Schoonover, M.D.

1. Introduction

In the emergency setting, the clinician must make decisions rapidly, often on the basis of limited historical data and without the advantages of an extended diagnostic evaluation. The patient may require containment of his behavior and immediate relief of his distress before he has established a working relationship with the clinician or before the underlying psychiatric disorder is defined. Therefore, the use of psychoactive drugs must be carefully tailored to the special requirements of the individual, the situation, and the setting.

2. Evaluating the Patient and Choosing Medication

The purpose of the initial phase of evaluation is to differentiate among life-threatening emergencies, urgent problems, and those not requiring immediate intervention.

2.1. Identify and Manage Life-Threatening Problems

Life-threatening presentations include out-of-control behaviors and medical emergencies either coexisting with or masquerading as a psychiatric problem. If the patient is out of control, physical restraint may be necessary to complete even the most preliminary assessment, including observing the patient's appearance and behavior (e.g., level of consciousness, pupil size and reactivity, skin color, motor movements and gait), asking critical questions, and administering relevant parts of the mental status examination (MSE) and the physical examination.

Ellen L. Bassuk, M.D. • Harvard Medical School, Boston, Massachusetts, 02115.   *Peter J. Panzarino, Jr., M.D.* • Harvard Medical School, Boston, Massachusetts 02115, and McLean Hospital, Belmont, Massachusetts 02178.   *Stephen C. Schoonover, M.D.* • Harvard Medical School, Boston, Massachusetts 02115.

Table 1. Medications Used in the Emergency Setting

Reason	Medication
To provide behavioral control	
Patients with functional disorders	High-potency antipsychotics
Patients with organic brain syndromes	High-potency antipsychotics in lower doses
To treat	
Functional disorders such as	
Acute psychoses	High-potency antipsychotics
Chronic psychoses	Antipsychotics
Acute anxiety	Short-term benzodiazepines if necessary
Insomnia	
Toxic disorders	
Wernicke's disease	Thiamine
Alcohol withdrawal	Chlordiazepoxide or diazepam
Alcohol hallucinosis	Antipsychotic drugs (e.g., trifluoperazine, chlorpromazine)
Opiate overdose	Narcotic antagonists such as naloxone (Narcan)
Opiate withdrawal	Detoxification with methadone
CNS depressants withdrawal	Detoxification with pentobarbital or phenobarbital
Amphetamine or cocaine psychosis	Antipsychotic drugs (e.g., haloperidol, chlorpromazine)
Hallucinogens	
Panic, flashbacks	Diazepam, if necessary
Toxic delirium	Antipsychotics or diazepam, if necessary
Drug-precipitated psychosis	Antipsychotics, only if necessary after 48 hours
Phencyclidine	
Intoxication	Diazepam, if necessary
PCP psychosis	Haloperidol, if necessary
Marijuana	
Panic, flashbacks	Diazepam, if necessary
Toxic delirium	Antipsychotics, if necessary
Chronic psychosis	Antipsychotics
Anticholinergic syndromes	Anticholinesterase therapy such as physostigmine

Sometimes the clinician may be able to make a definitive diagnosis, but more often he may be dealing with clusters of symptoms that may not obviously correspond to standard diagnostic categories. On the basis of his initial impressions and observations the clinician must decide if medication is indicated and if so, which one (see Table 1).

Generally, to provide behavioral control in patients with functional psychiatric disorders the clinician can administer high-potency antipsychotics. These same drugs should be given in lower doses to agitated patients with organic brain syndromes because of the likelihood of adverse reactions. The clinician should also know those toxic disorders that require specific drug treatments (see Table 1 and Chapter 9). Before deciding to medicate, however, the clinician should weigh the risks and benefits of medications against the use of physical restraints—either alone or in combination. Factors that he should consider include the degree of central nervous system (CNS) depression and the possibility of further CNS depression, the nature of the medical disorder, the patient's use of other medications or toxic substances, and the patient's response to physical restraint. Once the clinician decides to medicate, he should proceed quickly, explaining each step to the patient. (see Chapter 2 for a more detailed discussion).

2.2. Screen the Patient for Presence of Medical or Toxic Disorder

In less urgent situations, the clinician has more time to complete a thorough evaluation before administering medication. *The clinician should screen the patient for the presence of an underlying medical or toxic disorder* by taking a careful medical history (including medication, drug, and alcohol use), reviewing organ systems, completing vital signs (e.g., blood pressure, pulse, and temperature) and a physical examination, assessing specific physical complaints, and ordering laboratory studies to follow up positive findings.

Since psychiatric patients have a higher incidence of accompanying medical disorders than the general population, the clinician must always consider the possibility of the presence of both medical and psychiatric disorders.[1] Similarly, if a patient complains of a specific physical symptom, the clinician should not dismiss its authenticity until a medical evaluation has been completed. Remember that even severely hypochondriacal patients develop "real" disease.

2.3. Identify Those Disorders Requiring Medication during the Emergency Visit

2.3.1. Identify Medical or Toxic Disorders

Medical or toxic disorders that either coexist with or masquerade as functional disorders must be identified. Choice of medication may be determined by a well-established diagnosis or even by a high level of suspicion about the presence of a medical problem. For example, various toxic syndromes (e.g., anticholinergic delirium) have specific drug treatments (see Chapter 10.)

2.3.2. Differentiate Psychotic from Nonpsychotic Disorders

Although it may be difficult to differentiate among the psychoses, i.e., acute schizophrenia, acute psychosis accompanying an affective disorder (e.g., manic or depressive psychosis), and brief reactive psychosis,[2] the *acute* pharmacologic treatment of these disorders is the same.

To medicate patients who are out of control or who have an acute psychotic disorder, the clinician should choose a high-potency antipsychotic agent such

Table 2. Currently Available Antipsychotic Drugs[a]

Nonproprietary name	Trade name	Approximate potency[b]	Available as injectable
Phenothiazines			
Aliphatic			
Chlorpromazine	Thorazine	1:1	Yes
Triflupromazine	Vesprin	4:1	Yes
Piperidine			
Thioridazine	Mellaril	1:1	No
Mesoridazine	Serentil	2:1	Yes
Piperazine			
Trifluoperazine	Stelazine	30:1	Yes
Acetophenazine	Tindal	5:1	No
Butaperazine	Repoise	10:1	No
Fluphenazine	Permitil, Prolixin	50–100[c]:1	Yes
Perphenazine	Trilafon	10:1	Yes
Thioxanthenes			
Chlorprothixene	Taractan	1:1	Yes
Thiothixene	Navane	25:1	Yes
Butyrophenone			
Haloperidol	Haldol	50:1	Yes
Dibenzoxazepine			
Loxapine	Daxolin, Loxitane	7:1	Yes
Dihydroindolone			
Molindone	Lidone, Moban	10:1	No

[a] Adapted from Gelenberg.[5]
[b] Milligram equivalence to chlorpromazine.
[c] Oral only. Potency equivalences not established for long-acting injectable forms. Usual dosage for fluphenazine decanoate is 0.5 to 2.5 ml every three to five weeks.

as haloperidol (Haldol), trifluoperazine (Stelazine), fluphenazine (Permitil, Prolixin), perphenazine (Trilafon), or thiothixene (Navane).[2] (See Tables 2 and 3). The choice of a specific agent can depend, in part, on the patient's prior response to medication.[3] The usual dose is 5–10 mg haloperidol po or its equivalent, but it should be individualized according to the patient's condition.

Table 3. Spectrum of Adverse Effects Caused by Antipsychotic Drugs[a]

Low potency	High potency
Fewer extrapyramidal reactions (especially thioridazine)	More frequent extrapyramidal reactions
More sedation, postural hypotension	Less sedation, postural hypotension
Greater effect on the seizure threshold, electrocardiogram (especially thioridazine)	Less effect on the seizure threshold, cardiovascular toxicity
More likely skin pigmentation and photosensitivity	Fewer anticholinergic effects
Occasional cases of cholestatic jaundice	Occasional cases of neuroleptic malignant syndrome
Rare cases of agranulocytosis	

[a] From Gelenberg.[5]

Unless a specific drug treatment is indicated, agitated patients with an organic psychosis should be given lower doses of such high-potency antipsychotics as haloperidol. Starting doses generally range from 0.5 to 2.0 mg. If necessary, they can be administered safely in repeated parenteral doses. (See Chapter 2 for a discussion of rapid neuroleptization.[4])

Compared to low-potency antipsychotics, these drugs are safer in higher doses, have fewer adverse cardiovascular effects (such as postural hypotension and arrhythmias), and have fewer sedation and autonomic effects (see Table 3). However, they cause a high incidence of extrapyramidal reactions, especially acute dystonias. Dystonias are uncomfortable and frightening to the patient, but rarely dangerous. A rare manifestation, laryngospasm, may occasionally cause life-threatening respiratory compromise. The immediate treatment of acute dystonia is to administer either (1) diphenhydramine (Benadryl) IM or IV or (2) diazepam (Valium) IV injected slowly at the rate of 5 mg/min up to a maximum dose of 10 mg. The clinician should avoid accidental intraarterial injection or extravasation and should have equipment available for airway support.[5] After the patient's recovery from the acute dystonia the clinician can administer trihexyphenidyl hydrochloride (Artane) or benztropine mesylate (Cogentin) 1–2 mg once or twice per day for at least one week.

If the patient has a history of a poor response to high-potency agents, the clinician can administer a low-potency drug such as chlorpromazine (Thorazine and others). Postural hypotension occurs with higher doses. Treatment of severe hypotension consists of the following: keeping the patient supine, or in reverse Trendelenberg position, administering intravenous fluids to treat hypovolemia, and giving pressors with only alpha-noradrenergic stimulating properties such as levarterenol (Levophed) or metaraminol (Aramine). *Caution:* Never use isoproterenol (Iprenol, Isuprel), a beta stimulator, or epinephrine, a mixed alpha- and beta-acting drug, since they may further reduce blood pressure.[4]

2.3.3. Determine If Insomnia and Severe Anxiety Are Secondary to a Major Psychiatric Disorder

If there is such a disorder (e.g., organic brain syndromes, medical and toxic disorders, acute psychoses, severe depression), treat the primary illness. If not, other treatment aimed at symptom relief should be considered. For example, patients experiencing an acute situational crisis (e.g., rape, loss of a loved one) may present with severe insomnia and/or anxiety and may benefit by the short-term administration of a benzodiazepine. The clinician should determine if these patients can be managed effectively by sympathetic listening and supportive interviewing or if they require brief periods of medication for symptom relief. In patients with characterologic problems who present to the ER with chronic, severe anxiety, the clinician must assess other factors such as presence of psychosocial stressors, involvement in treatment, and motivation. Generally, the decision to medicate such patients should be made by their primary therapist and only within the context of ongoing treatment (see Chapters 12 and 13).

When anxiety and insomnia are not secondary to an acute psychosis, major affective disorder, or panic disorder, the clinician must decide whether or not to prescribe a sedative-hypnotic. Because the benzodiazepines have a very high therapeutic index (ratio of therapeutic to toxic doses) and few adverse effects, they are generally the drugs of choice. Unless combined with alcohol or other CNS depressants, they do not cause death.

Knowing the pharmacokinetics (absorption, distribution, metabolism and excretion) of these drugs should help the clinician choose a specific compound (see Tables 4 and 5). "The rate of drug absorption from the gastrointestinal tract, for example, largely determines the speed of onset of action after a single oral dose. Drugs that are absorbed rapidly produce a faster and more intense onset of clinical effects (e.g., diazepam), while the reverse is true for more slowly absorbed compounds (e.g., oxazepam). Termination of a drug's effects after a single dose is largely determined by the rate and extent of the drug's distribution. For example, highly lipid soluble compounds, such as diazepam, tend to be rapidly and extensively distributed throughout the body's tissues, indicating a relatively brief duration of clinical effect after a single dose. Distribution, rather than the elimination half-life, becomes clinically important. The elimination half-life determines the rate at which a drug accumulates in body tissues: Drugs with longer half-lives accumulate (steady-state concentrations are achieved after approximately four half-lives) and disappear from the body more gradually following discontinuation. Those with shorter half-lives are eliminated more rapidly (which for some drugs can result in the rapid appearance of an intense withdrawal syndrome). The half-life also can guide a clinician in choosing the frequency of doses; drugs whose half-lives exceed 24 hours usually can be administered once each day."[3] On the basis of these principles, the clinician should familiarize himself with a few short-acting and long-acting benzodiazepines. (See Tables 4 and 5 for a description of the benzodiazepines.)

2.3.4. Restart Medication in Patients Who Need Prescription Refills and Are Taking Maintenance Regimens

Assess the reasons why the patient decided to use the ER rather than returning to his primary therapist. Also, determine with the patient if his therapist should be called.

Since many patients who use the emergency department are taking psychotropic drugs, the clinician also should be familiar with the uses of other antipsychotics (see Table 1)—lithium, heterocyclic antidepressants, monoamine oxidase inhibitors, other sedative-hypnotics, and drugs for specific medical disorders (see Table 6, which describes the adverse reactions with MAO inhibitors, including the food restrictions).

Table 4. Benzodiazepine Antianxiety Drugs[a]

Drug	Approximate dose equivalents (Mg)	Available dosage forms	Rapidity of absorption	Active metabolites	Half-life (hr)
Alprazolam (Xanax)	0.5	0.25, 0.5, and 1.0-mg tablets	Intermediate	Alpha-hydroxy-alprazolam desmethylalprazolam, 4-hydroxy-alprazolam	6 to 20
Chlordiazepoxide (Librium and others)	10	5, 10, 25-mg tablets and capsules 100-mg/2-ml ampule	Intermediate	Desmethylchlordiazepoxide, Demoxepam, Desmethyldiazepam, Oxazepam	5 to 30
Clorazepate (Azene, Tranxene)	7.5	3.75, 7.5, and 15-mg capsules (Tranxene) 3.25, 6.5, and 13-mg capsules (Azene)	Fast	Desmethyldiazepam,[b] Oxazepam	30 to 200
Diazepam (Valium)	5	2, 5, 10-mg tablets 10-mg/2-ml ampules 50-mg/10-ml vials 10-mg/2-ml syringe	Fastest	Desmethyldiazepam, Oxazepam	20 to 100
Halazepam (Paxipam)	20	20, 40-mg tablets	Intermediate	Desmethyldiazepam	@ 14 (parent) 50 to 100 desmethyl-diazepam
Lorazepam (Ativan)	1	0.5, 1, 2-mg tablets 2 and 4-mg/ml syringes 2 and 4-mg/ml vials[c]	Intermediate	None	10 to 20
Oxazepam (Serax)	15	10, 15, 30-mg capsules 15-mg tablets	Slower	None	5 to 15
Prazepam (Centrax, Verstran)	10	5, 10-mg capsules 10-mg tablets	Slowest	Desmethyldiazepam,[b] Oxazepam	30 to 200

[a] From Gelenberg.[6]
[b] These drugs are pro drugs for desmethyldiazepam: The parent compound is rapidly converted to the active metabolite.
[c] As of this writing, approved by FDA only for preanesthetic use.

Table 5. Benzodiazepines Used to Treat Insomnia[a]

Drug	Usual bedtime dose for young adults	Available dosage forms	Active metabolites	Half-life (hr)
Flurazepan (Dalmane)	30 mg	15, 30-mg capsules	N-desalkyl flurazapam	40–250
Temazepam (Restoril)	30 mg	15, 30-mg capsules	None	5–25 (occasionally longer)

[a] From Gelenberg.[7]

2.4. Maintenance Regimens

Generally, the clinician should not begin maintenance regimens in the emergency setting unless he plans to become the ongoing therapist, can guarantee specific follow-up, and has completed an adequate medical evaluation. Drugs such as lithium and the heterocyclic antidepressants have a significant lag time before their clinical effects become apparent. Moreover, patients taking these medications often require extensive medical screening and careful monitoring. Before a maintenance regimen is implemented, the patient should have at least established the beginnings of a working relationship with the clinician.

2.4.1. Identify Major Depressive Disorders

Generally, the clinician should not begin antidepressant treatment in the emergency setting. A treatment plan should be initiated that will ensure appropriate medical screening, pharmacotherapy, and psychotherapy (see Chapter 12).

2.4.2. Identify Patients with Chronic Anxiety

Medicating patients for insomnia, anxiety, or panic issuing from a severe, chronic characterlogic problem should be avoided. These individuals often urgently demand pain medication or sedative-hypnotics. There are no data, however, to show that these medications help over time. Moreover, there is significant risk of dependence and abuse. Unfortunately, these drugs are injudiciously prescribed in large amounts for this type of clinical situation— either to placate a demanding patient, to avoid harm from a threatening individual, or to try to be helpful. The caretaker should acknowledge the covert agenda to himself and avoid acting on it. In general, administering medication should be avoided in the ER unless the clinician has established rapport with the patient and has planned adequate follow-up treatment.

3. Applying General Principles of Drug Use to the Emergency Setting

3.1. Choose Nonbiological Approaches When They Are as Effective as Pharmacotherapy[3]

Because of inherent pressures in the emergency setting, the clinician may tend to rely on medication as the first choice intervention. He should remember, however, that it is an intrusive form of treatment and can have significant physical and psychological morbidity. Medication is not necessarily effective for all emergency conditions, but for patients with a drug-responsive syndrome or symptoms, medication is essential.

3.1. Whenever Possible, Treat the Primary Psychiatric Disorder

Although absolute differential diagnosis is not always possible in the emergency setting, establishing probable diagnosis has important treatment implications in some cases. A patient with severe insomnia, for example, who presents with a thought disorder requires antipsychotic medication rather than a hypnotic.

3.3. Avoid Polypharmacy

Combinations of psychoactive drugs generally are not more effective than a single agent and indeed may increase the incidence of adverse reactions (because of their additive potential). Since some patients already on drugs complain about persistent symptoms and demand immediate relief, clinicians may feel compelled by their own frustration to dispense additional medications. Despite the evidence against polypharmacy, some patients are still given several agents at once. The average state hospital patient, for example, takes three different medications. In some situations, combinations of drugs are indicated, but usually because each drug addresses a different symptom. For example, extrapyramidal effects caused by antipsychotic medications may require treatment with antiparkinson agents[3] (see Chapter 10).

3.4. Whenever Possible, Administer the Medication Orally

"Parenteral preparations generally have a more rapid onset of action while all oral preparations, whether in capsules, tablets or liquid form provide equivalent amounts of medication with equal speed. Therefore, clinicians should avoid prescribing concentrates except for patients who have trouble swallowing medication. These preparations usually are more costly and may cause mucosal irritation and contact dermatitis."[3]

Using oral medication invites the patient to cooperate in treatment, allows him to exercise control, and supports his position as a respected and essential participant in treatment. In contrast, if a patient refuses medication or is paranoid and afraid of being poisoned, the medication should be administered

Table 6. Adverse Reactions with MAOIs[a]

Food and drugs that cause hypertension with MAOIs
  Cheeses
    1. High tyramine content: boursault, camembert, cheddar, gruyere, stilton
    2. Moderate tyramine content: gouda, parmesan
    3. Low tyramine content: American
  Other foods
    1. High tyramine content: lox, pickled herring
    2. Moderate tyramine content: salted herring, chicken liver, figs, raisins, broad beans (fava
       beans), yeast products, pickles, sauerkraut, coffee, chocolate, cocoa, soy sauce, sour
       cream, snails, avocado, banana peels, licorice
  Beverages
    1. High tyramine content: chianti
    2. Moderate tyramine content: sherry, beer
    3. Low tyramine content: champagne, Italian red wine, riesling, santeone, "hard" liquor
  Additives
    Cyclamates, monosodium glutamate
  Drugs
    1. Amphetamine (Benzedrine®), dextroamphetamine (Dexedrine®), methylamphetamine (De-
       soxyn®), ephedrine (Tedral® and others), procaine preparations (Novocain® and others)
       (which often contain epinephrine), epinephrine (Adrenalin® and others), methyldopa (Al-
       domet® and others), phenylpropanolamine (Dimetane®, Coricidin®, and others) or ephed-
       rine (in over-the-counter cold preparations), pseudoephedrine (Actifed®, Sudafed®, and
       others), dopamine (Intropin®), methylphenidate (Ritalin®), heterocyclic antidepressants, or
       another MAOI
  Drugs that cause severe hypotension with MAOIs (including occasional deaths reported from
    cardiovascular collapse)
    Narcotics, alcohol, analgesics, phenothiazines, thiazides, anesthetic agents, antihistamines,
       insulin (Iletin® and others), reserpine (Serpasil®, Diupres®, and others), antiparkinson
       agents, barbiturates
  Drugs that cause other adverse reactions with MAOIs
    1. Insulin and other hypoglycemics: hypoglycemia
    2. Heterocyclic antidepressants: severe anticholinergic syndrome marked by delirium, sei-
       zures, tremors and hypertonia, hyperpyrexia, and occasionally death
    3. Meperidine (Demerol® and others): enhanced narcotic effect, hyperpyrexia, and rigidity
       (may be very severe syndrome)
    4. Alcohol and phenothiazines: decreased monoamine oxidase inhibition
    5. Anesthetics, alcohol, chloral hydrate, cocaine, minor tranquilizers, barbiturates, codeine:
       significant CNS depression
  Surgical precautions
    1. If possible, discontinue MAO inhibitor 2 weeks prior to surgery
    2. When MAO inhibitor is being administered, warn the anesthesiologist about possible com-
       plications regarding the use of pressor agents

[a] From Schoonover.[8]

parenterally. When these patients are frightened and disorganized, they may
view oral medication as "forcing something down their throats" or injections
as physically intrusive. However, once the clinician has determined that pharmacologic intervention is required, it is in the patient's best interest to proceed
calmly and quickly.

3.5. Administer the Lowest Effective Doses

It is essential not to dispense or write a prescription for medication that exceeds the lethal dose or to provide automatic refills. Generally, the patient should be given enough medication to last until his next appointment or to effect symptom relief—which should be within a few days to a week. Particular care should be taken with patients evidencing self-destructive or substance abuse potential.

3.6. Provide the Most Cost-Effective Treatment

The clinician should help patients economize by prescribing drugs generically. However, the bioavailability (i.e., the amount of drug absorbed into the plasma) of different preparations may vary slightly within the same generic class. The clinician should try to prescribe the least expensive and most appropriate drug first unless problems of bioavailability dictate another choice. These considerations should be discussed with the patient.[3]

3.7. Exercise Special Care with Medically Ill and Elderly Patients

Special precautions should be taken when administering psychoactive drugs to medically ill and elderly patients. The risk of adverse effects increases, tolerance to medication decreases, and pharmacokinetics change. The elderly often are taking other medications that may potentiate the effects of psychoactive agents, or the medical condition itself may interfere with drug treatment. Because of these problems, the clinician should always assess the interplay of the medical disorder and the psychological symptoms, prescribe the lowest possible effective dose, and carefully follow the patient.[3]

3.8. Document in the Medical Record Assessment Findings, Treatment Plans, and Discussions with the Patient about Medication

The patient's chart should include notes about treatment, overall care, discussions about medication, potential problems, and any significant changes in the drugs (e.g., dosage changes, severe adverse reactions and their treatment) or in the patient (e.g., mental status changes, like suicidal ideation or psychotic symptoms). Detailed documentation in the chart facilitates transition from emergency care to follow-up treatment.

4. Forming a Relationship with the Patient

4.1. Establish a Working Relationship with the Patient

After assessing the characteristics of the patient and his illness and then selecting the appropriate drug, the clinician should encourage active cooperation. At the most basic level, this involves providing accurate information and discussing the patient's concerns openly. He should encourage the patient to acknowledge negative feelings and distorted beliefs about medication.[3] With an eye to developing a trusting relationship, the clinician must take time to clarify both his own and the patient's roles and responsibilities around the use of medication. On a pragmatic level, negotiating a collaborative medication plan with the patient means openly discussing potential risks (i.e., common and serious adverse reactions), potential benefits, and possible alternative treatments. Informed consent should not be obtained until the patient clearly understands his role and has developed legitimate expectations about the medication process. If a disorganized patient cannot give informed consent, the caretaker must involve relatives, friends, guardians, or lawyers (see Chapter 3).

The structure of follow-up treatment varies from patient to patient. However, the clinician should arrange for periodic review and be available at least by telephone during periods of distress. Even after the acute symptoms subside, a formal treatment program helps to increase medication compliance and may encourage the patient's participation.[3]

Focusing on drug-giving may sometimes cause the therapist to ignore the broader aspects of patient care. Just as psychiatric illnesses are often regarded as socially stigmatizing and the persons close to the patient become distant or unavailable, the same undercurrents of prejudice and interpersonal incompatability may operate in the therapeutic relationship. Sometimes, both transference and countertransference feelings compound the clinician's difficulties in establishing an empathic bond with the patient. Therefore, it is important to remember that pharmacotherapy is nested within a broader psychotherapeutic interaction.

4.2. If the Patient Is in Treatment Elsewhere, Discuss Plans for Pharmacologic and Psychosocial Management with the Patient's Primary Therapist

About one-third of emergency room patients are involved in treatment elsewhere at the time of their visit; use of the ER often reflects a crisis in their treatment. After obtaining consent from the patient, the primary therapist should be involved in immediate management and pharmacologic decisions.

4.3. Provide Adequate Follow-Up for All Patients Given Medication

The clinician should remain in contact with the patient to ensure continuity of care, to assess the need for additional medication, and to monitor possible adverse effects until he is transferred to a new treatment setting.

5. Conclusion

The emergency setting challenges the clinician's diagnostic skills in unparalleled ways. Crisis patients make poor historians, critical laboratory tests are sometimes unavailable, and symptom clusters with widely divergent etiologies may look very similar. The clinician must master a wide range of clinical skills: observing and listening, scrutinizing the available data, reflecting on personal reactions to patients, and treating the patient effectively, often without a clear diagnosis.

Because pharmacotherapy is such a potent therapeutic agent, the clinician's task is not only to decide whether or not to medicate, but to enlist the cooperation of patient, family members, and/or other physicians in the whole process. The meaning of medication to both the patient and the physician is an important, highly personalized issue and cannot be ignored. The success of any pharmacologic intervention ultimately depends on the patient's understanding of, and participation in, the medication process. Careful attention to these issues, as well as solid grounding in clinical psychiatry and psychopharmacology, is required to master the complex and demanding tasks of using medication in the psychiatric emergency room.

References

1. Bassuk E, Gerson S: Into the breach. Emergency psychiatry in the general hospital, *Gen Hosp Psychiatry* 1:31–45, 1979.
2. Pope H, Lipinski J: Diagnoses in schizophrenia and manic depressive illness, *Arch Gen Psychiatry* 35:811–828, 1978.
3. Schoonover SC: Introduction: The practice of pharmacotherapy, in Bassuk EL, Schoonover SC, Gelenberg AJ. (eds.): *The Practitioner's Guide to Psychoactive Drugs*, ed. 2. New York, Plenum Publishing Corp., 1983.
4. Gelenberg AJ: Psychiatric emergencies: The psychotic patient. *Drug Ther* May 1981, pp 25–36.
5. Gelenberg AJ: Psychosis, in Bassuk EL, Schoonover SC, Gelenberg A (eds.): *The Practitioner's Guide to Psychoactive Drugs*, ed 2. New York, Plenum Publishing Corp., 1983.
6. Gelenberg AJ: Anxiety, in Bassuk EL, Schoonover SC, Gelenberg AJ (eds.): *The Practitioner's Guide to Psychoactive Drugs*, ed 2. New York, Plenum Publishing Corp., 1983.
7. Gelenberg AJ: Insomnia, in Bassuk E, Schoonover SC, Gelenberg AJ (eds.): *The Practitioner's Guide to Psychoactive Drugs*, ed 2. New York, Plenum Publishing Corp, 1983.
8. Schoonover SC: Depression, in Bassuk EL, Schoonover SC, Gelenberg AJ (eds): *The Practitioner's Guide to Psychoactive Drugs*, ed 2. New York, Plenum Publishing Corp, 1983.

The Therapeutic Stance

Alvin Kahn, M.D.

There are many modalities of person-to-person interaction. Human beings can fight, feed, or play with each other. It is significant that one of the earliest references to another fundamental quality of many object relations appears in Genesis, 2:18; indeed, it is the first definition of a human relationship that is mentioned in the Bible. God creates woman as a *help*mate of Adam. More exactly, in the Hebrew, Eve is a *help meet* for Adam—a match for him, or someone to be *at his side*. It is a long way from the Creation to the busy workings of an emergency room, but the concept of one person helping another as equal partners in a mutually congruent relationship has been honored in all ages. The idea is captured in the modern theoretical construct of the therapeutic alliance, which we might appropriately rename the helping alliance. It is compounded of that part of the person in need that seeks, however awkwardly or even defiantly, some form of assisting contact with another; and that part of the therapist that is the matured distillation of his experience, his practical and theoretical knowledge, and those sublimations that have led him to his profession. This more or less rational aspect of the therapist's share in the helping relationship can be usefully designated as the *counteralliance*, much as the term countertransference is applied to that counterpart transference of the therapist that is analogous to the mostly irrational transference of the patient.

It is the counteralliance that is most severely stressed in crisis management, and for a period following the acute emergency. At other times in the course of ongoing therapy the alliance undergoes vicissitudes, but under conditions that permit more unhurried reflection as well as leisurely self-examination. This is hardly the case in the small hours of the morning when a patient presents in acute panic, with soft neurologic signs and a muddled history with hints of drug ingestion. Yet even in these circumstances it is clear that much will depend on the patient's willingness and ability to engage with the therapist, to muster those resources that are his unique contribution to the therapeutic endeavor.

In the ideal case—that is to say, in those clinical instances that are never observed—the patient has had previous rewarding experiences with helpful people. He understands the nature of his alliance with the therapist and is free of those defenses against closeness, interdependence, and submission that lace most relationships with difficult ambivalence. He brings a coalliance to the

Alvin Kahn, M.D. • Harvard Medical School, Boston, Massachusetts 02115.

therapeutic situation that sustains the work when the therapist's attention flags or his intuition and empathy fail. This ideal is most closely approached by those relatively normal individuals who come to the emergency room with acute drug reactions or suffering from emotionally traumatic external stress.

More often, of course, the ability of the patient to engage therapeutically is flawed to a significant degree. He would otherwise be receiving assistance from friends and relatives, or would otherwise have averted that culmination of fear, rage, and pain that precipitates a crisis condition. A special category here is that large group of emergency room patients who are currently in therapy elsewhere. They bring direct testimony of some breakdown in a helping alliance, where responsibility for the difficulties must be shared by both sides.

Finally, there are those particularly difficult people who come seeking relief but making every effort to thwart and reject help. It is here that more naive and simplistic attempts to be efficacious are distinguished from those informed and sophisticated engagements that put help-rejection in the context of early transference responses. A negative, antagonistic, or oppositional relationship is still a mode of engagement. When it can be understood and translated as such, one can sometimes make those clarifications that nourish, foster, and sustain the helping alliance by dissolving the transference resistance. It is all too common to find patients who cannot take in and use the observations of the therapist, or who cover this impediment with a subtly hostile compliance that defeats real progress. The therapist may, on his part, delude himself that a real rather than a false alliance exists, so that both therapist and patient are, in effect, playing at and talking about doing therapy when in actuality a stalemate exists. Focusing on this underlying problem in receiving thoughts and ideas from another is essential for engagement in treatment. In other individuals it soon becomes apparent that the therapist's words are absorbed with no effect other than a frustrating repetition of complaints or demands for direction. When the patient's feelings of starvation and wish for feeding by his helper are clarified, the issue is truly joined, an alliance is established, and the patient can relax. Especially in such situations is the vision of one insight worth a thousand words.

These are easy examples. Many chronic repeaters in emergency clinics are those individuals who defy all healing and are intent on reducing their helpers to impotence and defeat. They frustrate all the usual satisfactions that sustain the counteralliance. Understanding and exploration are blocked; competence and helpfulness are drained of all pleasure. Such patients seek the satisfaction of attack, rejection, victimization by their therapists, and they accept no substitutes for the real thing. It is particularly in these situations that one must be on guard for the regressive emergence of sadistic responses that follow the frustration of all sublimatory activity. Curiosity thwarted can result in too intrusive questioning or verbal harassment. Retaliatory rejection lurks beneath the guise of judicious limit-setting. The patient has truly defeated the therapist if he can evoke those angry and hurtful responses that compromise the helper's role as a compassionate interviewer.

The counteralliance is best maintained between those opposing bounds of optimism and pessimism, activity and passivity, where good judgment resides. One can be seduced by a honeymoon alliance into overlooking a flight into health. One can be tempted to avoid the work of engagement by prematurely deciding that there is little prospect of worthwhile psychotherapy. In the one instance, pathology is denied; in the other, the healthy ego is hidden by defenses. Such collusions of denial are not helping alliances. A special instance of this sometimes occurs shortly after a crisis has passed, when both patient and therapist reach a premature conclusion that a "breakthrough" has occurred or that the patient has emerged from his trials on a higher level of integration than before. On rare occasions this may be the case. More often, the need for considerable working through is being ignored.

The counteralliance is supported by a continual vigilance that focuses now on the immediate detail, at other times on a broader perspective. It is sometimes expressed through simple common sense, sometimes through articulations of a transference that had been almost taken for granted as a part of the therapeutic encounter. Much of the time, when clarity is obscured, ignorance must be borne and lack of understanding tolerated. The concept of therapeutic neutrality is of value in such circumstances. It is neutrality toward content and material, not toward the individual as a person in need. With due respect to each person's right to choose for himself his course in life, the therapist maintains in his counteralliance a bias in favor of relief from pain and overcoming distress. Therapeutic neutrality can be misused to buttress an inappropriate passivity or avoid indications for activity.

In addition to judgment, cognition, and the ability to form the case-specific object relationships, other ego functions contribute to the counteralliance in special ways. The therapist must be able to engage in that ineffable and creative regression, that suspension of his usual thought processes, that permits him to attend to the deeper aspects of the patient's communication. Understanding when a panic-stricken individual fears homosexual contact or when an acutely psychotic person is wrestling with murderous impulses has considerable bearing on management and disposition. Similarly, the therapist's ego must be able to tolerate the expression and the evocation of strong affect. Fear, rage, hate, and grief are draining passions, but they must be endured to a degree if proper assessment and diagnosis are to follow. It is essential that one not be a stranger to strong emotion if an alliance is to be effected and therapy pursued. The therapist must have the capacity to delay his own responses to such feelings, however. His own defenses must be sufficiently flexible to allow him to stay with the patient without shutting off his own ears or the patient's expression.

An old German proverb says that one may have many friends but few real helpers. The special aspect of the counteralliance that particularly distinguishes it from helping friendship and elevates it to the rank of knowledgeable professionalism is the ability both to permit and to scrutinize the emergence of countertransference responses. From this point of view, the countertransference is an evoked reaction whose derivatives may be either welcomed as observational data or opposed as dystonic interferences. One man's countertransference is another man's being manipulated. The patient who lies to get drugs may at a transferential level be communicating his experience of having had important supplies stolen from him by parental figures. The individual who attempts to set helping personnel against each other may be protecting early parental images by confirming that everybody fights and lives in discord.

To some extent, the task of the therapist includes accepting some measure of being his patient's victim. Certainly, his narcissistic equilibrium is under continual bombardment. It is as important sometimes to live with an overblown estimation of one's capacities as it is to acknowledge those real limitations that the devaluing patient does not hesitate to point out. Both positions imply a countertransference flexibility on the part of the therapist—to be the idealized parent or to be the inadequate and relatively helpless child: to be inflated out of hostility or to be diminished because of fear. This stress on the therapist's narcissism may be particularly onerous in those cases where a chronically repeating crisis patient maintains a positive transference to the institution rather than its employees. Working with this type of tenuous interpersonal relationship rather than merely viewing it as an indication of pathology may permit a more definitive resolution of the cycles of emergency visits.[1]

The therapist is on the spot in crisis situations. One patient demands a nurturant, all-accepting mother; another wants a benignly authoritarian, guiding father. One sees all therapists as depriving; another expects some form of hurtfulness. The accomplished therapist is not deterred when the patient's behavior is incongruent with his usual therapeutic stance. Ideally, he should neither fear nor need to be the nurturant mother. He should neither fear nor need to be the strong, potentially hurtful father.

Whatever his illusory role, he should be involved and in contact with his patient. The fact that the contact may be brief is not a good reason to avoid real commitment. It is often argued that the patient will be disappointed and forced to endure a new loss if the transient therapist fosters too much of a relationship. This consideration may particularly be used as an excuse to avoid closeness with those borderline individuals that constitute a majority of emergency room patients. Most of these patients are quite aware that their contact with a particular therapist will be limited. It is probably more beneficial for them to have made contact and lost it than not to have made contact at all. Patients remember those who have had an active interest in them, who have wanted to plumb their history, who have made some attempt to understand the disorder in their lives.

Similarly, strictures against making interpretations to emotionally fragile individuals can be misconstrued so that all painful material is avoided. Sensitivity to a patient's perilous distress does not mean not sharing his pain or clarifying what he is capable of understanding. It is here that one must distinguish the rhetoric of good intentions from the reality of effective intervention.

A special, and regularly important, instance of accepting and acting on a "good parent" countertransference occurs when it merges with an active, intervening counteralliance. Most emergency room patients need concrete help. Drugs must be prescribed, appointments made, support networks enlisted.

Jellinek[2] notes that many crisis patients who tend to be pushed off or referred in an offhand manner do not pursue treatment recommendations. A significant increase of positive responses occurs when prompt placement is pursued and the patient is aided in making necessary appointments. Here one is taking cognizance of the fact that the patient's coalliance, especially in borderline patients, may be very deficient in the capacity to care for, and take care of, the self. A form of heedlessness obtains, which may be obscured by the therapist's tendency to overidentify with his charge and impute the same caretaking concerns to the patient that he has for himself. It is important in this regard to help the patient to anticipate his own brand of difficulties and the repeated distress he may be called on to master in the future.

Complicating the task of the therapist in crisis situations is the wide range of indirect countertransference responses that arise toward colleagues and other hospital personnel in the emergency room, friends and relatives of the patient, and therapists of patients who are in ongoing treatment. The frustrations and excessive demands imposed on the therapist heighten the likelihood that these others will serve as convenient objects for the displacement of anger and hostility. They become adversaries rather than allies. Competitive stresses are never absent, nor is their propensity for invoking invidious comparisons. It is well to bear in mind that the patient is most likely to suffer in such polarized circumstances. Preoccupation with questions of who is right or wrong can retard the realization that there are differing degrees and styles of helpfulness in those concerned with the patient.

This is especially relevant for the patient who is in therapy at the time of his emergency room visit. A high proportion of crisis patients have outside therapists, and this fact exerts unusual pressure on the judgment and sensitivity of the therapist. One may recall that "it is an easy thing for one whose foot is on the outside of calamity to give advice and rebuke the sufferer." A judicious appraisal of the crisis in therapy requires first of all an appreciation of the many levels at which sins of omission and commission may have contributed to the difficulty. These are nicely detailed by Skodol.[3] Failures in communication may proceed entirely from the patient's deficient coalliance so that he has not communicated symptoms or concerns of importance. The therapist, on the other hand, may have missed underlying pathology or may have underestimated the patient's response to changes in hours, frequency of appointments, or vacations. From these relatively simple errors in the co- or counteralliance one may proceed to consideration of more complex failures in recognizing transference and countertransference issues, including impulses to act out on the part of both.

In general, it is important to be alert to the narcissistic seduction implicit in the rescuing therapist stance, and to the temptation to yield to a critical, professional superego in condemning the work of others. Sanctimony cloaked as professional concern helps neither patient nor therapist, and the opportunity to foster a better treatment situation may be lost. Most therapists welcome sensitive consultation. Most patients welcome validation of their concerns about the course of their therapy.

The crisis in the patient's life is frequently mirrored by an acute stress of lesser proportions in the therapist. Both may be inclined to cover over the period of disruption, or to assume that some emotional advance has been achieved when only the foundation for such growth has been laid. In general, the positive benefit that accrues to the patient from enduring a crisis situation is most likely to be the experience of a helpful relationship with another person—in learning that he can accept and profit from the sturdiness and understanding of another human being. This may occasion a limited, yet highly significant, shift in internal structure. It is sometimes only in concert with another that one learns to tolerate overwhelming affects of fear, rage, and grief.

Needless to say, "it is not enough to help the feeble up, but to support him after." Postcrisis therapy makes its special demands on the therapist's judgment. The need for continual working through of trauma must be balanced with the need to reintegrate and stave off unmanageable regressions. The therapeutic alliance at these times is always vulnerable. The crisis experience may be directly denied or avoided. Some individuals may throw themselves into a frenetic recollection and recounting of recent events in the vague hope that forceful, magical iteration will make them disappear. The therapist is misled if he confuses this attempt at denial with real working through. The specter of recent events that looms in the first days after a crisis is not the same as the ghost that needs exorcism a year later in therapy.

The weeks following the acute disruption may see the emergence of a general apathy in the patient that is normally part of a spontaneous healing following all severe pain. It is at this point that many therapists may be tempted to fall into a corresponding indifference, or to assume that the long-range prospects of therapy are bleak. Much patience is required to endure what may be pallid, unproductive encounters, and to recognize that the consistent interest of the therapist at these times affirms the solidity of the therapeutic commitment. At the same time, an eye must be kept to helping the patient review what was experienced at the time of crisis. The humiliation and shame of failure and regression must be borne, to recapture that part of reality that was intertwined with the emergency. This may be very difficult for both patient and therapist. *"Post calamitem memoria alia est calamitas*—after disaster, the memory of it is another disaster." Yet no real working through avoids the trauma, the losses, or the disappointments that precipitated crisis.

Ironically, those therapists most frequently called on to work with emergency patients are those with the least experience, those with the least seasoned professional knowledge. In the final analysis, when theory and clinical niceties fail, they are called on to exercise those simple virtues of courage, honesty, and caring that make them, in the broadest sense of the word, physicians.

References

1. Bassuk EL, Gerson S: Chronic crisis patients: A discrete clinical group. *Am J Psychiatry* 137:12–16, 1980.
2. Jellinek M: Referrals from a psychiatric emergency room: Relationship of compliance to demographic and interview variables. *Am J Psychiatry* 135:209–212, 1978.
3. Skodol A, Kass F, Charles E: Crisis in psychotherapy: Principles of emergency consultation and intervention. *Am J Orthopsychiatry* 49:585–597, 1979.

III

Patients and Clinical Syndromes 1
Potentially Life-Threatening

Emergency Management of Potentially Violent Patients

Andrew E. Skodol, M.D.

1. Introduction

The complexities of emergency psychiatric practice are especially dramatized by the agitated, threatening, or potentially violent patient. The need for decisive, accurate assessment and management must be balanced against the risk to personal safety. At the very core of this complicated intervention is the necessary, but virtually impossible, task of predicting the patient's potential for future violence. In essence, the emergency clinician must predict whether a patient who is now agitated or has a history of violence will sooner or later lose control. To this end, the clinician must assess the patient's history of aggression and the current psychological and environmental conditions aggravating or inhibiting his violent impulses, and must identify the precipitants of the current crisis. And yet there is no set of criteria based on etiologies, historical factors, syndromes, or symptoms with absolute predictive value. There is ultimately only an educated opinion. This chapter discusses the process of turning clinical impressions, historical data, and physical/psychological findings into just those sorts of seasoned judgments and management decisions.

2. General Assessment Issues

Violence is associated with a wide range of clinical pictures: the agitation of schizophrenia, rage attacks of the explosive disorder, chronic aggressive acts of the antisocial personality disorder, murder, child abuse, reckless driving, and drug-incited fury, to mention a few. Whatever its actual cause, violence occurs when the balance between impulse and control is disturbed (see Figure 1). When aggressive impulses are heightened, an individual may be preoccupied with violent thoughts, fears, or wishes. So long as the internal controls remain intact, however, the violent impulses will not give way to acts. If controls are weakened, increasing levels of agitation may accompany threats of violence,

Andrew E. Skodol, M.D. • College of Physicians and Surgeons of Columbia University, New York, New York 10032, and Biometrics Research Department, New York State Psychiatric Institute, New York, New York 10032.

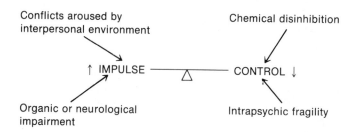

Figure 1. Mechanisms of violence.

but the patient will remain in control. When aggressive impulses are stimulated to a degree that they overwhelm normal controls, or when weakened controls cannot override even less potent aggressive drives, violence will erupt; aggression is acted out and discharged. Factors, therefore, that contribute to a heightened aggressive drive or a weakened set of internal controls should be considered. From an etiological viewpoint, these factors are commonly associated with functional psychiatric disorders, with organic or toxic disorders, or with compelling psychosocial stressors. Although the impulse–control relationship provides a model for understanding the internal balance of psychological forces, it does not in itself suggest a way of predicting violence.

There have been many attempts to define dangerousness: that is, to develop a set of predictive criteria for identifying the patient who will become violent. Solomon has suggested that the following factors have predictive value: the degree of intent to do violence, the presence of an identifiable victim, the frequency and openness of threats, the possession of a concrete plan, access to weapons, and a demonstrated incapacity to maintain control.[1] Kozol describes a dangerous patient as one who has already inflicted or attempted to inflict serious physical injury on another person; is chronically angry, hostile, or resentful; enjoys witnessing or inflicting suffering; lacks compassion; views himself as a victim; and resents or rejects authority.[2]

Others have suggested that various historical features are reliable predictors of future violence: childhood brutality or deprivation; homes lacking warmth and affection; early loss of a parent; violent triad of fire-setting, bed-wetting, and cruelty to animals; prior violent acts; military history; and reckless driving.[3-6] Some clinicians feel that the best predictor of future violence is past violence. In the final analysis, however, all attempts to correlate future behavior with historical factors or personality traits have uniformly low predictive reliability.[7] As psychiatric profiles, however, these correlations can serve as valuable indicators of increased risk for violence. One such formulation associates the potential for violence with the presence of any one of the following: preoccupation with, or fears of, acting violent; serious or repeated threats of

Table 1. DSM-III Classification of Disorders of Antisocial or
Aggressive Behavior[a]

Organic mental disorders
  Substance-induced
  Organic affective or personality disorder
  Deliria and dementias
  Intermittent explosive disorder
Mental retardation
Psychotic disorders
  Schizophrenia and psychotic disorders not elsewhere
    classified
  Paranoid disorder
  Major affective disorders
Intermittent or isolated explosive disorder
Personality disorders
  Antisocial
  Borderline
  Paranoid
  Narcissistic
Conduct disorders
  Socialized, aggressive
  Undersocialized, aggressive
Attention deficit disorder
Adjustment disorders
  Adjustment disorder with disturbance of conduct
V codes
  Childhood, adolescent, or adult antisocial behavior

---

[a] From American Psychiatric Association.[8]

assaultive or destructive behavior against specific people or property; past history of violence; and agitated, menacing demeanor.

The patient, however, does not always present with one of the signs mentioned above; he may in fact be relatively quiet, with an undramatic psychiatric history. Therefore, the clinician should be attentive to subtle or abrupt changes in mood, speech, or behavior, and must be ready to shift gears rapidly should violence erupt at any point during the interview (see Chapter 2).

3. Assessing and Managing the Potentially Violent Patient

In an emergency setting, evaluation must be rapid and accurate, and management decisive. Although definitive diagnosis by special tests and/or examinations is rarely possible, and may not even be necessary, it is desirable to evaluate the potentially violent patient for evidence of an organic, functional, or situational etiology (see Table 1).

Another aspect of the assessment of violent patients that is not traditionally diagnostic is an assessment of the patient's strengths and assets and the nature of his support network. The patient's adaptive functioning, interpersonal relations, motivation, and ego functions, including defenses and coping styles, will influence treatment decisions and prognosis (see Chapter 2). Although assessment is generally focused on pathology and intrapsychic conflict, adequate treatment planning requires that personal strengths and situational contingencies be noted as well.

3.1. Organic Etiology

Organic etiology is highly presumptive when characteristic mental status findings are present, including clouding of consciousness, disorientation, memory disturbance, or diminished cognitive capacity. Evidence of organicity may also come from the history (e.g., epilepsy or substance abuse), physical examination (e.g., head trauma or autonomic hyperactivity), or laboratory tests (e.g., low blood glucose level or presence of barbiturates in the blood). In other individuals, the manifestations of an organic brain syndrome (OBS) may be much softer and limited to a subtle, but abrupt, change in personality or to the violent behavior itself. Only careful observation, questioning, and physical examination will lead to the correct diagnosis.

Foremost among the organic causes of reduced impulse control is chemical disinhibition resulting from the use or abuse of various substances[9,10] (see Figure 1). Substance-induced states of intoxication (including idiosyncratic intoxication or delusional syndromes) and deliria (including withdrawal deliria) must always be considered by the emergency clinician who is evaluating an agitated, violent, or out-of-control patient (see Chapters 2 and 9).

> For example, an 18-year-old high school senior was brought to the emergency room by police after being picked up wandering in traffic on the Triborough Bridge. He was angry, agitated, and aggressive, reporting that various people were trying to "confuse" him by giving him misleading directions. His story was rambling and disjointed, but he admitted to the police officer that he had been using "speed." In the emergency room, he had difficulty focusing his attention and had to ask that questions be repeated. He was disoriented to time and place, and was unable to repeat a list of three names after five minutes. The family gave a history of the patient's regular use of "pep pills" over the past two years, during which time he was frequently "high" and did very poorly in school.[11]

In other patients, neurological impairment contributes to violent behavior.[12–15] These patients are often provoked by minor events, are characteristically explosive and unpredictable, and frequently are destructive of property or injurious to others. The term *episodic dyscontrol*[16] has been used to describe some of these patients. If a specific neurological disorder can be identified, treatment may reverse or at least control the associated rage attacks.

Epilepsy is the most common neurological diagnosis associated with violent behavior. Violence may occur in conjunction with seizure discharge (rare) or as an interictal or postictal phenomenon.[12,17] Patients often report a sense of rising tension—a physical wave flooding them with rage. Occasionally, a

patient can control the urge to strike out, but more often the expl
occurs. Afterwards, if the patient remembers the event, he may expe
extreme remorse and guilt. These features are particularly true of temp
lobe attacks occurring in adolescent or young adult males. However, not al
patients with a history of epilepsy are prone to violent behavior (range from
4.8% to 50%, with higher frequencies in temporal lobe epilepsy).[18-21] Abnormal
EEGs, although more common in epileptic patients with paroxysmal rage attacks, are not universal.[12,22] However, since the emergency clinician rarely
has immediate access to EEG data, he must rely on his clinical skills.

Another common neurological diagnosis associated with violence is minimal brain dysfunction syndrome (now referred to as Attention Deficit Disorder). It sometimes follows a perinatal trauma such as fetal anoxia, encephalitis, head injury, or febrile convulsions. Explosive behavior may also occur
in patients with frank cerebral palsy or mental retardation. In the latter two
cases, the clinician can usually identify the problem without tests.

3.2. Major Functional Psychiatric Disorders

These also may lead to reduced impulse control and violence. This is most
likely to occur with either psychotic disorders or severe personality disorders.

3.2.1. Psychoses

Psychotic illnesses are characterized by impaired reality testing evidenced
by delusions, hallucinations, or bizarre behavior. Since an accurate psychiatric
history may be impossible to obtain from the patient, it may be difficult to
discriminate among schizophrenia, schizoaffective illness, and major affective
disorder; any of these disorders can be associated with violent behavior. The
absence of such a diagnostic discrimination does not seriously hamper the
clinician, however, since the acute management in the ER is quite similar for
each of these patients (see Chapter 11).

> L.H., a 34-year-old Hispanic male, was brought by the police to the emer-
> gency room from the city welfare office. He was well known to emergency
> personnel since he had made over 100 visits in the course of the previous
> 10 years. He told the nurse on duty that he had been "getting the runa-
> round" from the case worker and had lost his temper. In fact, the case
> worker had called a few minutes before his arrival; in a very flustered tone
> she told the doctor that Mr. H. had threatened to kill her, shaking his closed
> fist and pounding repeatedly on her desk. When he would not leave her
> office she summoned the police.
>
> From the records, it was known that Mr. H. had been diagnosed as
> having chronic schizophrenia. He was followed in the outpatient clinic and
> was receiving fluphenazine enanthate (Prolixin) injections. Some of his ER
> visits had been prompted by angry outbursts or arguments, but many were
> made in the middle of the night when he had nowhere else to go. He had
> been hospitalized on psychiatric wards because of psychotic decompen-

previous 10 years. Nursing staff knew his story
⌐ who had been frequently abused by his foster
ng fires and shooting rats as a teenager.
events at the welfare center. His monthly check
⌐ a "computer breakdown." The social worker
ave to wait until next month to receive a double
⌐ way to process his case "out of sequence." Mr.
t on his furnished room was due next week, and
d. When he explained this to the case worker she
form for emergency funds, but that it would take
would receive any supplement. It was at this point
that he became angry and demanded that something be done. When the case worker said that there was nothing else that she could do, Mr. H. shook his fist at her and said, "I'm going to kill you." At this point in his story, Mr. H. turned to the doctor and said, "What am I supposed to do, Doc? I ain't got no money and if I don't pay my rent I ain't gonna have no place to go."

Mr. H. had several characteristics indicating that he might be "dangerous": he was frequently angry; he made a specific threat to a specific person; he appeared to be losing control; and he suffered from a psychotic disorder. Nonetheless, the on-call doctor felt that the context of the outburst had provoked the threat and that hospitalization was not required. Moreover, after the need for additional social assistance was discussed, Mr. H. calmed down considerably.

3.2.2. Personality Disturbance

The most common personality disturbance associated with violence is the antisocial personality disorder. It is characterized by a history of chronic antisocial and aggressive behavior dating back to childhood or early adolescence. The diagnosis is usually evident from the history, which confirms the presence of long-standing antisocial problems. The violent behavior of the antisocial personality is more organized and purposeful than that of a person with an organic brain syndrome or psychotic disorder. Often there is a clear motive. Other personality disturbances, such as the borderline, histrionic, narcissistic, or paranoid personality disorder, can have associated episodes of violent behavior.

In children and adolescents, repetitive, persistent patterns of aggressive antisocial behavior may indicate a conduct disorder. It is useful to distinguish the clearly aggressive child from the deliquent and to note the degree to which the child flouts social ties and obligations. Some children with Attention Deficit Disorder may manifest aggression during periods of hyperactivity. These children have impaired attention, increased impulsiveness, and increased motor activity.

3.2.3. Psychosocial Stressors

Not all causes of heightened impulsiveness are organic or neurological or related to functional psychiatric disorders. A thorough evaluation of the particular context in which violence occurs or is threatened becomes a critical part of the emergency assessment. Numerous studies have confirmed that violence commonly occurs in close or intimate social contexts.[23] The focus of treatment in these cases is the contextual precipitant: the violent system or dyad, not the patient's organic or functional pathology *per se*.

In assessing the nature and severity of psychosocial stressors associated with violent behavior, it is important to consider several parameters: the source—parental, conjugal, financial, or legal—and the chronicity—is the stress related to a single event, repetitive pattern, or persistent condition? Violent behaviors directly attributable to situational stress have a better prognosis than those seemingly autonomous behaviors attributable to intrapsychic or organic etiology. Of course, stress may not be the sole determinant of violence and may also complicate the course of mental disorder. For example, it may precipitate violent behavior in an individual with a personality disorder or it may lead to the development of a transient conduct disturbance.

3.2.4. Unspecifiable Etiology

Society, in general, regards violence as closely linked to mental illness.[24–26] Persons with impulse control problems are therefore customarily brought to emergency psychiatrists at the insistence of third parties—in some cases by family members, but in others by representatives of social agencies such as the police. A majority of these patients are brought to the ER involuntarily and are consequently either uncooperative or deliberately evasive and misleading. They are not generally motivated for treatment. In some instances, violence and the failure to see it as socially unacceptable are due to impaired reality testing—the product of a psychotic disorder. In other instances, however, the violence stems not from mental disorder but from intolerable social or political conditions. There is finally also the category of individuals for whom violence represents a way of life—not necessarily a character style or even a "last-resort" response to social injustice, but a chronic exploitation of society's vulnerable members. For these individuals, a violent way of life involves a profound failure of conscience of, undoubtedly, unspecifiable etiology. The treatability of violence of this type within the context and constraints of contemporary psychiatry is controversial at best, for although the demography of violence is well defined, the social situation is not. The ER clinician should, therefore, not attempt to act as judge and jury on complex social issues but rather should consider what assistance he has to offer to an individual who is brought for evaluation. The clinician must be aware of his therapeutic options as well as his limitations.

Most clinicians, when confronted with a violent individual in the emergency room, tend to accept responsibility for management and treatment without considering the appropriateness of this role. Few clinicians take into account, for example, that to restrain, medicate involuntarily, or hospitalize a person against his will can be an infringement of the person's civil liberties unless demonstrable benefits can be achieved by such measures. Treatment without such provisions is a form of preventive detention. On the other side of the dilemma, however, is the responsibility for releasing the violent or potentially violent patient who then harms another person, property, or himself. Combined moral and social concerns contribute to the clinician's willingness to let safety override patients' rights (see Chapter 3).

The following case illustrates this thorny dilemma:

> A 29-year-old man was brought to the emergency room accompanied by police from the local county jail. He had been arrested two weeks previously, following a mugging at knife point of an elderly woman on a dark residential street. On three occasions, when authorities attempted to bring him before a judge for arraignment, he began to scream and struggled with the police until they had to restrain him forcibly and return him to his cell. Following the third occurrence, the judge ordered that the man be taken to the local hospital for psychiatric evaluation. In obtaining the history from police, the emergency doctor discovered that the man had an extensive criminal record involving several arrests and convictions for car theft, robbery, assault, and possession of weapons. He had served three relatively short terms in the state penitentiary. He allegedly told the arresting policemen that they would never get him back in jail again.
>
> When interviewed by the psychiatrist, the man was sullen. He answered questions but provided only a minimum of information. He admitted his previous crimes but denied having been involved in the current robbery. He stated that he had been approximately one-half block away from the scene; when police approached he began to run, and they pursued him instead of the actual assailant. He denied any past psychiatric history or treatment and denied experiencing mood disturbance, delusions, hallucinations, seizures, or drug use. When asked why he raised such a ruckus at the arraignment hearings he first looked at the interviewer defiantly, then gave a brief, muffled laugh as if telling himself a private joke, and turned away to stare out the window. Then he was silent. He denied wanting to be hospitalized. The psychiatrist told the police that there were no symptoms of an emotional disturbance that he could treat and that he felt the individual was using uncooperative behavior as a strategy to avoid being tried for this crime. The police responded, "But, Doc, can't you take him? What are we supposed to do with him? He'll just keep doing this." The psychiatrist wrote a lengthy letter to the judge acknowledging the problem, but reiterating that the individual was neither treatable nor detainable by psychiatric standards, and that the courts would have to work out another arrangement for completing the man's arraignment.

In this case, the psychiatrist recognized the individual's pattern of antisocial behavior and sympathized with the court's plight. He resisted the temptation, however, to act as if psychiatry had an answer; he determined that the man had no mental disorder requiring treatment in a general hospital setting. It is clear from the man's history that the onset of antisocial behavior occurred before the age of 15, consistent with the diagnosis of antisocial personality disorder. But even so, he was very unlikely to benefit from treatment in a general hospital inpatient psychiatric unit. Although some criminals feign mental illness to avoid being confined in jail, this man had no such desire. He was merely resisting, in the only way he knew how, being processed for another potential jail term.

4. Treatment Options

Treatment plans for a potentially violent person should be based on the etiology (functional vs. organic vs. situational) of the disorder, psychological status of the patient, and availability of resources. Options actually available to the emergency clinician include those used during the immediate context (physical restraint, medication, and brief psychotherapeutic intervention) and those approaches considered for postemergency treatment (hospitalization and referral).

4.1. Psychopharmacology

In the emergency setting, medication is frequently used to achieve behavioral control. Most often, high-potency antipsychotic medications such as haloperidol (Haldol) are administered (see Chapters 2 and 4). In general, maintenance medication regimens should not be initiated in the ER unless firm plans for follow-up have been made, the patient is motivated and cooperative, and he has been medically evaluated. Table 2 describes the pharmacologic treatment of acute and chronic violence.

4.2. Psychotherapy

Psychotherapy with potentially violent patients is rarely a short-term affair. The emergency setting may be especially appropriate for the initial phases, but the clinician should try to establish sufficient rapport to effect a successful transition to longer-term treatment. During crisis management in the ER, the therapist can help the patient begin to reestablish internal controls and, when possible, to mobilize environmental resources that will also help to calm the patient. The clinician should encourage the patient to link precipitating factors, such as the use of drugs or alcohol, situational stresses, and interpersonal conflicts, with the violent outburst so that he can exert more effective controls or avoid the identified causes of violence. The short-term goal of psychotherapy in the ER should be to contain the aggressive impulses and move toward longer-term resolution.

5. Disposition

The ER clinician must make three major dispositional decisions about the violent patient: (1) Should the patient be hospitalized? (2) Does the patient need

Table 2. Schematic Differential Diagnosis and the Pharmacologic Treatment of Violence

——— Psychotic dimension ———	——————— Organic dimension ———————		——————— Characterologic dimension ———————		
Functional	Toxic-metabolic → OBS		Structural	Episodic dyscontrol	Other
	Drug → ETOH		→ Epilepsy	→ Intermittent explosive	↗ Antisocial ↘ Emotionally unstable character
Schizophrenia Mania	↘ Intoxication ↗ Withdrawal	Deliria	Attention deficit disorder		
		Dementias	Retardation		
	Benzodiazepines	Antipsychotics	Benzodiazepines		
	Antihistamines				
	Antipsychotics				
	Physostigmine				
Acute Depression Antipsychotics					
Chronic Antipsychotics Lithium Antidepressants	Benzodiazepines Antabuse	Antipsychotics Cerebral vasodilators	Anticonvulsants Benzodiazepines Barbiturates Stimulants Antidepressants	Anticonvulsants Lithium Antipsychotics	

continued treatment such as crisis intervention? (3) If outpatient treatment is indicated, is it urgent or elective?

5.1. Hospitalization

Deciding whether or not to hospitalize a violent patient is often difficult. Hospitalization may prevent further violence by restricting the opportunity for its occurrence, even when it does not necessarily resolve the clinical problem. Although there are no reliable guidelines for predicting dangerousness, "dangerousness to others" is still considered a criterion for hospitalization and overrides patients' rights (see Chapter 3). Peszke and Wintrob[27] conducted a survey of emergency commitment procedures indicating that psychiatrists' attitudes toward involuntary hospitalization were individualized and subjective, and often had little correlation with state statutes. Fifty percent of psychiatrists listed potential harm to others as a legitimate reason for hospitalizing someone against his will. In one study[28] 47% of patients were involuntarily hospitalized because of dangerousness to others, while in another the authors concluded that "if a person had been assaultive, this almost invariably played a role in hospitalization whether voluntary or involuntary."[29]

Most clinicians, in the "heat of battle" in the ER, subordinate questions about the patients' legal rights and society's use of psychiatry as a "cure-all" for social ills and allow a perceived threat to determine the decision to hospitalize. This attitude persists in spite of the unreliability of predictive indicators, including the presence of a threat. In this context, medical and legal decision making are different processes. The physician is trained to explore and attend to low probability events, e.g., the less likely possibilities in a differential diagnosis. In contrast, the courts demand high levels of certainty ("beyond a reasonable doubt" = 90% certain; "clear and convincing proof" = 75% certainty) in their evidentiary tests.[30] There is no simple solution to this dilemma—clinicians will undoubtedly continue to make decisions based on "a threat of violence" as long as they feel the pressure of conscience and have no other reliable predictors.

Although additional studies are necessary to define specific "hospitalization criteria" and evaluate their appropriateness, the literature suggests that diagnostic considerations—specifically the detection of a psychotic disorder among violent patients—may constitute a valid reason for hospitalization.[28,29,31] Skodol and Karasu,[32] for example, studied assaultive patients in the ER and found a high incidence of disturbed perception, cognition, and reality testing due to psychosis, organic mental disorders, and intoxicating drugs in conjunction with violent ideation and behavior. They also found that the diagnosis of a psychotic disorder, specifically schizophrenia, influenced the clinician's decision to hospitalize more than factors such as the degree of premeditation, the degree of intent expressed by the patient, or the potential lethality of a violent act.[33]

Not all violent patients require involuntary hospitalization. Sometimes it is possible to enlist the cooperation of the patient and to encourage a voluntary admission. Such an approach promotes the individual's sense of responsibility for his actions and bolsters his self-esteem—which is often at a low point following the loss of control. Unfortunately, it is not rare for the patient to refuse hospitalization, even if it is in his best interests. Another consideration is whether or not the psychotic patient understands the nature of his contract. In such cases, involuntary hospitalization might protect the patient's rights by guaranteeing requisite reviews and documentation that, in turn, might support the need for hospitalization.

Hospitalization of patients who are psychotic and/or intoxicated need not be long. Well-equipped emergency departments often have an overnight or holding unit either as a physical part of their service or on the inpatient unit.[34,35] Given the transient nature of many substance-induced deliria and substance-related psychotic syndromes, and the effectiveness of rapid neuroleptization, it is reasonable to expect that many assaultive or violent patients will require nothing more than admission to a short-stay unit.

Criteria for hospitalizing violent patients with personality or character disturbances are still controversial. Many patients with major character pathology do poorly in the usual inpatient settings of the general hospital psychiatry service. Some patients who do require hospitalization derive more benefit and do less to impede the care of other patients when they are treated on specialized units, such as prison hospital units.

5.2. Psychotherapy/Outpatient Treatment

If the patient does not need hospitalization, what additional measures are indicated? If continued treatment is necessary, how can the ER clinician ensure that future treatment will indeed occur? For patients whose violent outbursts or thoughts arose from environmental or interpersonal circumstances or for patients where controls have been transiently impaired by chemical or psychological processes, short-term psychotherapy may be particularly helpful. When the problem arises from a family conflict, referral for family therapy is appropriate. Continued crisis intervention has the following advantages: (1) The situations that push the patient beyond the limits of his tolerance into a violent outburst are not allowed to continue or consolidate; (2) in focused therapy the violent individual and the violent network learn new modes of resolving conflict and new coping skills.

For patients with difficulties in impulse control who cannot use either a systems approach or introspective psychotherapy, referral to specialty clinics for violent patients, such as that offered by Lion and his associates,[36] has distinct advantages. Not only is there more flexibility in routine procedures and therapeutic style, but the normative behavior for the patients and the expectations of the staff are specifically geared to the potentially violent patient who is generally poorly organized and poorly motivated.

The final point concerns the possibility of giving no care. Violence *per se* does not always indicate a psychiatric disorder; it may constitute a social problem of devastating proportions, but the psychiatrist is not in a position to solve it alone, even under ideal circumstances.

6. Conclusion

Although violence is among the most difficult clinical problems encountered by the clinician working in the emergency setting, it is also among the most compelling because of its social impact. The clinician must search for the sources of the individual's violent inclinations under the severely restrictive conditions of the emergency setting. He must then carefully assess what assistance he can give, keeping in mind the need to balance his obligations to the individual and to society.

References

1. Salamon I: Violent and aggressive behavior, in Glick R, Meyerson A, Robins E, et al (eds.): *Psychiatric Emergencies*. New York, Grune and Stratton, 1976, pp 109–119.
2. Kozol HL, Boucher RJ, Gawfalo RF. The diagnosis and treatment of dangerousness. *Crime and Delinquency* 18:371–392, 1972.
3. Duncan, GM, Frazier SH, Litin EM, et al: Etiological factors in first degree murder. *JAMA* 168:1755–1758, 1958.
4. Hellman DS, Blackman N: Eneuresis, firesetting and cruelty to animals: A triad predictive of adult crime. *Am J Psychiatry*, 122:1431–1435, 1966.
5. Silver JB, Dublin CC, Lourie RS: Does violence breed violence? Contributions from a study of the child abuse syndrome, *Am J Psychiatry* 126:404–407, 1969.
6. Justice B, Kraft IA: Early warning signs of violence: Is a triad enough? *Am J Psychiatry* 131:457–459, 1974.
7. *APA Task Force on Clinical Aspects of the Violent Individual*. Washington D.C., American Psychiatric Association, 1974.
8. American Psychiatric Association: *Diagnostic and Statistical Manual of Mental Disorders* (DSM III), ed 3. Washington, D.C., American Psychiatric Association, 1980.
9. Lion, JR, Bach-y-Rita G, Ervin FR: Violent patients in the emergency room. *Am J Psychiatry* 125:1706–1711, 1969.
10. Tuason VB: The psychiatrist and the violent patient. *Dis Nerv Syst* 32:764–768, 1971.
11. Spitzer RL, Skodol AE, Gibbon M, et al: *DSM-III Case Book*. Washington, D.C., American Psychiatric Association, 1981.
12. Williams D: Neural factors related to habitual aggression. *Brain* 92:503–520, 1969.
13. Mark VH, Ervin FR: *Violence and the Brain*. New York, Harper & Row, 1970.
14. Fields WS, Sweet WH (eds): *Neural Bases of Violence and Aggression*. St. Louis, Warren H. Green, Inc., 1975.
15. Elliott FA: The neurology of explosive rage. *Practitioner*, 217:51–60, 1976.
16. Bach-y-Rita, G, Lion JR, Climent C, et al: Episodic dyscontrol: A study of 130 violent patients. *Am J Psychiatry* 127:1473–1478, 1971.
17. Stevens JR: Interictal clinical complications of complex partial seizures, in Penry JK, Daly DD (eds.): *Advances in Neurology*, vol 2. New York, Raven Press, 1975.
18. Bingley T: Mental symptoms in temporal lobe epilepsy and temporal lobe glioma. *Acta Psychiatr Neurol Scand* 33 (Supp 120):1–151, 1958.
19. Curry S, Heathfield KW, Henson RA, et al: Clinical course and prognosis of temporal lobe epilepsy: A survey of 666 patients. *Brain* 94:173–190, 1971.
20. Rodin EA: Psychomotor epilepsy and aggressive behavior. *Arch Gen Psychiatry* 28:210–213, 1973.

21. Elliott FA: Neurological factors in violent behavior: The dyscontrol syndrome. *Bull Am Acad Psychiatr Law* 4:297–315, 1976.
22. Monroe RR: *Episodic Behavioral Disorders: A Psychodynamic and Neurophysiologic Analysis.* Cambridge, Harvard University Press, 1970.
23. Field MH, Field HF: Marital violence and the criminal process: Neither justice nor peace. *Soc Sci Rev* 47:221–240, 1973.
24. Grunberg F, Klinger BI, Gurmet B: Homicide and the deinstitutionalization of the mentally ill. *Am J Psychiatry* 134:685–687, 1977.
25. Lagos JM, Perlmutter K, Saexinger H: Fear of the mentally ill: Empirical support for the common man's response. *Am J Psychiatry* 134:1134–1137, 1977.
26. Tardiff K, Sweilamm A: Assault, suicide and mental illness, *Arch Gen Psychiatry* 37:164–169, 1980.
27. Peszke MA, Wintrob RM: Emergency commitment: A transcultural study. *Am J Psychiatry* 131:36–40, 1974.
28. Spensley J, Barter JT, Werme PH, et al: Involuntary hospitalization: What for and how long? *Am J Psychiatry* 131:219–223, 1974.
29. Gove, WR, Fain T: A comparison of voluntary and committed psychiatric patients. *Arch Gen Psychiatry* 34:669–676, 1977.
30. Ennis BJ, Litwack TR: Psychiatry and the presumption of expertise: Flipping coins in the courtroom. *California Law Rev.* 62:693–752, 1974.
31. Flynn R, Henisz JE: Criteria for psychiatric hospitalization: Experience with a checklist for chart review. *Am J Psychiatry* 132:847–850, 1975.
32. Skodol AE, Karasu TB: Emergency psychiatry and the assaultive patient. *Am J Psychiatry* 135:202–205, 1978.
33. Skodol AE, Karasu TB: Toward hospitalization criteria for violent patients. *Compr Psychiatry* 21:162–166, 1980.
34. Rhine MW, Mayerson P: Crisis hospitalization within a psychiatric emergency service. *Am J Psychiatry* 127:1386–1391, 1971.
35. Schwartz DA, Weiss AT, Milner JM: Community psychiatry and emergency service. *Am J Psychiatry* 129:710–714, 1972.
36. Lion JR, Madden DJ, Christopher RL: A violence clinic: Three years' experience. *Am J Psychiatry* 133:432–435, 1976.

Emergency Care of Suicidal Patients

Ellen L. Bassuk, M.D.

1. Introduction

Suicide is the ninth leading cause of death in the United States and currently accounts for 60 to 70 deaths per day. Its rate has increased slightly since the turn of the century and is now approximately 12.7 per 100,000 population.[1] Many more people attempt suicide than succeed. In recent years the number of attempts, especially by drug overdosage, has climbed to epidemic proportions and has led to a rise in the number of associated hospital admissions. The reported ratio of eight attempts to one completed suicide is significantly underestimated.[2] In addition, countless people seriously contemplate the act without carrying it out. Many of these individuals require professional help. Taken together, the entire range of suicidal feelings, impulses, and acts constitutes a major health care problem and reflects the untold suffering of large numbers of people.

The emergency clinician faces the challenging task of evaluating suicidal patients both to determine the degree of risk and to develop an appropriate management and treatment plan. Unfortunately, many persons do not present with an explicit chief complaint related to suicide, nor do they reveal their self-destructive intent. Thus, the evaluator should elicit information from all patients about suicidal thoughts and preoccupations and should be alert to indicators of increased risk.

Since the suicidology literature is voluminous, diverse, and sometimes contradictory, caretakers may have difficulty determining the relative importance of various factors when assessing an individual. This chapter describes a clinical checklist for evaluating suicide that integrates both statistical and clinical indicators of risk. The approach evolved from extensive experience in an emergency setting in an urban general hospital where approximately one-third of the psychiatric patients present with suicidal thoughts and behaviors.[3]

It should be borne in mind that although this chapter discusses suicidal impulse, behavior, and ideation as if they are classifiable phenomena, it is

This chapter is condensed from material on the assessment and emergency care of suicidal patients, in Bassuk EL, Schoonover S, Gill A (eds): *Lifelines: Clinical Perspectives on Suicide*. New York, Plenum Publishing Corp, 1982.

Ellen L. Bassuk, M.D. • Harvard Medical School, Boston, Massachusetts 02115.

not assumed that suicide is predictable. In fact, for the individual, suicide is generally not predictable. The assessment grids that follow should be construed only as guidelines, and not as rigorous or reliable predictive criteria.

The checklist for assessment includes the following categories: demographics, presenting symptoms, severity of suicidal ideas or behaviors, circumstances and meaning of the act, the nature of the suicidal crisis, and history. The choice of other items (i.e., quality of relationship, nature and availability of the support network, and the interaction with the interviewer) is based on the assumption that patients who are connected solidly with other people, agencies, and meaningful belief systems are less likely to commit suicide. Utilizing the checklist as a general guideline for gathering information from the patient and persons close to him will ensure a comprehensive evaluation. However, the specific sequence and structure of the interview depends on the patient's needs and the evaluator's clinical style.

To ensure consistency in classifying suicidal thoughts and behaviors, we have adopted a simple, descriptive terminology proposed by suicidologists. In the subsequent discussion three patient vignettes will illustrate this categorization and the use of the checklist:

1. Completed suicides include all deaths resulting from a "willful, self-inflicted, life-threatening act"[4] (p. 36).

> John D. is an elderly white male who was brought into the emergency ward by ambulance and pronounced dead on arrival. He lived alone in a single room in a large city and had not been seen for several days by other residents of the rooming house. Finally, the superintendent called the police, who broke into his room and found two empty bottles of aspirin and a suicide note on the bed next to his body. His only living relative, a son, was notified of his death.

2. Suicide attempts are any acts that are life-threatening or have that appearance. Some attempters with an intense wish to die use a highly lethal method, but somehow still survive. Other individuals, who are more ambivalent about dying and make "object-related" attempts, are labeled "manipulative" or "hysterical." These acts are commonly called "gestures." Because of the negative connotations associated with these terms, this chapter refers only to attempts.

> Mary R. is a 22-year-old graduate student who was taken to the emergency department by her worried boyfriend after she had ingested 10 unidentified yellow pills during an argument.

3. Suicidal ideas are thoughts and/or behaviors (such as a suicide note) which indicate that the individual is considering suicide.

> Vera L., a middle-aged housewife, presented to the emergency room with symptoms of depresson and persistent thoughts of dying by carbon monoxide poisoning in her car.

Table 1. Demographics of Completed Suicides[a]

Age	Older than 40 years old (Peak: 75 to 79 years old)
Sex	Male:Female = 2:1 to 7:1
Race	American Indians > white > black
Marital status	Single, widowed, divorced (living alone)
Occupation	Professional persons, especially health-care personnel and business executives
Geographic area	Urban or transitional
Method	Firearms or explosives or hanging > toxic substances

[a] From Frederick.[1]

2. Clinical Checklist for Assessment

2.1. Demographics (see Tables 1 and 2)

The case of John D. typifies the group of patients who, on the basis of demographic factors, are at highest risk for successful suicide: a white or Indian, separated, divorced, or widowed male 45 years or older who is either unemployed or retired and lives alone in a transitional or metropolitan geographic area.[1] Clinicians should be alert to the statistically greater possibility that a patient with these characteristics will die by suicide and should pursue the indicators included in the checklist. In contrast, a common demographic profile of a suicide attempter is Mary R., a young single student in her 20s. While the estimated ratio of males to females who successfully commit suicide ranges between 2:1 and 7:1, the ratio for attempts is reversed and is 2:1 to 3:1, females to males.[2]

Patients who have made a serious attempt are at much greater risk of dying by suicide during the subsequent two to four years, with a peak occurring during the initial three months.[5] Characteristics of high lethality attempters include symptoms of depression and/or insomnia and any of the following: 40 years or older, married or separated within the previous month, middle class with good work history.[6] In general, "the more closely suicide attempters approximate completed suicides with respect to age, sex or method, the higher their risk."[2]

Table 2. Demographics of Suicide Attempters[a]

Age	Young 20 to 30 years old (Peak: 20 to 24 years old)
Sex	Female:Male = 2:1
Race	Inconclusive
Marital status	Divorced
Occupation	Unemployed among males
Geographic area	Urban
Method	Drug ingestion

[a] From Weissman.[2]

2.2. Presenting Symptomatology/Diagnostic Assessment

The case of Vera L., a 39-year-old married mother of two adolescent sons illustrates a patient who, on the basis of demographic predictors alone, is not in a statistically high-risk group for attempted suicide. A comprehensive clinical evaluation is necessary to identify other indicators of increased risk.

> Vera L. presented to the emergency room with a chief complaint of rest-lessness, early morning wakening, a 15-pound weight loss, lack of interest in her usual routine, and ruminations about death of approximately two months' duration. She had no prior history of emotional disturbance and no symptoms of mania such as irritability, euphoria, racing thoughts, or hyperactivity.

The evaluator concluded that Vera's presenting symptoms were the manifestations of a major affective disorder (unipolar depression), placing her in a high-risk category. In fact, 15% of patients with a severe depressive illness successfully complete suicide.[7] During a lengthy interview, the evaluator supportively questioned Vera about her wish to die. With reluctance, she revealed feeling preoccupied with disturbing fantasies of her own death by suicide.

Although John D. may not have had a major affective disorder, his symptoms suggested that he too was at high risk for suicide.

> John D.'s son reported that his father had become increasingly "hopeless and despondent" since the death of his wife one year ago. As a younger man he was energetic and handled adversity with a great deal of strength. However, since the failure of his business at age 62, 10 years prior to his death, he gradually had exhausted all his resources. More recently, he seemed emotionally spent, despondent over the loss of his business and the death of his wife, and hopeless about his future. He was a heavy drinker, but for many years was able to control it without any major impairment of his ability to work. His wife had been tolerant of his problem until his business failed and he remained at home drinking large quantities of whiskey. Since that time she had repeatedly threatened to leave, and his physician had warned him of progressive liver damage. After his wife's death, he drank even more.

Like patients with a major affective disorder, 15% of alcohol abusers eventually die by suicide.[8] Moreover, alcoholics suffering an interpersonal loss are at even greater risk within the six weeks following the loss.[9]

Another group at a higher risk are patients with depressive or paranoid delusions accompanied by suicidal ideation or behavior. A follow-up study of wrist-slashing in psychotic patients with delusional guilt suggests that they should be hospitalized.[10]

Groups at lower risk for completing suicide include drug addicts, compulsive gamblers, schizophrenics, and, to an even lesser degree, personality disorders.[11] Patients at the lowest end of the suicide risk continuum often manifest anxiety, guilt, rage, and poor impulse control. Clinicians generally categorize these latter individuals as borderline or primitive personality disorders. Mary R., for example, expressed feelings of abandonment, emptiness, frustration, and anger when her boyfriend refused to stop dating other women. The presenting symptoms alone indicate that her suicide intent was not associated with greatly increased risk. In fact, little correlation exists between specific diagnosis and suicide attempts. Although attempters generally do not have major affective disorders, they may have some symptoms of depression.[2]

2.3. Suicidal Ideas or Acts

Clearly, the clinician must assess the seriousness of the suicidal thought or behavior. Three dimensions are important: *intent*, or the subjective wish to die; *lethality*, or the objective danger to life; and *mitigating circumstances*, or factors such as toxicity or dementia that might interfere with an individual's ability to assess the consequences of his act.[4]

> On three previous occasions, Mary R. was brought to the emergency room by her boyfriend after a deliberate overdose. During two of these visits the attempt was rated low for both intent and lethality. On each occasion she had ingested small amounts of diazepam (Valium), claiming that she only wanted to sleep for a long time to escape her misery. However, six months earlier, after ingesting a small number of tricylic antidepressants, she developed an arrhythmia requiring inpatient medical treatment.

Intent and lethality, for both current and previous attempts, must be evaluated carefully. Mary R.'s third suicide attempt differs significantly from the first two. Her wish to die was minimal, but her unpredictable sensitivity to the tricyclics resulted in a moderate to high lethality attempt. Because of accidental circumstances—unpredictable medication or late arrival of an individual unconsciously designated as rescuer—a suicidal act in which the patient has a covert agenda or is ambivalent about dying can be very serious. Because of inherent difficulties in assessing lethality, all individuals who use suicidal behavior as a way to interact with others are potentially at risk whatever their intent. Furthermore, the probability of a successful suicide increases significantly with a history of prior attempts of high lethality.

2.4. Circumstances and Meaning of the Act

2.4.1. Evaluation of Attachments

Theories of attachment offer insight into the meaning of a suicidal crisis and deepen our understanding of suicidal behavior.[12] Each individual has a view about the meaning of his life that usually involves an assessment of his attachments to other persons, ideas, beliefs, activities, and aspirations. The loss or threatened loss of major attachments can precipitate a suicidal crisis in some patients. Physical illness, financial reversals, transitional phases of life such as retirement, and interpersonal failures are common precipitants.

2.4.1.a. Interpersonal Relationship. Various authors have emphasized the importance of understanding suicide as an interpersonal event and have focused on the extent, quality, and meaning of the individual's major interactions.[13,14] Impairment of an individual's capacity to form and maintain relationships that provide mutual warmth and support may result in chronic feelings of loss, disappointment, and alienation, and may contribute to the development of suicidal preoccupations.

Mary R.'s difficulty in forming close, trusting relationships illustrates a set of problems common to many suicide attempters. She is unable to negotiate a comfortable interpersonal distance without feeling alienated or to develop a sense of intimacy without feeling engulfed. In each of her multiple, short-lived relationships, usually with married or emotionally unavailable men, she was caught in the same repetitive pattern. Magical expectations of each new lover gave way to feelings of intense disappointment and rejection. She could not satisfy her needs and feel supported and loved. To ward off loss of the relationship with her lover, Mary resorted to suicidal behavior. Despite the "object-related" property of this attempt, the clinician had to view it as serious and possibly life-threatening.

It is important to elicit information about the quality of interactions, extent of participation, and degree of satisfaction and benefit from shared pleasures, roles, and responsibilities, as illustrated in the following case:

> Vera married her high school sweetheart. Over the past 20 years they had gradually become more distant and uncommunicative. Her husband was a demanding, self-involved, hard-driving individual while she was hard-working, self-effacing, and long-suffering. She rarely expressed her own needs and saw the family's wishes as more important than her own. Direct questioning about their relationship revealed the following: Her husband's recent business successes required that he spend over 12 hours per day at work and many weeks overseas, usually without his wife. As he became increasingly unavailable to his family, Vera totally absorbed herself in her children's activities. However, with the departure of her youngest child to college, the discord in her marriage became more apparent and disturbing. Two months prior to her presentation, Vera became suspicious that her husband was involved with another woman and shortly thereafter developed symptoms of depression. She was unable to function in her usual role of homemaker and her household became markedly disorganized.

2.4.1.b. Support System. An individual's support system includes not only major interpersonal relationships (i.e., family, friends, and psychotherapist) but also interactions with people at work, school, church, and recreational organizations. The nature and availability of these resources and the patient's ability to use them should be assessed carefully. Lack of a meaningful network or decreasing participation and satisfaction in relationships should alert the clinician to the possibility of serious emotional difficulty.

The three patients described above had significant problems with their support network. For example, although Mary R. had extensive supports consisting of her family, boyfriend, school friends, and psychotherapist, she became involved in a destructive cycle of exaggerated help-seeking, disappointment, and help-rejection with her therapist and hospital personnel. Vera also had an extensive network, but her severe depressive symptoms interfered with a satisfying and beneficial use of these relationships.

In contrast to Vera and Mary R., John D. had gradually depleted his support network. John D.'s son recognized that his father had become increasingly hopeless and took his father to a community mental health center for treatment. Despite the efforts of his social worker, however, John D. remained apathetic and skeptical about treatment, refusing to participate actively or to assume responsibility for himself. When hospitalization was suggested, he discontinued contact with the social worker. His son visited every week and attempted to involve him in some activity, but without success. Several weeks before John D.'s death, his son had discussed a possible job transfer to another city.

The case of John D. illustrates the evolution of the "presuicidal syndrome," a final common pathway that correlates highly with successful suicide. It is characterized by three components: the progressive constriction of many aspects of the patient's life, the redirection of aggression toward the self, and the elaboration of suicidal fantasies.[15] John D. manifested this constriction by a loss of spontaneity, passive behavior, and inhibition. According to his son, he deprecated most aspects of his life, felt worthless, and described feelings of meaninglessness and monotony. Shneidman would have described the uniformity of the patient's behavior and his single-minded pessimistic outlook as the "frozen perspective" of a person who moves only in the direction of suicide.[16] John D.'s recent history, characterized by gradual immobilization, emotional exhaustion, and depletion of his supports, illustrates the course of a patient who is presuicidal. His son's feelings also reflect the evolution of a corresponding syndrome; he experienced emotional fatigue and anger caused by his father's demands and his own feelings of intense concern. This left John D.'s son exhausted, unable to detect or respond to specific clues of his father's impending death.

2.4.2. Evaluation of the Suicidal Crisis

If not worked through, any crisis state may result in a regression and the crystallization of emotional symptoms into a psychiatric disturbance. A history of an individual's previous capacity to cope with crisis may indicate how the patient will manage the current stress. However, if multiple efforts at problem-solving have been unsuccessful, the patient may develop a prolonged crisis state sometimes accompanied by depressive and suicidal symptoms. To understand the potency of a suicidal crisis, the possible disruption of attachments should be examined against the backdrop of (1) the precipitating stress, (2) relevant past history, and (3) life-stage issues. Factors from each in combination with immediate or perceived loss can form a lethal nexus.

2.4.2a. The Precipitating Stress. The evaluator should determine the precipitating stress and try to link it to the current suicidal crisis. The question

"Why now?" should be answered carefully. Life stresses leading to an increase in emotional disturbance include the loss of a loved person by either death or divorce, problems in major relationships, changes in roles, or serious physical illness. When compared with depressives and the general population, suicide attempters have been shown to experience a greater number of situational crises in the previous six months, with the peak occurring in the month prior to the suicidal act.[17] Because interpersonal or role disappointments are not always based on realistic expectations, they may appear less evident to the evaluator and require knowledge of the context of a person's life and a sense of the individual's current priorities, involvements, and motivations. Careful questioning should elicit the extent, nature, and stability of a person's attachments and major life activity or role (e.g., worker, housewife, or student). Difficulties in coping in any of these areas prior to the onset of the symptoms should be compared to the current ability to function; the discrepancy will give the evaluator some clue to the onset of the crisis and its impact. Often, explicitly linking the precipitant with the suicidal feelings may relieve the patient's distress and clarify the meaning of the crisis.

2.4.2b. Relevant Past History. It is necessary to understand the historic context of the current stress to appreciate how a specific event threatens the stability of an attachment. For example, Mary's difficulties in forming close relationships were based on a disturbed early mother–child interaction. As the middle child of seven in a family with an absent, alcoholic father and a young, depressed, unavailable mother, Mary grew up feeling abandoned, unloved, and rejected. Her current style of relating to men replicated aspects of her relationship with her parents and resulted in not unfamiliar feelings of emptiness, loneliness, frustration, and rage.

2.4.2c. Life-Stage Issues. In each of the three patients, the losses and disappointments were superimposed on a life-stage crisis—late adolescence for Mary, midlife for Vera, and retirement for John. Delineating the impact of these developmental issues may help to clarify the interplay of factors precipitating the current crisis. For example, Vera's youngest son's departure for college precipitated her depression and highlighted the chronic problems with her husband. She had concealed these marital difficulties by becoming overly involved with her children. Now that her sons had left, she was faced with an "empty nest," an absent husband, and role disruption. For most people, midlife issues lead to a review and questioning of values, roles, and accomplishments and a renewed confrontation with life's limitations. However, because of Vera's chronic difficulties, this process became intolerable. Like her mother before her, she sought to resolve these issues by suicide.

2.5. History

2.5.1. Psychiatric History

To identify the presence of disorders correlated with increased risk such as depression, alcoholism, and previous suicide attempts (particularly of high lethality), the patient should be questioned about prior psychiatric illness. Assessing a patient with a past history of a major affective disorder who now presents with a seemingly unrelated chief complaint poses a difficult problem. Does the patient have a masked depression or a depressive equivalent? For example, patients presenting with somatic complaints and hypochondriacal preoccupations, who have been medically worked up with no resultant finding of physical disease, should be evaluated for depression and questioned about suicidal ideation.

2.5.2. Medical History

A medical history should be obtained from every patient. An individual currently in poor health, particularly with chronic, debilitating, or terminal illness, may be at high risk for suicide. The meaning of the illness to the patient and the patient's capacity to cope successfully with its impact must be ascertained. How does the patient function in usual roles both currently and before the onset of the disease? A marked difference in functioning, inconsistent with the severity of the medical illness, shoud alert the clinician to the possibility of depression and increased suicidal potential. Similarly, inability to adjust to a severe medical illness or handicap may signal presuicidal morbidity.

The majority of patients who successfully complete suicide have sought medical and/or psychiatric care within one year before their death.[18,19] Nevertheless, patients far more commonly express their preoccupation with suicide to their spouse and close relatives than to their physician.[20] Further complicating the interpretation of these communications is the fact that most patients who discuss suicidal ideas do not translate them into behavior.

2.5.3. Family History

When evaluating a suicidal patient, determine if the patient has a family history of illnesses associated with increased risk such as a major affective disorder or alcoholism. If a close family member has committed suicide, the evaluator should assess the patient's identification with the deceased. This may be a central factor in a person's decision to commit suicide.

> For example, Vera spoke tearfully of her mother's death by suicide, which occurred when Vera was an adolescent preparing to leave for college. She described her initial shock, disbelief, inability to cry, and long-standing feelings of abandonment, isolation, and emptiness. Since her mother's death, she had intermittent fantasies of rejoining her. Recently those thoughts had become persistent and troublesome.

The similarity between Vera's current situation and her mother's concerned the evaluator. Vera, like her mother, was just 39 years old and had recently enrolled her youngest child in an out-of-town college. Sometimes, the quality of an anniversary reaction to a family member's suicide indicates that the patient's relationship with this individual is troubled. For example, Vera's inability to mourn her mother and to integrate her memory suggested that they had had an ambivalent relationship. Indeed, during the interview Vera was unable to acknowledge feelings of sadness, neediness, guilt, or anger, but was able to report compelling thoughts of joining her mother.

2.6. Interaction with the Interviewer

The development of positive rapport and a therapeutic relationship with the suicidal patient provides the context for the evaluation. The clinician must be empathic, introspective, knowledgeable, and technically skilled—qualities that constitute the "art of interviewing." Havens eloquently summarized both the verbal and nonverbal tasks in a psychologic examination and emphasized the importance of identifying "how the patient makes us feel"[21] (p. 213).

The interviewer may experience a wide range of intense, discomforting emotions, depending on the nature of the suicidal behavior, the underlying psychopathology, and the manner in which the patient relates. The therapist must acknowledge the nature of these feelings to himself without acting on them, use them as a barometer of the patient's distress, and understand them as a reflection of dynamics and history. Often, the patient's feelings are expressed indirectly. For example, Vera conveyed a sense of hopelessness, helplessness, and a wish to be rescued. At the same time, she felt apathetic, immobilized, and unable to take responsibility for herself. She was verbally compliant during the interview, but her withdrawal, distance, and desperation indicated the need for the therapist to take an active, protective stance.

In contrast, Mary R. related in a manipulative, help-rejecting manner. While she actively sought support, she devalued her caretakers and refused to follow through on realistic treatment plans, evoking considerable hostility. Her poor self-regard and chronic feelings of disappointment in all relationships lead her to attempt suicide repeatedly. The interviewer's frustration, anger, and helplessness mirrored similar feelings in the patient, her family, and friends.

3. Management

The first priority in the emergency management of acutely suicidal patients is to protect them from immediate self-harm. The patient should not be left alone—even for a few minutes. Emergency personnel should try to "suicide-proof" the interviewing area by defining specific security areas and ensuring that screens are impenetrable and glass shatterproof.

The psychologic management of the suicidal patient is fundamentally similar to the care of other emergency patients. The same principles apply as those discussed in the sections on crisis intervention. Based on the assessment, the primary disorder (e.g., psychosis, unipolar depression) should always be treated (see Part V). Involving persons close to the patient in his intensive care

Table 3. Criteria for Intensive Treatment

 I. Unequivocally dangerous—moderate to high intent and/or lethality
 II. Questionably dangerous and exhibiting one of the following:
   a. Lack of an effective support system
   b. Disruption of attachments
   c. Significant psychopathology associated with increased risk such as:
      1. Major affective disorders
      2. Suicidal symptoms in response to delusions and hallucinations
      3. Presuicidal syndrome
      4. Pathological identification with suicidal person(s)
   d. Need for intensive diagnostic evaluation and/or special treatments such as electroshock therapy, medications, detoxification
   e. Involvement in a pathological system promoting a suicidal crisis (e.g., family, psychotherapy)
   f. Recent escalation of suicidal behaviors
   g. Inability to be engaged in an ongoing treatment process
   h. Inability to assess dangerousness

---

may be very beneficial. Pathological family relationships, however, may exacerbate the patient's symptoms.

4. Treatment Planning

4.1. Introduction

Treatment planning actually begins during the initial contact with the patient and continues throughout the emergency intervention and referral process. On the basis of the assessment, the patient's response to immediate management, his requests, and the availability of community resources, the clinician should develop a treatment plan. It should include recommendations for immediate care, the specific disposition, and a statement about follow-up. In part, its successful implementation depends on whether or not the clinician and the patient can agree about the treatment plan.[22]

4.2. Intensive Treatments

Rather than describing each specific modality such as hospitalization, day care, or residential placements, general criteria for intensive treatments as a group are presented. For example, the decision to hospitalize can be used interchangeably with other approaches. This section discusses criteria that can guide the clinician in his choice of disposition (see Table 3).

Important indicators of the need for intensive treatment include assessment findings, previous treatment history, and current motivation for help. In addition, the patient's interaction with the interviewer provides important clues about the difficulty of engaging the patient and forming a therapeutic relationship. If a patient cannot cooperate with a recommended disposition (e.g., crisis intervention psychotherapy), hospitalization may offer an effective short-term alternative. Patients with characterologic problems who attempt suicide in response to minor stress are particularly difficult to engage in ongoing treatment and often require brief hospitalization.[23]

All patients considered dangerous to themselves at the time of evaluation should have 24-hour protection, even if involuntary admission is the only alternative. This includes suicidal patients who are intent on dying and who may have performed an act of high lethality and survived only by chance. Other patients requiring intensive treatment may be more ambivalent in their intent but are concerned about the compelling strength of their impulses. For example, the departure of Vera's children, superimposed on chronic marital difficulties, precipitated a major affective illness requiring treatment. Although she had supports, she was unable to utilize them and felt helpless and despairing, strongly identifying with her mother's suicidal resolve. The evaluator felt that despite Vera's apparent compliance, she made little real contact, remaining distant and preoccupied. On the basis of this assessment, the interviewer concluded that inpatient treatment was indicated. Vera and her husband agreed.

For patients who might be dangerous to themselves, problems in major relationships can potentiate the need for intensive treatment. Conflicted interactions, decreasing participation in relationships, real or fantasied losses may precipitate a suicidal crisis and may cause the patient to feel alienated, hopeless, and worthless. This may lead to progressive disengagement and retreat from help, hallmarks of the presuicidal syndrome.[15]

The clinician should refer those patients with major psychiatric illnesses and increased suicidal risk to the hospital or for other intensive treatment. These include persons with major affective disorders, psychotic patients who perform bizarre suicidal acts or develop suicidal symptoms in response to delusions and hallucinations, and those with a pathological identification with an individual who died by suicide. In others, the risk of suicide may be lower, but intensive diagnostic evaluation or special treatments, such as electroshock therapy, pharmacotherapy, or detoxification, are necessary. Also, suicidal patients who are unable to give a history and have no available family or friends should be referred for intensive treatment.

Sometimes, involvement in a pathologic system such as a family, marital, or psychotherapy relationship may provoke suicidal behavior. Recent escalation of suicidal activity may reflect increasing distress in the system and may require removal of the patient. If trouble in the psychotherapy relationship is increasing suicidal risk, hospitalization may help work through and resolve a patient–therapist bind and provide consultation to the outpatient therapist. For other psychotherapy patients, however, hospitalization might lead to marked regression and interfere with therapeutic goals. To ensure an integrated approach toward management, the planning process should involve the patient's primary caretakers.

Whenever possible, the clinician should choose the "least restrictive alternative" that fulfills treatment objectives. Many factors, not only the location of care, determine the restrictiveness of the setting. These include type of facility, staffing, patient characteristics, and available treatment modalities.[24] Leeman illustrates this when he comments: "Consider, too, that for some actively psychotic or suicidal patients, safe treatment on an unlocked unit may mean being confined to a small single room with a staff member stationed at the door, while on a locked unit, the patient could be allowed much greater mobility and freedom"[25] (p. 231).

However, if the patient requires involuntary hospitalization, the reasons for the decision should be discussed openly with the patient and the persons close to him. The interviewer should maintain a firm but reassuring stance, using details of the patient's chief complaint and history to support the need for admission. Many patients and their families respond with relief, but others adamantly protest. The interviewer should remain calm and supportive when discussing the patient's objections.

Emergency clinicians should know the criteria and steps for commitment in their state. For certain high-risk patients who do not fulfill the criteria for involuntary admission or when a bed is unavailable, alternative approaches can include (1) arranging for persons close to the patient to take interim responsibility, (2) arranging for partial hospitalization, or (3) structuring an intensive crisis intervention program.

4.3. Outpatient Treatments

Certain suicidal patients can be treated safely and effectively in outpatient crisis psychotherapy. A program tailored to meet the patient's needs may be an appropriate alternative to hospitalization. Of course, this presupposes that treatment is readily available and that the patient is motivated and cooperative.

Outpatient treatment should be considered for patients who make suicide attempts that are low in intent, sometimes repetitive, but not escalating in severity. Mary R. typifies the patient whose multiple attempts were unconsciously designed to effect interpersonal change, not suicide. Like Mary, many emergency patients are involved in psychotherapy at the time of their visit. Often, the attempt defends against intense transference feelings about the therapist. For example, Mary's argument with her boyfriend was superimposed on chronic, although predictable, difficulties in the therapeutic relationship. When informed of her therapist's month-long summer vacation, the patient retreated into the current affair. The overdose coincided with the therapist's return. For patients like Mary, the use of the emergency room to deal with feelings stirred up by therapy is a predictable part of treatment and should be managed by contacting the therapist, clarifying the meaning of the attempt, referring the patient back for continued treatment, and developing an integrated program for containing future suicidal behavior. Specific details of the treatment plan should be in accord with the meaning of the suicidal behavior as it pertains to both the real and the transference relationship with the therapist.

Some patients, who are not involved in ongoing treatment, make single or repetitive low-risk attempts. Despite the efforts of emergency clinicians to refer these patients for definitive care, the rate of completed referrals remains very low. In fact, this group follows through on treatment recommendations less often than patients who are not suicidal. In one study, only 35.6% of attempters received follow-up treatment, and the rate of repeated attempts was high. Of the group that was referred for outpatient care (32% of the total), only 3% completed the referral.[26] Similarly, other authors have reported high rates of attrition and uncooperative behavior among attempters.[27]

To deal with this problem, Spitz proposed the formation of a psychiatric-medical suicide care team.[28] To prevent fragmentation of care and lack of follow-through, the crisis intervention team was staffed by the same personnel as those running the emergency service. Another creative approach to the outpatient management of the suicidal patient is the continuing relationship maintenance program (CRM). It offers high-risk individuals who have telephoned a hotline the possibility of weekly telephone contact with a paraprofessional or a volunteer for a two-year period. In addition, this program provides home visits, "befriending contacts," and other activities. The relationship diminishes the patient's sense of isolation and facilitates the use of community resources.[29]

Unfortunately, many emergency services do not have the manpower to provide ongoing treatment or outreach. Therefore, to increase the rate of completed referrals, a general approach toward implementing outpatient treatment should be developed. When a disposition is made, the evaluator should contact the outpatient facility before the patient leaves the emergency room and, whenever possible, obtain a date and time for an appointment with a specific clinician. The patient should be given this information in writing along with directions to the clinic.

Understanding the nature of the patient's expectations about both the emergency visit and continued treatment will also increase compliance. Efforts should be made to work through any discrepancy between the dispositional plan and the patient's verbal or nonverbal requests. Direct discussion of the seriousness of the attempt and the necessity for ongoing therapy may resolve the patient's objections. Involving family and/or friends in the initial planning also will improve the rate of follow-up. Support, encouragement, and even pressure in certain situations help to increase motivation. For example, persons with major depressive reactions are notoriously poor at completing referrals. Although these patients appear compliant and aggreeable, they often lack the energy and optimism to follow through on treatment recommendations.[30]

For all attempters, the evaluator should follow up the disposition to determine if it was successful. If the patient did not complete the referral, he should be contacted and encouraged to become involved in treatment. Persistent outreach, including home visits, is sometimes necessary. If other treatment alternatives are not available, the telephone can be used as a "therapeutic medium to provide continuing contact with high-risk groups."[31]

5. Conclusion

The unique requirements and structure of the emergency setting compound the challenging task of providing treatment and formulating dispositional plans

Table 4. Assessment of Suicidal Idea or Act: The Rating Scales

1. Scale for Suicide Ideation[33]
   19-item scale "to quantify and assess suicidal intention"[33] (p. 343) by focusing on "the intensity, pervasiveness and characteristics of the ideation"[33] (p. 344). Most relevant variables are active and passive suicidal desire and concrete plans.
2. Hopelessness Scale[34]
   Hopelessness operationalized as "negative expectations of the future." Positive correlation with suicidal intent.
3. Suicide Intent Scale[35]
   Evaluates circumstances of act. Also self-report by patient of feelings about attempt.
4. Risk-Rescue Rating[36]
   Quantitatve and descriptive method for determining lethality of implementation.
5. Suicide Risk among Attempters[37]
   Assessment of demographic charcteristics and the circumstances of the act. Identified characteristics associated with the highest risk of death by suicide.
6. Scale for Assessing Suicide Potential/Los Angeles Suicide Prevention Center Scale[11]
   Overall assessment instrument for all patients. Focuses on both demographic and clinical factors.

for the suicidal patient. Major objectives of the emergency intervention include assessing the level of risk, providing protection, and involving patients in treatment. Engaging the patient in an ongoing therapeutic relationship requires patience, persistence, and outreach. Involving members of the patient's support network, collaborating with all caretakers, and designating a clinician with primary responsibility for the patient are essential therapeutic maneuvers. Their success, in part, depends on the development of specialized programs reflecting the general principles of care described in this chapter and yet realistically accounting for the limitations of manpower and community resources.

Appendix
The Rating Scales

Introduction (see Table 4)

Various rating scales focusing on the feelings, circumstances, and plans related to the idea or act and on demographic and clinical factors have been developed for the assessment of suicide. While these scales cannot accurately predict patients at greatly increased risk of suicide without including a large number of false positives, they are useful for highlighting "issues that are of significance in prediction" and for determining "levels of risk"[32] (p. 408). In addition, the items on the rating scales can help the clinician gather information by suggesting specific questions about the patient's suicidal thoughts, feelings, and behavior.

Six rating scales describe different aspects of the suicidal act and diverse characteristics of the patient. By using the scale for suicidal ideation (Figure 1),[33] the hopelessness scale (Figure 2),[34] and the suicide intent scale (Figure 3),[35] the interviewer can assess either directly or indirectly the seriousness of the patient's *intent* or subjective wish to die. In contrast, the risk-rating scale

Scale for Suicide Ideation (for Ideators)[33]

Name _____ Date _____

Day of
Interview

Time of Crisis/
Most Serious
Point of Illness

I. Characteristics of Attitude toward Living/Dying

( ) 1. Wish to Live   ( )
     0. Moderate to strong
     1. Weak
     2. None

( ) 2. Wish to Die   ( )
     0. None
     1. Weak
     2. Moderate to strong

( ) 3. Reasons for Living/Dying   ( )
     0. For living outweigh for dying
     1. About equal
     2. For dying outweigh for living

( ) 4. Desire to Make Active Suicide Attempt   ( )
     0. None
     1. Weak
     2. Moderate to Strong

( ) 5. Passive Suicidal Attempt   ( )
     0. Would take precautions to save life
     1. Would leave life/death to chance (e.g., carelessly
        crossing a busy street
     2. Would avoid steps necessary to save or maintain
        life (e.g., diabetic ceasing to take insulin)

If all four code entries for Items 4 and 5 are "0," skip sections II, III, and IV and enter
"8"—"Not Applicable" in each of the blank code spaces.

II. Characteristics of Suicide Ideation/Wish

( ) 6. Time Dimension Duration   ( )
     0. Brief, fleeting periods
     1. Longer periods
     2. Continuous (chronic), or almost continuous

( ) 7. Time Dimension: Frequency   ( )
     0. Rare, occasional
     1. Intermittent
     2. Persistent or continuous

( ) 8. Attitude toward Ideation/Wish   ( )
     0. Rejecting
     1. Ambivalent; indifferent
     2. Accepting

( ) 9. Control over Suicidal Action/Acting-Out Wish   ( )
     0. Has sense of control
     1. Unsure of control
     2. Has no sense of control

( ) 10. Deterrents to Active Attempt (e.g., family; religion;   ( )
     serious injury if unsuccessful; irreversible)
     0. Would not commit suicide because of a
        deterrent
     1. Some concern about deterrents
     2. Minimal or no concern about deterrents
        (indicate deterrents, if any: _____

Figure 1. Copyright © 1978 and © 1979 by Aaron T. Beck, M.D. Reproduction without the author's express written consent is forbidden. Further information about these scales and/or permission for their use may be obtained from Center for Cognitive Therapy, Room 602, 133 South 36th Street, Philadelphia, Pennsylvania 19104.

Name _____   Date _____

<table>
<tr><td>Day of
Interview</td><td></td><td>Time of Crisis/
Most Serious
Point of Illness</td></tr>
</table>

( )   11. Reason for Contemplated Attempt   ( )
        0.   To manipulate the environment, get attention, revenge
        1.   Combination of "0" and "2"
        2.   Escape, surcease, solve problems
            III. Characteristics of Contemplated Attempt

( )   12. Method: Specificity/Planning   ( )
        0.   Not considered
        1.   Considered, but details not worked out
        2.   Details worked out/well formulated

( )   13. Method: Availability/Opportunity   ( )
        0.   Method not available; no opportunity
        1.   Method would take time/effort; opportunity not really available
       2a. Method and opportunity available
       2b. Future opportunity or availability of method anticipated

( )   14. Sense of "Capability to Carry out Attempt"   ( )
        0.   No courage, too weak, afraid, incompetent
        1.   Unsure of courage, competence
        2.   Sure of competence, courage

( )   15. Expectancy/Anticipation of Actual Attempt   ( )
        0.   No
        1.   Uncertain, not sure
        2.   Yes
            IV. Actualization of Contemplated Attempt

( )   16. Actual Preparation   ( )
        0.   None
        1.   Partial (e.g., starting to collect pills)
        2.   Complete (e.g., had pills, razor, loaded gun)

( )   17. Suicide Note   ( )
        0.   None
        1.   Started but not completed or deposited, only thought about
        2.   Completed; deposited

      18. Final Acts in Anticipation of Death (insurance, will,
( )   gifts, etc.)   ( )
        0.   None
        1.   Thought about or made some arrangements
        2.   Made definite plans or completed arrangements

( )   19. Deception/Concealment of Contemplated Attempt   ( )
        0.   Revealed ideas openly
        1.   Held back on revealing
        2.   Attempted to deceive, conceal, lie
            V. Background Factors

Items 20 and 21 are not included in total score.

( )   20. Previous Suicide Attempts   ( )
        0.   None
        1.   One
        2.   More than one

Figure 1. (*continued*)

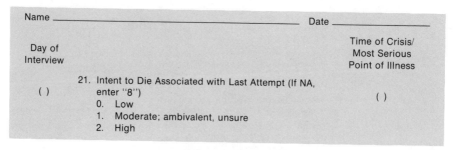

Name _____ Date _____

Day of Interview

Time of Crisis/ Most Serious Point of Illness

( )

21. Intent to Die Associated with Last Attempt (If NA, enter "8")
    0. Low
    1. Moderate; ambivalent, unsure
    2. High

( )

Figure 1. (*continued*)

(Figure 4) measures *lethality* of implementation.[36] The remaining two scales focus on demographic and clinical characteristics of the patient. These include Tuckman and Youngman's scale (Table 5), which measures risk among attempters,[37] and the Los Angeles Suicide Prevention Center Scale (Figure 5).[11]

Clinical Applications

Vera's suicide intent can be evaluated by using Beck's scales of suicidal ideation and hopelessness as general guidelines.

> Although Vera had been ruminating about leaving the car engine running in her garage when her husband was away on a business trip, her attitude toward implementing this was ambivalent. She was fearful that she would be unable to maintain control. Her expressed reason for wanting to die was to escape from "sick, empty feelings" and despair about the future.

The interviewer asked Vera for her view of the future. Vera's replies were similar to many positive items on the hopelessness scale, such as "I might as well give up because there's nothing I can do about making things better for myself," "It is very unlikely that I will get any real satisfaction in the future," and "The future seems vague and uncertain to me."[34] On the basis of these and other questions about her suicidal thoughts, the evaluator concluded that Vera's intent was moderate to high.

Mary R.'s attempt could be similarly evaluated using Beck's scales of hopelessness and suicidal intent and Weisman's scale of lethality. Because Mary R. initially refused to discuss her behavior, her boyfriend related the following: During a bitter argument about his involvement with another woman, Mary R. ran into the bathroom, grabbed a handful of yellow pills, and dramatically ingested them in front of him while screaming that she no longer wanted to live. A nurse knew Mary from a previous admission. She commented that Mary's first attempt was precipitated by a similar disagreement but had resulted in her lover terminating his other relationship. Her current overdose was impulsive, aimed at changing her boyfriend's mind by using a previously effective strategy. On the basis of questions from the suicidal intent scale, which

Hopelessness Scale[34]

Name _____ Date _____

This questionnaire consists of a list of 20 statements (sentences).
Please read the statements carefully one by one.

If the statement describes your attitude *for the past week, including today,* write TRUE
next to it. If the statement if false for you, write FALSE next to it. You may simply write T
for TRUE and F for FALSE.
Please be sure to read each sentence.

_____ A. I look forward to the future with hope and enthusiasm.
_____ B. I might as well give up because there's nothing I can do about making
            things better for myself.
_____ C. When things are going badly, I am helped by knowing that they can't stay
            that way forever.
_____ D. I can't imagine what my life would be like in 10 years.
_____ E. I have enough time to accomplish the things I most want to do.
_____ F. In the future I expect to succeed in what concerns me most.
_____ G. My future seems dark to me.
_____ H. I happen to be particularly lucky and I expect to get more of the good things
            in life than the average person.
_____ I. I just don't get the breaks, and there's no reason to believe I will in the
            future.
_____ J. My past experiences have prepared me well for my future.
_____ K. All I can see ahead of me is unpleasantness rather than pleasantness.
_____ L. I don't expect to get what I really want.
_____ M. When I look ahead to the future I expect I will be happier than I am now.
_____ N. Things just won't work out the way I want them to.
_____ O. I have great faith in the future.
_____ P. I never get what I want so it's foolish to want anything.
_____ Q. It is very unlikely that I will get any real satisfaction in the future.
_____ R. The future seems vague and uncertain to me.
_____ S. I can look forward to more good times than bad times.
_____ T. There's no use in really trying to get something I want because I probably
            won't get it.

Key
True   2. I might as well give up because I can't make things better for myself.
           4. I can't imagine what my life would be like in 10 years.
           7. My future seems dark to me.
           9. I just don't get the breaks, and there's no reason to believe I will in the
               future.
          11. All I can see ahead of me is unpleasantness rather than pleasantness.
          12. I don't expect to get what I really want.
          14. Things just won't work out the way I want them to.
          16. I never get what I want so it's foolish to want anything.
          17. It is very unlikely that I will get any real satisfaction in the future.
          18. The future seems vague and uncertain to me.
          20. There's no use in really trying to get something I want because I probably
               won't get it.

False   1. I look forward to the future with hope and enthusiasm.
           3. When things are going badly, I am helped by knowing they can't stay that
               way forever.
           5. I have enough time to accomplish the things I most want to do.
           6. In the future, I expect to succeed in what concerns me most.
           8. I expect to get more of the good things in life than the average person.
          10. My past experiences have prepared me well for my future.
          13. When I look ahead to the future, I expect I will be happier than I am now.
          15. I have great faith in the future.
          19. I can look forward to more good times than bad times.

Figure 2. Copyright © 1978 by Aaron T. Beck, M.D. Reproduction without the author's express written consent is forbidden. Further information about these scales and/or permission for their use may be obtained from Center for Cognitive Therapy, Room 602, 133 South 36th Street, Philadelphia, Pennsylvania 19104.

Suicide Intent Scale (for Attempters)[35]

Name _____ Date _____

For all items in this scale, use code number "8" for "Not applicable." "8's" are *not* counted when calculating the total score.

I. Objective Circumstances Related to Suicide Attempt

1. Isolation
   0. Somebody present
   1. Somebody nearby, or in visual or vocal contact
   2. No one nearby or in visual or vocal contact
2. Timing
   0. Intervention is probable
   1. Intervention is not likely
   2. Intervention is highly unlikely
3. Precautions against discovery/intervention
   0. No precautions
   1. Passive precautions (as avoiding others but doing nothing to prevent their intervention; alone in room with unlocked door)
   2. Active precautions (as locked door)
4. Acting to get help during/after attempt
   0. Notified potential helper regarding attempt
   1. Contacted but did not specifically notify potential helper regarding attempt
   2. Did not contact or notify potential helper
5. Final acts in anticipation of death (e.g. will, gifts, insurance)
   0. None
   1. Thought about or made some arrangements
   2. Made definite plans or completed arrangements
6. Active preparation for attempt
   0. None
   1. Minimal to moderate
   2. Extensive
7. Suicidal note
   0. Absence of note
   1. Note written, but torn up; note thought about
   2. Presence of note
8. Overt communication of intent before the attempt
   0. None
   1. Equivocal communication
   2. Unequivocal communication

II. Self-Report

9. Alleged purpose of attempt
   0. To manipulate environment, get attention, revenge
   1. Components of "0" and "2"
   2. To escape, surcease, solve problems
10. Expectations of fatality
    0. Thought that death was unlikely
    1. Thought that death was possible but not probable
    2. Thought that death was probable or certain
11. Conception of method's lethality
    0. Did less to self than he thought would be lethal
    1. Wasn't sure if what he did would be lethal
    2. Equaled or exceeded what he thought would be lethal

Figure 3. Copyright © 1978 by Aaron T. Beck, M.D. Reproduction without the author's express written consent is forbidden. Further information about these scales and/or permission for their use may be obtained from Center for Cognitive Therapy, Room 602, 133 South 36th Street, Philadelphia, Pennsylvania 19104.

12. Seriousness of attempt
    0. Did not seriously attempt to end life
    1. Uncertain about seriousness to end life
    2. Seriously attempted to end life
13. Attitude toward living/dying
    0. Did not want to die
    1. Components of "0" and "2"
    2. Wanted to die
14. Conception of medical rescuability
    0. Thought that death would be unlikely if he received medical attention
    1. Was uncertain whether death could be averted by medical attention
    2. Was certain of death even if he received medical attention
15. Degree of premeditation
    0. None; impulsive
    1. Suicide contemplated for three hours or less prior to attempt
    2. Suicide contemplated for more than three hours prior to attempt
            III. Other Aspects (Not Included in Total Score)
16. Reaction to attempt
    0. Sorry that he made attempt; feels foolish, ashamed (circle which one)
    1. Accepts both attempt and its failure
    2. Regrets failure of attempt
17. Visualization of death
    0. Life-after-death, reunion with descendants
    1. Never ending sleep, darkness, end-of-things
    2. No conceptions of, or thoughts about death
18. Number of previous attempts
    0. None
    1. One or two
    2. Three or more
19. Relationship between alcohol intake and attempt
    0. Some alcohol intake prior to but not related to attempt, reportedly not enough to impair judgment, reality testing
    1. Enough alcohol intake to impair judgment, reality testing and diminish responsibility
    2. Intentional intake of alcohol in order to facilitate implementation of attempt
20. Relationship between drug intake and attempt (narcotics, hallucinogens, etc., when drug is *not* the method used to suicide)
    0. Some drug intake prior to but not related to attempt, reportedly not enough to impair judgment, reality testing
    1. Enough drug intake to impair judgment, reality testing and diminish responsibility
    2. Intentional drug intake in order to facilitate implementation of attempt

(Intent Scale)

CLINICIAN'S ESTIMATE OF RELIABILITY[35]

Estimated reliability of patient
      0. Uncertain
      1. Poor
      2. Fair
      3. Good

VARIABLES INFLUENCING RELIABILITY OF PATIENT

Confusion as a medical consequence of attempt
      0. None   1. Some   2. Moderate   3. Severe
Disorientation at time of attempt due to alcohol or drug abuse
      0. None   1. Some   2. Moderate   3. Severe
Disorientation at time of attempt due to emotional state
      0. None   1. Some   2. Moderate   3. Severe

Figure 3. (*continued*)

VARIABLES INFLUENCING RELIABILITY OF PATIENT

Lack of truthfulness or reluctance to disclose information

      0. None   1. Some   2. Moderate   3. Severe

Current memory impairment, amnesia, "blocking" regarding attempt

      0. None   1. Some   2. Moderate   3. Severe

Current withdrawal, partial mutism, inability to verbalize

      0. None   1. Some   2. Moderate   3. Severe

"Objective items that patient didn't explicitly answer (list by #)
_____

Clinician's confidence in his inferences about above questions:

      0. N/A   1. Low   2. Moderate   3. High

"Self-report" items that patient didn't explicitly answer (list by #)
_____

Clinician's confidence in his inference about above questions:

      0. N/A   1. Low   2. Moderate   3. High

Clinician's overall estimate of the scale's validity as a measure of suicidality, in view of all above factors:

      0. Low   1. Moderate   2. High

(Intent Scale)

SUPPLEMENT TO INTENT SCALE[35]

Why did the patient choose this particular method? (Enter patient's verbatim response and then enter appropriate category)

Patient's response: _____
_____
_____

0.   Most immediately accessible
1.   Believed to be most lethal
2.   Least painful
3.   Method suggested by another person
4.   Imitation of suicide attempt by another person
5.   Method suggested or demanded by voices
6.   Method has particular psychological or symbolic significance to this patient
7.   Other

If the patient took a drug overdose and had ingested alcohol, was he or she aware of the fact that the combined effects of alcohol and certain drugs are greater than the total of their separate effects?

0.   Yes, patient was aware of it
1.   No, he/she was not aware of it
2.   Question is not applicable to this case

What is the relationship between alcohol ingestion and the attempt?

0.   No alcohol ingestion
1.   Alcohol ingestion was normal for this patient, and unrelated to the suicide attempt
2.   Alcohol ingestion was excessive and may have impaired judgment, but patient did not drink in order to facilitate the attempt
3.   Patient drank excessively to gain courage for the attempt
4.   Patient drank in order to add to the effects of an overdose
5.   Patient took alcohol in combination with a drug overdose, knowing that this would produce an extra lethal effect
6.   Alcohol ingestion was related to the attempt in another way.
    (Specify) _____
_____
_____

Figure 3. (*continued*)

Risk-Rescue Rating[36]

Patient_____ Age _____Sex _____ Risk score _____
Circumstances _____ Rescue score _____
_____ Risk–rescue
                                                           rating   _____

RISK FACTORS	RESCUE FACTORS
1. Agent used:	1. Location:
1. Ingestion, cutting, stabbing	3. Familiar
2. Drowning, asphyxiation, strangulation	2. Nonfamiliar, nonremote
3. Jumping, shooting	1. Remote
2. Impaired consciousness:	2. Person initiating rescue[a]
1. None in evidence	3. Key person
2. Confusion, semicoma	2. Professional
3. Coma, deep coma	1. Passerby
3. Lesions/toxicity:	3. Probability of discovery by a rescuer:
1. Mild	3. High, almost certain
2. Moderate	2. Uncertain discovery
3. Severe	1. Accidental discovery
4. Reversibility:	4. Accessibility to rescue:
1. Good, complete recovery expected	3. Asks for help
2. Fair, recovery expected with time	2. Drops clues
3. Poor, residuals expected, if recovery	1. Does not ask for help
5. Treatment required:	5. Delay until discovery:
1. First aid, emergency ward care	3. Immediate, 1 hour
3. Intensive care, special treatment	1. Greater than 4 hours

Total risk points: _____   Total rescue points: _____

RISK SCORE	RESCUE SCORE[b]
5. High risk (13–15 risk points)	1. Least rescuable (5–7 rescue points)
4. High moderate (11–12 risk points)	2. Low moderate (8–9 rescue points)
3. Moderate (9–10 risk points)	3. Moderate (10–11 rescue points)
2. Low moderate (7–8 risk points)	4. High moderate (12–13 rescue points)
1. Low risk (5–6 risk points)	5. Most rescuable (14–15 rescue points)

[a] Self-rescue automatically yields a rescue score of 5.
[b] If there is undue delay in obtaining treatment after discovery, reduce final rescue score by one point.

Figure 4. Risk-Rescue Rating.[36]

evaluates both the circumstances related to the act and the patient's reported feelings, the evaluator concluded that Mary R.'s wish to die at the time of the attempt was low.

For some patients, questions from Weisman's risk-rescue scale can be used to assess the lethality of implementation, i.e., "the probability of inflicting irreversible damage. . . . [It] may be expressed as a ratio of factors influencing risk and rescue."[36] (p. 553). Mary's overdose in front of her boyfriend guaranteed rescue; the small amount ingested did not endanger her physical health. However, in contrast to the current attempt, which was low on both intent and

COMPUTATION OF RISK–RESCUE SCORES[a]

Risk score	Rescue score	Risk–rescue score
1	5	17
1	4	20
1	3	25
1	2	33
1	1	50
2	5	29
2	4	33
2	3	40
2	2	50
2	1	66
3	5	38
3	4	43
3	3	50
3	2	60
3	1	75
4	5	44
4	4	50
4	3	57
4	2	66
4	1	80
5	5	50
5	4	56
5	3	63
5	2	71
5	1	83

[a] These ratings have been computed on the basis of $(A/A + B) \times 100$, where A = risk score and B = rescue score.[36]

Figure 4. (*continued*)

lethality, the previous overdose with tricyclics was more serious. Although rescue was still possible, the drug ingestion was moderately toxic and led to a medical admission. A formula provided by the authors (factors are scored and converted into a composite rating) assesses the immediate lethality of the attempt, although it does not predict continued risk.

Unlike Mary's attempt, which was "impulsive, manipulative, and discoverable," 20% of suicide attempts are carefully planned and reflect an intense wish to die. Tuckman and Youngman state that attempters most similar to patients who complete suicide are at increased risk.[37] Some patients with low to moderate intent are not realistic about the consequences of their action and "mistakenly" complete a suicidal act. Both groups of attempters and completed suicides include patients with varying degrees of intent and are not homogeneous categories. Therefore, it is always important to assess the danger of each individual act.

On the basis of information gathered from John D.'s son and from the circumstances of his death, it appeared that John D. had an intense wish to die and had carefully planned a method with little possibility of rescue. His suicide note described feelings of worthlessness and despair and included in-

Table 5. Suicide Rate per 1000 Population among 3800 Attempted Suicides by High- and Low-Risk Categories of Risk-Related Factors[a]

Factor	High-risk category	Suicide rate	Low-risk category	Suicide rate
Age	45 years of age and older	24.0	Under 45 years of age	9.4
Sex	Male	19.9	Female	9.2
Race	White	14.3	Nonwhite	8.7
Marital status	Separated, divorced, widowed	12.5	Single, married	8.6
Living arrangements	Alone	48.4	With others	10.1
Employment status[b]	Unemployed, retired	16.8	Employed[c]	14.3
Physical health	Poor (acute or chronic condition in the 6-month period preceding the attempt)	14.0	Good[c]	12.4
Mental condition	Nervous or mental disorder, mood or behavioral symptoms including alcoholism	19.1	Presumably normal, including brief situational reactions	7.2
Medical care (within 6 months)	Yes	16.4	No[c]	10.8
Method	Hanging, firearms, jumping, drowning	28.4	Cutting or piercing, gas or carbon monoxide, poison, combination of other methods, other	12.0
Season	Warm months (April–September)	14.2	Cold months (October–March)	10.9
Time of day	6:00 a.m. to 5:59 p.m.	15.1	6:00 p.m. to 5:59 a.m.	10.5
When attempt was made	Own or someone else's home	14.3	Other type of premises, out of doors	11.9
Time interval between attempt and discovery	Almost immediately, reported by person making attempt	10.9	Later	7.2
Intent to kill (self-report)	No[c]	14.5	Yes	8.5
Suicide note	Yes	16.7	No[c]	12.3
Previous attempt or threat	Yes	25.2	No[c]	11.0

[a] From reference 37.
[b] Does not include housewives and students.
[c] Includes cases for which information on this factor was not given in the police report.

Los Angeles Suicide Prevention Center Scale

Age and Sex (1–9)	Rating for Category
Male	
50 plus (7–9)	( )
35–49 (4–6)	( )
15–34 (1–3)	( )
Female	
50 plus (5–7)	( )
35–49 (3–5)	( )
15–34 (1–3)	( )
Symptoms (1–9)	
Severe depression: sleep disorder, anorexia, weight loss, withdrawal, despondency, loss of interest, apathy (7–9)	( )
Feelings of hopelessness, helplessness, exhaustion (7–9)	( )
Delusions, hallucinations, loss of contact disorientation (6–8)	( )
Compulsive gambling (6–8)	( )
Disorganization, confusion, chaos (5–7)	( )
Alcoholism, drug addiction, homosexuality (4–7)	( )
Agitation, tension, anxiety (4–6)	( )
Guilt, shame, embarrassment (4–6)	( )
Feelings of rage, anger, hostility, revenge (4–6)	( )
Poor impulse control, poor judgment (4–6)	( )
Other (describe)	( )
Stress (1–9)	
Loss of loved person by death, divorce or separation (5–9)	( )
Loss of job, money, prestige, status (4–8)	( )
Sickness, serious illness, surgery, accident-loss of limb (3–7)	( )
Threat of prosecution, criminal involvement, exposure (4–6)	( )
Change(s) in life, environment, setting (4–6)	( )
Success, promotion, increased responsibilities (2–5)	( )
No significant stress (1–3)	( )
Other (describe):	
Acute versus Chronic (1–9)	
Sharp, noticeable, and sudden onset of specific symptoms (1–9)	( )
Recurrent outbreak of similar symptoms (4–9)	( )
No specific recent change (1–4)	( )
Other (describe):	
Suicidal Plan (1–9)	
Lethality of proposed method—gun, jumping, hanging, drowning, knife, pills, poison, aspirin (1–9)	( )
Availability of means in proposed method (1–9)	( )
Specific detail and clarity in organization of plan (1–9)	( )
Specificity in time planned (1–9)	( )
Bizarre plans (1–9)	( )
Rating of previous suicide attempt(s) (1–9)	( )
No plans (1–3)	( )
Other (describe):	

Figure 5. Los Angeles Suicide Prevention Center Scale.[11]

	Rating for Category
Resources (1–9)	
No sources of support (family, friends, agencies, employment (7–9)	( )
Family and friends available, unwilling to help (4–7)	( )
Financial problems (4–7)	( )
Available professional help, agency or therapist (2–4)	( )
Family and/or friends willing to help (1–3)	( )
Stable life history (1–3)	( )
Physician or clergy available (1–3)	( )
Employed (1–3)	( )
Finances no problem (1–3)	( )
Other (describe):	
Prior Suicidal Behavior (1–7)	
One or more prior attempts of high lethality (6–7)	( )
One or more prior attempt of low lethality (4–5)	( )
History of repeated threats and depression (3–5)	( )
No prior suicidal depressed history (1–3)	( )
Other (describe):	
Medical Status (1–7)	
Chronic debilitating illness (5–7)	( )
Pattern of failure in previous therapy (4–6)	( )
Many repeated unsuccessful experiences with doctors (4–6)	( )
Psychosomatic illness e.g., asthma, ulcer, hypochondria (1–3)	( )
No medical problems (1–2)	( )
Other (describe)	
Communication Aspects (1–7)	
Communication broken with rejection of efforts to reestablish by both patient and others (5–7)	( )
Communications have internalized goal, e.g., declaration of guilt, feelings of worthlessness, blame, shame (4–7)	( )
Communications have interpersonalized goal, e.g., to cause guilt in others to force behavior, etc. (2–4)	( )
Communications directed toward world and people in general (3–5)	( )
Communications directed toward one or more specific persons (1–3)	( )
Other (describe):	
Reaction of Significant Others (1–7)	
Defensive, paranoid, rejected, punishing attitude (5–7)	( )
Denial of own or patient's need for help (5–7)	( )
No feelings of concern about the patient; does not understand the patient (4–6)	( )
Indecisiveness, feelings of helplessness (3–5)	( )
Alternation between feelings of anger and rejection and feelings of responsibility and desire to help (2–4)	( )
Sympathy and concern plus admission of need for help (1–3)	( )
Other (describe):	

Figure 5. (*continued*)

structions to his son about his belongings. Although he seemed to realize the consequences of his behavior, the clinician should not ignore mitigating circumstances such as alcohol intoxication, Korsakoff's syndrome, or senile dementia. Identifying such factors in the attempter group is particularly important since action can then be taken to protect the patient.

References

1. Frederick C: Current trends in suicidal behavior in the United States. *Am J Psychotherapy* 32:172–201, 1978.
2. Weissman M: The epidemiology of suicide attempts, 1960 to 1971. *Arch Gen Psychiatry* 30:737–746, 1974.
3. Bassuk E: The impact of deinstitutionalization on the general hospital psychiatric emergency ward. *Hosp Comm Psychiatr* 31:623–627, 1980.
4. Pokorny A: A scheme for classifying suicidal behaviors, in Beck A, Resnik H, Lettieri D (eds.): *The Prediction of Suicide.* Bowie, Md, Charles Press Publications, 1974, pp 29–45.
5. Stengel E: *Suicide and Attempted Suicide.* Baltimore: Penguin Books, 1964.
6. Rosen D: The serious suicide attempt: Epidemiological and follow-up study of 886 patients. *Am J Psychiatry* 127:764–770, 1970.
7. Guze S, Robins E: Suicide and primary affective disorders. *Br J Psychiatry* 117:437–438, 1970.
8. Mayfield R, Montgomery D: Alcoholism, alcohol intoxication and suicide attempts. *Arch Gen Psychiatry* 27:349–353, 1972.
9. Murphy G, Armstrong J, Hernele S, et al: Suicide and alcoholism. *Arch Gen Psychiatry* 36:65–69, 1979.
10. Nelson S, Grunebaum H: A follow-up study of wrist slashers. *Am J Psychiatry* 127:81–85, 1971.
11. Los Angeles Suicide Prevention Center Scale, in Beck A, Resnik H, Lettieri D (eds.): *The Prediction of Suicide.* Bowie, Md, Charles Press Publications, 1974, pp 76–78.
12. Bowlby J: *Attachment.* New York, Basic Books, 1969.
13. Fawcett J, Leff M, Bunney W: Suicide—Clues from interpersonal communication. *Arch Gen Psychiatry* 21:129–137, 1969.
14. Murphy G, Robins E: The communication of suicidal ideas. in Beck A, Resnik H, Lettieri D (eds.): *The Prediction of Suicide.* Bowie, Md, Charles Press Publications, 1974, pp. 164–170.
15. Ringel E: The presuicidal syndrome. *Suicide Life Threat Behav* 6:131–149, 1976.
16. Shneidman E, Farberow N (eds.): *Clues to Suicide.* New York, McGraw-Hill, 1957.
17. Paykel E, Prusoff B, Myers J: Suicide attempts and recent life events. *Arch Gen Psychiatry* 32:327–333, 1975.
18. Dorpat T, Ripley H: A study of suicide in the Seattle area. *Comp Psychiatry* 1:349–359, 1960.
19. Robins E, Gassner S, Kayes J, et al: The communication of suicidal intent: A study of 134 consecutive cases of successful (completed) suicide. *Am J Psychiatry* 115:724–733, 1959.
20. Kovacs M, Beck A, Weisman A: The communication of suicidal intent. *Arch Gen Psychiatry* 33:198–201, 1976.
21. Havens L: Recognition of suicidal risks through the psychologic examination. *N Engl J Med* 276:210–215, 1967.
22. Lazare A, Eisenthal S, Wasserman L, et al: Patient requests in a walk-in clinic. *Compr Psychiatry* 16:467–477, 1975.
23. Hankoff L: Categories of attempted suicide: A longitudinal study. *Am J Public Health* 66:558–563, 1976.
24. Bachrach L: Is the least restrictive environment always the best? Sociological and semantic implications. *Hosp Comm Psychiatry* 31:97–103, 1980.
25. Leeman C: The "least restrictive environment": From rhetoric to practice. *Gen Hosp Psychiatry* 3:229–232, 1980.

26. Bogard H: Follow-up study of suicidal patients seen in emergency room consultation. *Am J Psychiatry* 126:1017–1020, 1970.
27. Paykel E, Hallowell C, Dressler D: Treatment of suicide attempters. *Arch Gen Psychiatry* 31:487–491, 1971.
28. Spitz L: The evaluation of a psychiatric emergency crisis intervention service in a medical emergency room setting. *Comp Psychiatry* 17:99–113, 1976.
29. Litman R, Wold C, Graham M: Beyond emergency services: The continuing relationship maintenance program, in Parad H, Resnik H, Parad L (eds.): *Emergency and Disaster Management.* Bowie Md, Charles Press Publications, 1976, pp 55–67.
30. Craig T, Huffine C, Brooks M: Completion of referral to psychiatric services by inner city residents. *Arch Gen Psychiatry* 31:353–357, 1974.
31. Waltzer H, Hankoff L: One year's experience with a suicide prevention telephone service. *Comm Mental Health J* 1:309–315, 1965.
32. Sletten I, Barton J: Suicidal patients in the emergency room: A guide for evaluation and disposition. *Hosp Comm Psychiatry* 30:407–411, 1979.
33. Beck A, Kovacs M, Weisman A: Assessment of suicidal intention: The scale for suicide ideation. *J Consult Clin Psychol* 47:343–352, 1979.
34. Beck A, Weisman A, Lester D, et al: The measurement of pessimism: The hopelessness scale. *J Consult Clin Psychol* 42:861–865, 1974.
35. Beck A, Schuyler D, Herman I: Development of suicidal intent scales. in Beck A, Resnik H, Lettieri D (eds.): *The Prediction of Suicide.* Bowie Md, Charles Press Publications, 1974, pp 76–78.
36. Weisman A, Worden W: Risk-rescue rating in suicide assessment. *Arch Gen Psychiatry* 26:553–560, 1972.
37. Tuckman J, Youngman W: A scale for assessing suicide risk of attempted suicides. *J Clin Psychol* 24:17–19, 1968.

IV

Patients and Clinical Syndromes 2
Medication-Related/Toxic Origins

8

Alcohol Use and Abuse

W. R. Cote, R.N.C., C.A.C., and F. D. Lisnow, M.Ed., C.A.C.

1. Introduction

Alcohol is the most widely used mood-altering agent in America. One need only walk down a city street or peruse a popular magazine to gain an idea of how important alcohol is in our society. It is both a social lubricant and a pharmacological tool for tension relief. Unfortunately, in more than 10% of all Americans who drink, alcohol will eventually be abused, adversely affecting the health, family life, or legal status of these individuals.

Alcoholism is multicausal. Researchers speculate that its development might be related to genetic predisposition, social and/or environmental factors, personality characteristics, and/or biochemical determinants. Specific epidemiological factors associated with increased risk of alcohol abuse include having low socioeconomic status, belonging to a particular ethnic group (Irish, American Indian), coming from a family in which there are other alcoholics, and being divorced. However, membership in other socioeconomic, ethnic, or family groups offers no immunity from this disorder.

2. Definitions

Although the precise definition of alcoholism remains controversial, the World Health Organization describes an alcoholic as a person whose repetitive drinking significantly interferes with health, work, and/or family relationships. The *Diagnostic and Statistical Manual* (DSM-III) subdivides pathological drinking into two distinct categories: alcohol abuse and alcohol dependence. Table 1 summarizes these distinctions. Either may be complicated by acute intoxication, idiosyncratic intoxication, withdrawal phenomena, and the organic sequelae of chronic use. Alcohol abuse may also complicate the clinical course of other psychiatric disorders, especially affective illness and panic disorder.

W. R. Cote, R.N.C., C.A.C., and F. D. Lisnow, M.Ed., C.A.C. • Northeast Kingdom Mental Health Services, St. Johnsbury, Vermont 05819.

Table 1. DSM III Criteria for Alcohol Abuse and Alcohol Dependence[a]

Criteria for Alcohol Abuse

1. *Pattern of pathological alcohol use*: need for daily use of alcohol for adequate functioning; inability to cut down or stop drinking; repeated efforts to control or reduce excess drinking by "going on the wagon" (periods of temporary abstinence) or restricting drinking to certain times of the day; binges (remaining intoxicated throughout the day for at least two days); occasional consumption of a fifth of spirits (or its equivalent in wine or beer); amnesic periods for events occurring while intoxicated (blackouts); continuation of drinking despite a serious physical disorder that the individual knows is exacerbated by alcohol use; drinking nonbeverage alcohol.

2. *Impairment in social or occupational functioning due to alcohol use*: e.g., violence while intoxicated, absence from work, loss of job, legal difficulties (e.g., arrest for intoxicated behavior, traffic acidents while intoxicated), arguments or difficulties with family or friends because of excessive alcohol use.

3. Duration of disturbance of at least one month.

Criteria for Alcohol Dependence

Either a pattern of pathological use or impairment in social or occupational functioning due to alcohol use.

Pattern of pathological alcohol use: daily use of alcohol as a prerequisite for adequate functioning; inability to cut down or stop drinking; repeated efforts to control or reduce excess drinking by "going on the wagon" (periods of temporary abstinence) or restriction of drinking to certain times of the day; drinks nonbeverage alcohol; goes on binges (remains intoxicated throughout the day for at least two days); occasionally drinks a fifth of spirits (or its equivalent in wine or beer); has had two or more "blackouts" (amnesic period for events occuring while intoxicated); continues to drink despite a serious physical disorder that the individual knows is exacerbated by alcohol use.

Impairment in social or occupational functioning due to alcohol use: e.g., violence while intoxicated, absence from work, loss of job, legal difficulties (e.g., arrest for intoxicated behavior, traffic accidents while intoxicated), arguments or difficulties with family or friends because of excessive alcohol use.

Either tolerance or withdrawal.

[a] Adapted from *Diagnostic and Statistical Manual of Mental Disorders* (DSM-III), ed. 3. Washington, D.C., American Psychiatric Association, 1980, p 169.

3. Pharmacology

Alcohol is absorbed quickly from the gastrointestinal tract. Approximately 20% of the alcohol consumed is absorbed in the stomach. The remainder is absorbed in the upper sections of the small bowel. Absorption may be affected by such factors as rate of consumption, concentration of alcohol, and concurrent ingestion of food.

Once absorbed into the bloodstream, ethyl alcohol is distributed uniformly throughout body tissues, including the brain. An equilibrium between tissue concentrations and plasma level is reached rapidly. The drug is oxidized in the liver at an average rate of 10 ml/hr, with a maximum of 375-480 ml/day. The degree of intoxication is directly associated with the blood alcohol level, which, in turn, is a function of the above-noted factors. The following sections describe some of the common complications of acute and chronic intoxication and their management.

4. Acute Intoxication

4.1. Simple Alcohol Intoxication

Alcohol acts as a CNS depressant. Decreased inhibition in the cerebral cortex is thought to account for its initial stimulatory effects. The early stages of intoxication are characterized by giddiness, increased talkativeness, and a general loosening of social inhibitions. For most users, this is, in fact, the desired effect. It is usually achieved at a blood alcohol concentration (BAC) of 30–60 mg/deciliter (dl). At higher BACs, noticeable impairment begins.

In most states the legal definition of intoxication (with other supporting evidence) is a BAC of 100 mg/dl. At this level, an individual's ability to operate a motor vehicle is assumed to be impaired. It should be emphasized, however, that even in milder states of intoxication, concentration, verbal and motor performance, insight, judgment, and recent memory may be impaired. At 200 mg/dl most users are grossly intoxicated. Levels above 400 mg/dl are potentially lethal. The stages of alcohol intoxication are described in Table 2.

4.2. Idiosyncratic "Pathological" Intoxication

Pathological intoxication occurs in susceptible individuals after the ingestion of relatively small amounts of alcohol. It seems to occur most commonly in persons with chronic anxiety and impaired impulse control. Episodes usually last a few hours and are characterized by impaired consciousness, confusion, disorientation, delusions, and even visual hallucinations. These patients also exhibit increased aggressiveness, rage, agitation, and violence. Episodes usually terminate with a deep sleep, after which there is total amnesia for the events that took place during the period of intoxication.

5. Sequelae of Chronic Intoxication

5.1. Tolerance and Physical Dependence

Chronic alcohol ingestion fosters the development of both metabolic and pharmacodynamic tolerance. Metabolic tolerance refers to the increased activity of liver enzymes (e.g., alcohol dehydrogenase) in oxidizing ingested alcohol. Pharmacodynamic (tissue) tolerance refers to cellular changes that occur in response to the chronic presence of alcohol. The rate at which both types of tolerance develop varies among individuals. Within three weeks after stopping drinking, both types of tolerance are markedly reduced. Tolerant individuals require increased amounts of alcohol to produce the same degree of intoxication previously achieved at a lower BAC. Tolerance, however, does not develop to the lethal dose of alcohol.

The development of tolerance to alcohol is accompanied by the development of physical dependence on the drug. An individual who is physically

Table 2. Stages of Alcohol Intoxication

Blood-alcohol level (mg/dl)[a]	Effects on feeling and behavior	Time required for all alcohol to leave the body
0.02–0.03%	Absence of obvious effects; mild alteration of feelings; slight intensification of existing moods; minor impairment of judgment and memory	2 hours
0.03–0.06%	Feeling of warmth, relaxation, mild sedation; exaggeration of emotion and behavior; slight impairment of fine motor skills; slight increase in reaction time	4 hours
0.08–0.09%	Visual and hearing acuity reduced; slight speech impairment; minor disturbance of balance; increased difficulty in performing motor skills; feeling of elation or depression; desire for more to drink; speaks louder and becomes more argumentative	6 hours
0.11–0.12%	Difficulty in performing many gross motor skills; uncoordinated behavior; definite impairment of mental facilities, i.e., judgment and memory, decreased inhibitions; becomes angered if he cannot have another drink or is told he has had enough	8 hours
0.14–0.15%	Major impairment of all physical and mental functiona; irresponsible behavior; general feeling of euphoria; difficulty in standing, walking, talking; distorted perception and judgment; feels confident of driving skills; cannot recognize impairment	10 hours
0.20%	Feels confused or dazed; gross body movements cannot be made without assistance; inability to maintain a steady upright position	12 hours
0.30%	Minimum perception and comprehension; general suspension or diminution of sensibility	
0.40%	Nearly complete anesthesia, absence of perception; state of unconsciousness, coma	
0.50%	Deep coma	
0.60%	Death is possible following complete anesthesia of the respiratory center	

[a] Milligrams per deciliter.

dependent on alcohol will develop a characteristic abstinence syndrome of varying severity when the drug is discontinued abruptly. Abstinence phenomena and their management are described in Section 6.

5.2. Central Nervous System Pathology

Chronic alcohol abuse may lead to the development of central nervous system pathology. In *Wernicke's disease*, the result of an alcohol-induced thiamine (Vitamin B1) deficiency, nystagmus, bilateral sixth cranial nerve palsies, and paralysis of conjugate gaze are frequently seen, along with ataxia and various mental disturbances. Most common among the latter is a "quiet delirium,'' characterized by apathy, lassitude, disorientation, and drowsiness. A less common syndrome, *Korsakoff's psychosis* (alcohol amnestic disorder), presents with profound anterograde and retrograde amnesia in an otherwise alert individual. Confabulation also may be present. Wernicke's disease and Korsakoff's psychosis are not separate entities; rather, the latter is a variably present component of the former. When both are present, the disease is called *Wernicke-Korsakoff syndrome*. Postmortem brain examination of these patients often reveals structural lesions in the mammillary bodies.

Prompt diagnosis and treatment of Wernicke's disease is imperative. Immediate administration of thiamine, 50 mg IV and 50 mg IM, followed by 50 mg IM or po each day until the patient is eating well, should improve the ocular difficulties within hours to days. The ataxia also may improve during this time period. Delirium, when present, is also reversible, but as confusional symptoms recede, the symptoms of Korsakoff's psychosis may become more evident. In Korsakoff patients, recovery may take a year or more and may be incomplete.

5.3. Alcoholic Hallucinosis

Alcoholic hallucinosis occurs in some chronic alcoholics after the cessation of prolonged drinking. The most observable and pronounced features of this syndrome are persistent and/or recurrent auditory hallucinations, frequently of a threatening nature. Paranoid ideas of reference are also noted. Unlike other toxic disorders, there is no clouding of consciousness or disorientation to time, place, or person. Because of the menacing nature of the hallucinations, these patients may seek to protect themselves and may be dangerous. Episodes last from a few hours to a week. In 10% of patients the disorder persists. Treatment with antipsychotic drugs like trifluoperazine (Stelazine) or chlorpromazine (Thorazine) is often helpful.

5.4. Accidental Injury/Concurrent Medical Problems

The emergency evaluation of a patient with a history of alcohol abuse should include a careful evaluation for both injuries and medical problems. Because of alcohol's disruptive effect on coordination, judgment, response time, and motor control, people who drink excessively are especially susceptible to accidental injury. The problem may be further compounded by the drinker's lack of awareness of his injuries.

6. Alcohol Withdrawal

6.1. Clinical Manifestations

The symptoms of alcohol withdrawal vary in intensity from mild tremors, headache, and gastric irritability to delirium tremens (DTs), which may be life-threatening. Most symptoms can be attributed to CNS hyperirritability and occur primarily after prolonged ingestion of high doses.

6.1.1. Stage I: Minor Abstinence Syndrome

Mild to moderate withdrawal is essentially a severe "hangover" that begins several hours after the last drink. The patient usually presents with tremors, agitation, and abdominal distress. He may also appear restless and startle easily. Complaints of insomnia, nausea, vomiting, anorexia, muscle weakness, and general malaise are also frequent. Physiological changes include tachycardia, diaphoresis, and increased blood pressure. Occasionally, grand mal seizures ("rum fits") occur, usually within 48 hours after the last drink.

6.1.2. Stage II: Impending Delirium Tremens

This is a transitional stage in the development of a major abstinence syndrome. It is characterized by many of the above symptoms, but in more severe form. Pulse, blood pressure, and respiratory rate will be markedly elevated during this stage. Agitation, panic, visual and auditory hallucinations, and paranoid delusions also occur, along with a sense of "losing control." Patients left to their own devices will often drink to relieve such symptoms.

6.1.3. Stage III: Major Abstinence Syndrome/Delirium Tremens

About 5% of patients who manifest a minor abstinence syndrome will go on to develop a state characterized by confusion, disorientation, agitation, and delirium. This severe form of alcohol withdrawal is called delirium tremens (DTs). Symptoms generally begin 72 to 96 hours after the last drink and may last from a few hours to a few weeks. Hallucinations (usually visual), tremulousness, disorientation, insomnia, and nightmares are common, as are signs of autonomic nervous system hyperactivity, including fever, sweating, tachycardia, hypertension, and increased respirations.

In most cases the patient with delirium tremens has a history of excessive drinking for at least five years, along with recent heavy drinking. The severity of the syndrome depends on the degree of prior intoxication, general health of the patient, and adequacy of preventive treatment. Once delirium develops, drug treatment and other management efforts may not alter its course. The mortality rate, even in treated cases, is approximately 10%. Death may occur either as the result of hyperthermia or cardiovascular collapse. Autopsy examinations in such patients have failed to elucidate the exact pathophysiology of the problem.

6.2. Treatment

Tables 3A–3C provide general guidelines for patient care during each stage of alcohol withdrawal. In Stage I, treatment is geared toward reducing CNS irritability and preventing the progression of the withdrawal syndrome. The Stage II regimen is designed to arrest a deteriorating condition and prevent further increase in the severity of symptoms. In Stage III, the emphasis is on

Table 3A. Treatment of Alcohol Withdrawal

Stage I: Mild to moderate withdrawal

1. Regular diet as tolerated.
2. Encourage physical activity.
3. Assess hydration (i.e., skin turgor, change in normal body weight, urine specific gravity); force
   fluids as necessary (120 ml O.J. or milk Q 30 min × 8 then 120 ml O.J. or milk Q 1 hr × 6).
4. Vital signs Q 4 hr × 48 hr, then during each shift.
5. PPD intermediate strength.
6. CBC, urinalysis, prothrombin time, fasting glucose, BUN, electrolytes, alk phos., bilirubin,
   SGOT, CPK, LDH, uric acid, total protein, albumin, globulin, stool for occult blood, VDRL,
   serum calcium, magnesium, amylase.
7. Chest X ray, EKG as soon as possible.
8. Urine toxicology for other drugs of abuse.
9. Chlordiazepoxide 25–100 mg PO on admission, repeat in 1 hr.[a]
10. Chlordiazepoxide 25–100 mg PO Q 6 hr × 24 hr.[a]
    Day 2: Cut day 1 dose in half.
    Day 3: Cut day 2 dose in half.
    Day 4: DC.
11. Thiamine HCl 100 mg IM stat and 100 mg po tid and Qhs × 10 days.
12. Folic acid 1 to 5 mg IM or PO Qd.
13. Berocca C of Solu B Forte, 2 cc IM or IV on admission, then daily × 2 days (IM administered
    in gluteal muscle only).
14. After third dose of Berocca, stress caps bid × stay.
15. Vitamin K 5 to 10 mg IV (only if protime 3 sec control).

[a] Diazepam (DZ) may be substituted for chlordiazepoxide (CDX); 1 mg DZ = 2.5 mg CDZ.

maintaining vital functions, controlling, correcting, and preventing injury due
to seizures. In all three stages, medical problems resulting from, or independent
of, alcohol withdrawal should be promptly treated. These may include pneumonia, malnutrition, cirrhosis, gastritis, and anemia. Subdural hematomas and
meningitis also occur with increased frequency in this population.

6.2.1. Minor Abstinence Syndrome

In treating minor abstinence symptoms, the clinician can take advantage
of the cross-tolerance between alcohol and other CNS depressants by substi-

Table 3B. Treatment of Alcohol Withdrawal Seizures

1. Diazepam 10 mg IV (stat) given slowly.[a]
2. Diazepam 5 mg IV Q5 min until calm but awake; then
3. Diazepam 5 mg IV or po Q4 hr until delirium clears, then decrease dose by 50% Qd until patient
   is withdrawn completely.
4. Optional prophylaxis. Phenytoin loading dose 1 gm IV undiluted given slowly over 4 hours (rate
   no higher than 50 mg/min). EKG monitoring is helpful during IV administration.
5. IV loading followed by phenytoin 100 mg po tid through withdrawal period. Maintain blood
   level between 10 and 20 mg/ml.

[a] Chlordiazepoxide 2.5 mg may be substituted for each 1 mg of diazepam.

Table 3C. Treatment of Alcohol Withdrawal

Treatment of Stage II withdrawal
(impending delirium tremens)[a]

1. Strict bedrest with side rails and physical restraints as needed.
2. Vital signs Q 1 hr.
3. Force fluids if possible (at least 180 ml milk or O.J. Q 30 min × 8 then Q 1 hr × 6).
4. Magnesium sulfate 2 cc IM (50% solution) Q 12 hr × 2 days.
5. If vomiting or diarrhea, give 1000 ml 5% D/W with 1 amp. Berocca C at 150 cc/hr.
6. Follow with 1000 ml 5% D/NaCl with amp. Berocca C at 150 cc an hour until hydration is adequately maintained.
7. Diazepam 10 mg PO Q 1 hr–2 hr prn agitation.
8. Diazepam 10 mg PO Q 4 hr × 2 hr days, then 10 mg PO tid × 2 days, then 5 mg PO tid × 2 days, then D/C.

Treatment of Stage III withdrawal
(delirium tremens)

1. Monitor input and output.
2. Liquids by mouth ad lib.
3. Check bladder for distention Q 3 hr and catheterize with indwelling Foley if necessary.
4. If serum K^+ is low and urinary output is adequate give 20 meq KCl/hr in 1000 cc 5% dextrose or NaCl solution.
5. Magnesium sulfate 2 cc (50% solution) IM Q 8 hr × 3 days.
6. Haloperidol (Haldol) 5 mg IM/PO (concentrate) Q 1 hr until calm. Not to exceed 30 mg and only if bp 90/60.
7. Haloperidol (Haldol) 2–5 mg IM/PO (concentrate) prn to maintain calmness but only if bp 90/60.

[a] Chlordiazepoxide 2.5 mg may be substituted for each 1 mg of diazepam.

tuting a longer-acting depressant drug for alcohol and then gradually reducing the dose of the latter. Generally, chlordiazepoxide (Librium) 25–100 mg PO is administered and the dose repeated in 1 hour and then every 4 hours until signs and symptoms of alcohol withdrawal are suppressed or the maximum dose of 400–600 mg is reached in the first 24 hours. Intramuscular administration should not be used because of poor absorption. If symptoms are adequately controlled, the dose can then be reduced by 50% per day, and the drug discontinued by the fourth day of treatment. Concurrently, the patient's nutritional status should should be assessed and appropriate dietary supplements given.

For patients who are being detoxified at home, written instructions detailing the dosage and adverse effects of the prescribed medication should also be provided, along with a follow-up appointment and the phone number and address of an emergency alcohol treatment facility. If a responsible friend or relative is available, they, too, should be given this information.

6.2.2. Treatment of Seizures Related to Alcohol Withdrawal

Seizures ("rum fits") are infrequent in withdrawing alcoholics, but when they occur they are typically grand mal in type and begin 48–72 hours after the last drink. They are usually self-limited and rarely exceed one to four in number. The prophylactic use of antiseizure medications in alcohol withdrawal is controversial. Some have recommended that anticonvulsants not be prescribed, even for patients with a past history of withdrawal seizures. Others feel that in patients with a seizure history, combined treatment with phenytoin (Dilantin) and a benzodiazepine [i.e., chlordiazepoxide (Librium) or diazepam (Valium)] offers better protection against seizures than a benzodiazepine alone. Table 3B outlines a suggested regimen for the treatment of withdrawal seizures using diazepam (or chlordiazepoxide).

6.2.3. Treatment of Delirium Tremens

As described in Table 3C, patients who have had a seizure or are thought to be entering a state of delirium should receive vigorous treatment. These patients are seriously ill and require intensive inpatient care. The major objectives of treatment are prevention of exhaustion, reduction of CNS irritability, and correction of potentially fatal fluid and electrolyte imbalances. Vitamin replacement and treatment of concurrent illnesses also are important considerations. Careful monitoring of vital signs is necessary to avoid respiratory depression or hypotension.

Patients who enter Stage III (DTs) need even more careful monitoring of fluid and electrolyte balance. In addition, some have suggested that haloperidol may be useful in controlling agitation and hallucinosis. Phenothiazines lower seizure threshold and should be avoided. Dystonias due to haloperidol can be treated with benztropine mesylate (Cogentin).

7. General Approach to Treatment Planning

The recommendations outlined in Tables 3A–3C should be regarded only as guidelines and should be individualized to specific patient needs, particularly for elderly and/or medically fragile individuals. As nursing staff and physicians gain sophistication in the treatment of alcoholic patients, some flexibility may be introduced. In deciding whether to hospitalize the alcoholic patient, the following guidelines may be helpful:

A patient with alcoholism should be admitted if he or she has been drinking recently, and

- has an infectious disease that is likely to become aggravated by continued alcohol abuse.
- has a systemic disease of known or unknown cause with fever of 101°F (38.3°C) or above, or hypothermia below 95°F (35°C).
- has an alcohol-induced disorder (e.g., alcoholic hepatitis, acute pancreatitis, Wernicke's disease) that is likely to progress in severity with continued alcohol use.
- has a significant metabolic problem, such as acidosis with or without ketosis, uncontrolled diabetes mellitus, or hypoglycemia.

- is in congestive heart failure, or has significant hypertension, tachycardia, or arrhythmia.
- has active gastrointestinal bleeding, significant vomiting or dehydration.
- has a significant anemia.
- has a serious disulfiram-alcohol reaction with hyperthermia, chest pain, arrhythmia, or hypotension.
- has hallucinations (visual, auditory, or tactile) or manifests serious confusion.
- manifests signs of impending or active delirium tremens.
- has a history of convulsions.
- is comatose, stuporous, or has a fluctuating level of consciousness.
- has severe depression, expressed hopelessness, or suicidal ideation.

8. Conclusion

The acute treatment of alcohol-abusing patients should be followed by efforts to promote long-term rehabilitation. Referral to Alcoholics Anonymous, individual, couples, and family therapy, and maintenance on disulfiram (Antabuse) are among the treatment modalities that may be useful in promoting a stable abstinence. Recognition and effective treatment of coexistent psychiatric disorders (e.g., major depression, manic-depressive disease) is also crucial if rehabilitation efforts are to succeed.

Bibliography

1. Bean M: Alcoholics Anonymous, Chapter I: Principles and methods, *Psychiatr Ann* 5:7–21, 1975.
2. Bibb RE: The outpatient treatment of the alcoholic. *Ohio State Med J* 66:686–689, 1970.
3. Cohen S: *The Substance Abuse Problems*. New York, Haworth Press, 1981.
4. Feldman OJ, Pattison E, Sobell C, et al: Outpatient alcohol detoxification: Initial findings on 564 patients. *Am J Psychiatry* 132:407–412, 1975.
5. Fuller, RK, Roth HP: Disulfiram for the treatment of alcoholism. *Ann Intern Med* 90:901–904, 1979.
6. Gitlow SE, Peyser HS: (eds): *Alcoholism: A Practical Treatment Guide*. Plenum Press, 1976, pp 103–129.
7. Goodwin DW: Alcoholism and heredity. *Arch Gen Psychiatry* 36:57–61, 1979.
8. Hanson JE, Jones KL, Smith DW: Fetal alcohol syndrome: Experience with 41 patients. *J Am Med Assoc* 235:1458–1460, 1976.
9. Jones RW, Helrich AR: Treatment of alcoholism by physicians in private practice, a national survey. *Q J Stud Alcohol* 33:117–131, 1972.
10. Kisin B, Begleiter H (eds): *The Biology of Alcoholism, Vol. I: Biochemistry*. New York, Plenum Press, 1971.
11. Kissin B, Begleiter H (eds): *The Biology of Alcoholism, Vol. II: Physiology and Behavior*. New York, Plenum Press, 1972.
12. Kissin B, Begleiter H (eds): *The Biology of Alcoholism, Vol. III: Clinical Pathology*. New York, Plenum Press, 1974.
13. Kissin B, Begleiter H (eds): *The Biology of Alcoholism, Vol. IV: Social Aspects of Alcoholism*. New York, Plenum Press, 1976.

14. Kissin B, Begleiter H (eds): *The Biology of Alcoholism, Vol. V: Treatment and Rehabilitation of the Chronic Alcoholic.* New York, Plenum Press, 1977.

15. Lieber S: The metabolism of alcohol. *Sci Am* 234:3, 1976.

16. Mayer J, Myerson J: Outpatient treatment of alcoholics: Effects of status, stability and nature of treatment. *Q J Stud Alcohol* 32:620–627, 1971.

17. Mendelson JH, Mello NK: Biologic concomitants of alcoholism. *N Engl J Med* 301:912–921, 1979.

18. Mendelson JH, Mello NK: *The Diagnosis and Treatment of Alcoholism.* New York, McGraw-Hill, 1979.

19. Miller R: *The Addictive Behaviors. The Treatment of Alcoholism, Drug Abuse, Smoking and Obesity.* New York, Pergamon Press, 1980.

20. O'Connor J, Morgan DW: Multidisciplinary treatment of alcoholism. *Q J Stud Alcohol* 29:903–908, 1968.

21. Parker M: The effects of ethyl alcohol on the heart. *JAMA* 228:741–742, 1974.

22. Pattison EM: Nonabstinent drinking goals in the treatment of alcoholism: A clinical typology. *Arch Gen Psychiatry* 33:923–930, 1976.

23. *Second Special Report to the U.S. Congress on Alcohol and Health, New Knowledge*, E. Chafetz (chair). Rockville, Md, National Institute on Alcohol Abuse and Alcoholism, 1974.

24. Silberfarb PM: Recognizing alcoholism early by physical signs. *Postgrad Med* 59:79–81, 1976.

25. Sollers EM, Kalant H: Alcohol intoxication and withdrawal. *N Engl J Med* 294:757–762, 1976.

26. Stinson DJ, Smith WG, Amidjaya I, et al: Systems of care and treatment outcomes for alcoholic patients. *Arch Gen Psychiatry* 36:535–539, 1979.

27. Vaillant GE: Natural history of male psychological health: VIII. Antecedents of alcoholism and orality. *Am J Psychiatry* 137:181–186, 1980.

28. Victor M, Adams RD: Alcohol, in Isselbacher KJ, Adams RD, Braunwald E, et al (eds): *Harrison's Principles of Internal Medicine*, ed 9. New York, McGraw-Hill, 1980, pp 969–977.

29. Weissman MM, Myers JK: Clinical depression in alcoholism. *Am J Psychiatry* 137:372–374, 1980.

9

Drug Use and Abuse

Steven M. Mirin, M.D., and Roger D. Weiss, M.D.

1. Abuse of Opiate Drugs

1.1. Introduction

Estimates of the prevalence of narcotic addiction vary considerably but probably include 0.3% of the population, or about 600,000 heroin addicts. They present to the emergency room for the following reasons: serious medical problems resulting from overdose or intoxication, medical complications of their addictions, and/or withdrawal symptoms and signs resulting in drug-seeking behavior.

1.2. Classification

We can divide the opiates into the following categories:

- Natural alkaloids of opium derived from the resin of the opium poppy such as opium, morphine, and codeine.
- Semisynthetic derivatives of morphine such as diacetyl morphine (heroin), hydromorphone (Dilaudid), and oxycodone (Percodan).
- Purely synthetic opiates, which are not derivatives of morphine, such as meperidine (Demerol), methadone (Dolophine), and propoxyphene (Darvon).
- Opiate-containing preparations such as elixir of terpin hydrate with codeine and paregoric.

The most commonly abused substances are the semisynthetic and pure derivatives.

1.3. Pharmacology

The opiate drugs are readily absorbed from the gastrointestinal tract, nasal mucosa, and lung, but parenteral administration more rapidly elevates blood

---

This chapter, reprinted here with permission, is condensed and adapted from a similar chapter in Bassuk EL, Schoonover SC, Gelenberg AJ. (eds): *The Practitioner's Guide to Psychoactive Drugs*, ed 2. New York, Plenum Publishing Corp, 1983.

Steven M. Mirin, M.D. • Harvard Medical School, Boston, Massachusetts 02115, Westwood Lodge Hospital, Westwood, Massachusetts 02090, and McLean Hospital, Belmont, Massachusetts 02178. *Roger D. Weiss, M.D.* • Harvard Medical School, Boston, Massachusetts 02115, and McLean Hospital, Belmont, Massachusetts 02178.

levels and produces intoxication. For example, following intravenous administration of heroin, the drug is almost immediately hydrolyzed to morphine by the liver, with peak plasma morphine levels attained in approximately 30 minutes. The drug then rapidly leaves the blood and is concentrated in body tissues. Only small quantities of injected opiates cross the blood-brain barrier, but plasma levels correlate directly with the level of intoxication. Morphine is metabolized primarily by conjugation in the liver. Its half-life (i.e., the amount of time necessary for one-half of a given dose to be cleared from the blood) is approximately 2 1/2 hours, and 90% of the total dose administered is excreted in the urine within the first 24 hours. The remainder is excreted through the biliary tract and appears in the feces.

1.4. Clinical Effects

1.4.1. Acute Effects/Central

Acute administration of heroin, especially intravenously, produces an orgasmlike "rush" lasting 30 to 60 seconds, followed by a brief period of euphoria and a profound sense of tranquility. This latter state may last for several hours, depending on the dose administered and the plasma level of morphine attained. It is characterized by drowsiness ("nodding"), lability of mood, mental clouding, apathy, and motor retardation. Respiratory depression (i.e., diminished volume and slower rate) secondary to inhibition of the brainstem respiratory center also occurs. Stimulation of the brainstem chemoreceptor trigger zone for emesis may produce nausea and vomiting. However, with repetitive use tolerance develops to this effect.

1.4.2. Acute Effects/Peripheral

In the healthy patient, the cardiovascular effects of opiates are minimal. In some patients, however, peripheral vasodilation may contribute to orthostatic hypotension. These drugs also decrease secretions in the stomach, biliary tract, and pancreas, and inhibit the contractility of smooth muscle. As a result of the latter effect, opiate use may be accompanied by constipation; diminished smooth muscle tone in the ureters and bladder may produce urinary hesitancy. Inhibition of the smooth muscle of the iris results in pupillary constriction, an important sign of opiate intoxication in man.

1.4.3. Tolerance and Physical Dependence

Tolerance to some effects of opiate drugs begins to develop after only a week of regular use. Tolerance to other effects develops more slowly. Thus, patients become tolerant rather quickly to the euphoric, analgesic, sedative, respiratory depressant, and emetic effects, while continuing to exhibit pupillary constriction and constipation. In most persons receiving therapeutic doses of morphine four times a day for two or three days, some degree of physical dependence occurs.

1.5. Patterns and Abuse

1.5.1. Acute Intoxication and Overdose

1.5.1a. Etiology. Among chronic opiate abusers overdose is relatively common; it may be accidental or reflect suicidal intent. Unintentional overdose stems from two basic preconditions: (1) The user does not know the dose of opiate actually administered—street drugs have widely fluctuating concentrations; 2) opiate users vary considerably in their level of drug tolerance. Overdose deaths probably result from respiratory depression and anoxia, although anaphylactoid reactions to heroin or its common adulterants also may play a role.

1.5.1b. Clinical Manifestations. Patients who overdose on illicitly obtained opiate drugs usually are alone, and the untoward effects are immediate. Thus, diagnosis and medical intervention are often too late. When these patients present for treatment, they may be in stupor or coma, with constricted pupils and diminished pulse and respiration. Hypothermia and pulmonary edema (usually noncardiogenic) are seen in severe cases.

The clinician must differentiate opiate overdose from other causes of respiratory depression and coma. While pupillary constriction usually is a reliable sign, it also occurs in severe barbiturate intoxication. Moreover, in the event of circulatory collapse and cyanosis, the pupils become dilated. The treating physician should look for dermatologic evidence of repeated intravenous injections (i.e., needle tracks). Signs of other medical illnesses often associated with chronic opiate use (e.g., hepatitis, infectious endocarditis, and multiple abscesses) also may help make the diagnosis.

1.5.1c. Management/General Life-Support Measures. The first task in treating acute opiate poisoning is to establish an adequate airway. Aspiration can be prevented either by placing the patient on his side or by using a cuffed endotracheal tube. Gastric lavage should be performed if the clinician suspects recent oral intake of opiates or other drugs. If hypoglycemia complicates the clinical picture, the physician should establish a reliable intravenous route and slowly infuse a 50% solution of glucose in water. Pulmonary edema, if present, can be treated with positive-pressure respiration.

1.5.1d. Management/The Use of Naloxone. Narcotic antagonists can dramatically reverse respiratory depression and other symptoms associated with acute opiate toxicity. The current drug choice is *naloxone (Narcan)*, a pure, potent narcotic antagonist with no agonistic (i.e., opiatelike) effects of its own. Naloxone, 0.4 mg (1 ml) administered intravenously, should reverse manifestations of overdose within two minutes. Increase in respiratory rate and volume, rise in systolic blood pressure, and dilation of the pupils indicate a favorable response. If the initial response is unsatisfactory, the same dose may be given twice more at five-minute intervals. Failure to respond after three doses of naloxone suggests either that the diagnosis of opiate poisoning is erroneous or that another problem (e.g., barbiturate poisoning, head injury) is complicating the clinical picture. Unfortunately, the duration of action of naloxone is much shorter (one to four hours) than most opiate drugs. For this reason, patients with severe overdoses should be hospitalized and monitored closely for a least 24 to 48 hours. A significant decrease in respiratory rate or level of consciousness should prompt additional antagonist treatment and prevent relapse into opiate-induced coma.

Most patients who overdose on drugs like heroin or methadone are also physically dependent on these agents. Repeated administration of naloxone, which displaces opiates from their receptor sites in the brain and elsewhere, may precipitate an acute abstinence syndrome. Signs and symptoms of opiate withdrawal may appear within minutes and last for several hours. Moreover, they cannot be easily overcome by giving additional opiates. The severity and duration of abstinence symptoms depend upon the degree of opiate dependence and the dose and route of administration of naloxone. The use of a small dose (0.4 mg IV) at five-minute intervals may help to avoid this unwelcome complication.

1.5.1e. Management/Other Considerations. Since patients who use opiates tend to abuse other drugs as well, overdoses may be accompanied by alcohol, barbiturates, antidepressants, and antianxiety drugs. For this reason, the clinician should obtain blood and urine from all patients for toxicologic screening. Upon recovery, the degree of suicidal intent associated with overdose should be assessed; prior to discharge, patients can be offered referral to an appropriate treatment facility.

1.5.2. Opiate Withdrawal

The opiate-dependent patient sometimes comes to the emergency ward when the quality or availability of heroin or other opiates declines on the street, making it difficult to stave off symptoms of withdrawal. When abstinence symptoms occur, their severity depends upon the type of opiate previously used, degree of tolerance, time elapsed since the last dose, and emotional meaning of the symptoms. The symptoms themselves reflect increased excitability in organs previously depressed by chronic opiate use. Despite the discomfort experienced during withdrawal, however, this syndrome is rarely life-threatening.

In the *early stages of withdrawal* from heroin (i.e., 6 to 12 hours after the last dose), the patient may yawn and sweat, his nose and eyes may run, and he may experience considerable anxiety. Craving for opiates and drug-seeking behavior intensify. As withdrawal progresses, pupils dilate and the patient may develop gooseflesh, hot and cold flashes, loss of appetite, muscle cramps, tremor, and insomnia or restless tossing sleep. Eighteen to 24 hours after the last dose of heroin, nausea, vomiting, and elevations in blood pressure, pulse, respiratory rate, and temperature occur. After 24 to 36 hours, diarrhea and dehydration may develop.

In the case of heroin or morphine, abstinence symptoms generally peak 48 to 72 hours after the last dose. By this time, laboratory alues reflect the clinical process. Leukocytosis is common, while ketosis and electrolyte imbalance may develop due to dehydration. In untreated cases, clinical symptoms usually disappear within 7 to 10 days, although physiologic disturbances may be detected for several months afterward. Withdrawal from methadone is characterized by slower onset (24 to 48 hours after the last dose) and more gradual resolution of symptoms (three to seven weeks). Indeed, patients often complain of fatigue, weakness, and insomnia for several months after stopping the drug.

The emergency clinician must know the federal laws governing the administration of methadone. Generally, only licensed facilities can dispense methadone "to maintain and addict." "In an emergency situation, at the *time of hospitalization*, it may be necessary to provide a dose to avoid the painful withdrawal symptoms . . ." (p. 182)* If the patient doesn't require immediate hospitalization he should be referred to a licensed detoxification facility.

The use of methadone in the treatment of opiate withdrawal is based on several factors. As a result of the strong cross-dependence between methadone and the other opiates, sufficient doses (*10 to 40 mg/day*) *of methadone will prevent abstinence symptoms* in patients who are physically dependent on other opiate drugs. In addition, methadone is well absorbed from the gastrointestinal tract and is effective orally, thus avoiding the hazards of intravenous opiate use. Since the drug is more slowly metabolized than heroin or morphine, it has a longer duration of action (24 to 36 hours), allowing for once-per-day administration. Finally, oral administration of therapeutic doses to tolerant individuals does not produce the euphoria that follows intravenous use of shorter-acting opiates like heroin. The acute effects include sedation, analgesia, and respiratory depression. Table 1 describes detoxification with methadone.

1.5.3. Chronic Opiate Abuse

A wide variety of medical and psychosocial complications accompanies the chronic use of opiate drugs. These, coupled with poor living conditions and a deviant life-style, combine to produce significant morbidity and mortality. The death rate among urban addicts is estimated at 1% per year. Drug overdose and violence account for many deaths, but medical complications take their toll as well. These are reviewed briefly.

1.5.3 a. Medical Complications. Hepatitis B (serum hepatitis) is a frequent and sometimes lethal complication of chronic intravenous drug use. Up to 65% of urban heroin addicts will develop hepatitis B at some time in their drug-using career. Infected individuals transmit the blood-borne virus by sharing contaminated needles. Recurrent infection and chronic persistent hepatitis also are common. About 60% of current heroin users have chronically elevated

---

*Slaby AE, Lieb J, Tancredi LR: *Handbook of Psychiatric Emergencies.* New York, Medical Examination Publishing Co, 1981.

Table 1. Detoxification with Methadone

Due to the variable reliability of patients and the uncertainty about the percentage of active drug contained in street samples (3–10%), the following detoxification method can be used:

1. Observe the patient for objective signs of opiate withdrawal (i.e., 20% rise over baseline blood pressure and pulse, sweating, pupillary dilation).
2. When 2 of the above signs present give 10 mg dissolved methadone orally.
3. Signs of withdrawal should abate—at least temporarily—within an hour.
4. Repeat above as often as necessary within the next 24 hours, but the amount (stabilization dose) should not exceed 40 mg.
5. Over the next 24 hours give the stabilization dose in two divided doses.
6. Beginning on the 3rd day, taper methadone by 5 mg per day, beginning with the morning dose, until the patient is completely withdrawn.
7. Dispense all methadone in liquid form.
8. Monitor patients' urines on a daily or twice-weekly random schedule.
9. Course of outpatient detoxification takes from 3 to 21 days.
10. During and after detoxification, patients may complain of fatigue, muscle pain, and insomnia.

---

serum transaminase levels, possibly related also to a high incidence of alcoholism.

Intravenous drug users, even those with no known history of heart disease, also are prone to develop infectious endocarditis, often from *Staphylococcus aureus*. Other medical complications include foreign body emboli, pulmonary fibrosis, pneumonia, lung abscess, and tuberculosis. In patients who inject these drugs subcutaneously or intramuscularly, abscess formation may occur with infection, ulceration, and, occasionally, gangrene as sequelae.

1.5.3b. Treatment Approaches. Chronic opiate users who present themselves for treatment are often both physically ill and psychosocially disabled. In addition to the pharmacologic effects of these drugs, the addict life-style itself may be reinforcing, particularly for individuals with low self-esteem and limited opportunities for success in the mainstream of society. The clinician should view opiate dependence as a chronic relapsing illness. Patients often require a wide range of medical and rehabilitative services. Remedial education, job training and placement, legal assistance, and individual, group, and family counseling, when appropriate, should supplement biological intervention.

Successful treatment of chronic opiate use hinges on motivating the patient to seek an alternative life-style—a task that any single treatment modality, whether it be intensive long-term psychotherapy or methadone maintenance, cannot accomplish by itself. Moreover, successful treatment usually incorporates some element of control over patient behavior, whether it be chemical control (e.g., methadone maintenance), custodial control (e.g., civil commitment), the control exercised by an autocratic peer group (e.g., therapeutic communities), or the self-control provided by regular administration of a narcotic antagonist. While the nature of the controls may differ, all attempt to counteract the patient's high degree of impulsivity and covert self-destructiveness. The ER clinician should refer the patient to programs that offer one

or a combination of the following: methadone maintenance, narcotic antagonists, outpatient drug-free treatment, or a therapeutic community.

2. Abuse of Central Nervous System (CNS) Depressants

2.1. Introduction

Although less publicized, the prevalence of sedative abuse probably exceeds that of the opiates. In 1976, 128 million prescriptions were written for
sedative-hypnotic drugs in the United States. Most physicians would agree that
at times these drugs are grossly overprescribed, often without adequate evaluation. Federal legislation has eliminated "open-ended" prescriptions for most
of these agents.

Unlike opiate abusers, the vast majority of depressant abusers do not belong to a drug-using subculture and an illicit system of drug distribution. Instead, they are primarily individuals who have received legitimate prescriptions
to treat insomnia or anxiety. With prolonged administration, however, tolerance develops to the hypnotic and anxiolytic effects of these drugs, often
prompting either an increase in dosage or a switch to another drug in the same
general class. At the same time, the cross-tolerance that develops among the
various CNS depressants limits the effectiveness of this therapeutic maneuver.
Eventually, the patient may become physically dependent upon one or more
of these agents, and subsequent attempts at withdrawal may result in abstinence
symptoms.

A second group of sedative abusers are younger, tend to abuse other drugs
(e.g., stimulants or heroin), and generally depend on illicit sources of supply.
Intravenous drug use is much more common in this group. Generally, they
prefer the short-acting barbiturates like pentobarbital, sedatives like methaqualone, and anxiolytics like diazepam (Valium). They may use these drugs
regularly (i.e., daily) or during sprees of intoxication lasting several days. In
either situation, they may consume massive doses (e.g., 300 mg of diazepam
per day).

Finally, many stimulant abusers use CNS depressants to "come down"
after a prolonged period of amphetamine or cocaine use. Others take phar-
maceutical preparations that combine a stimulant like dextroamphetamine with
a short- or intermediate-acting barbiturate, and some develop physical dependence on the CNS depressant component. These individuals are more likely
to administer depressants intravenously, increasing their risk of fatal overdose.

2.2. Classification

The central nervous (CNS) depressants have widely varied chemical structures and include the barbiturates, the benzodiazepines, and sedative-hypnotics, like methaqualone, glutethimide, meprobamate, chloral hydrate, paraldehyde, methyprylon, ethchlorvynol, and alcohol (see Chapter 8).

2.2.1. Barbiturates

The barbiturates are usually classified by their duration of action into ultra-short-, short-to-intermediate-, and long-acting types. The ultra-short-acting barbiturates, like methohexital (Brevital) and thiopental (Pentothal), are used primarily as intravenous anesthetics. The short-to-intermediate-acting drugs, like amobarbital (Amytal), pentobarbital (Nembutal), and secobarbital (Seconal), are employed primarily for their sedative and hypnotic properties. The relatively long-acting barbiturates, like phenobarbital (Luminal and others), may be employed as sedative-hypnotics but are most useful in the control of some seizure disorders. The may also be used to facilitate withdrawal from other sedative-hypnotics.

2.2.2. Benzodiazepines

To a larger extent, the benzodiazepines (e.g., diazepam, chlordiazepoxide, oxazepam) have replaced the barbiturates for the pharmacological treatment of anxiety. In addition, the hypnotic effects of these compounds have contributed to their increasing popularity. Taken for brief periods in therapeutic doses, the benzodiazepines are safe and effective; however, chronic use may result in the development of tolerance and physical dependence.

2.2.3. Other Sedative-Hypnotics

In addition to the barbiturates and benzodiazepines, a number of other drugs depress CNS functioning and therefore have potential utility (and abuse liability) as sedative-hypnotics. Though they vary considerably in their chemical structure and pharmacologic properties, the clinical picture in both intoxication and withdrawal is quite similar. Some of the more commonly used (and abused) agents are described below.

Chloral hydrate (Noctec), the oldest and best known drug of this group, will induce sleep at doses of 0.5 to 1.0 g PO. Habitual use may produce tolerance and physical dependence. Abrupt withdrawal may result in delirium, seizures, and death. Patients may occasionally display a "break in tolerance," leading to sudden unexpected death by overdose.

Methaqualone (Quaalude, Sopor) is a drug that has achieved wide popularity among drug abusers, who enjoy the sense of well-being, disinhibition, paresthesias, and ataxia that characterize intoxication ("luding out"). In addition, methaqualone has been purported to have aphrodisiac properties, a claim that has not been substantiated. Many users find that methaqualone, unlike the barbiturates, does not make them drowsy. The usual hypnotic dose is 150 to 300 mg po, but some abusers may take up to 2 g per day. Death has been reported after intravenous injection of 8 g, but most deaths occur in abusers who also have been drinking alcohol.

Glutethimide (Doriden) in an oral dose of 500 mg rapidly induces sleep in most nontolerant individuals. Doses of greater than 2 mg per day for a month produce physical dependence. In these individuals, abrupt discontinuation of the drug may result in a general depressant withdrawal syndrome. When taken in large doses, glutethimide is stored in the body's fatty tissue and is thus difficult to dialyze. In cases of overdose, episodic release from body stores may occur so that the patient's degree of intoxication may fluctuate widely. Therefore, the patient must be monitored for at least 24 hours. Serum concentration may not correlate well with the level of consciousness. Unlike other CNS depressants, dilated pupils may accompany glutethimide poisoning. Overdose with this drug has been implicated in many suicides.

Methyprylon (Noludar) in doses of 200 to 400 mg will induce sleep. As in the case with other sedatives, prolonged use of large doses will result in physical dependence. Death has been reported following the ingestion of as little as 6 g, but individuals vary greatly in their degree of tolerance.

Ethchlorvynol (Placidyl) is a sedative-hypnotic with a rapid onset and short duration of action. Ingestion of 2 to 4 g per day over several months can produce physical dependence. As in the case with methyprylon, the potentially lethal dose widely varies. Ingestion of more than 10 g at once is usually fatal.

Meprobamate (Miltown, Equanil) is a carbamate derivative that had been widely used as an antianxiety agent and a skeletal muscle relaxant. The benzodiazepines have largely supplanted this drug as both a therapeutic compound and a drug of abuse. The usual therapeutic dose is 400 mg three or four times per day. Chronic administration of slightly higher doses will produce physical dependence, with the possibility of seizures upon withdrawal. The lethal dose varies between 12 and 40 g.

2.3. Tolerance and Physical Dependence

With repetitive administration, three types of tolerance develop to the central nervous system depressants. They include (1) *dispositional tolerance*, in which the enzyme systems of the liver become more capable of rapidly metabolizing these drugs; (2) *pharmacodynamic tolerance*, in which the cells of the CNS adjust themselves to the presence of increasing doses of these drugs; and (3) *cross-tolerance* to the effects of other central nervous system depressants, including alcohol.

Tolerance to the hypnotic effects of a short-acting barbiturate like pentobarbital (Nembutal) begins to develop within a few days, even when administered in therapeutic doses. After two weeks, the therapeutic effectiveness of a given dose may be reduced by 50%. Moreover, the simultaneous development of cross-tolerance to other CNS depressants makes substitution of a second drug in this general class therapeutically ineffective since the patient will likely be tolerant to its effects. On the other hand, since some CNS depressants (including barbiturates and alcohol) compete for hepatic metabolism, concurrent use of two or more of these agents will result in clinical effects far greater than any of the drugs alone. Heightened toxicity and accidental overdose are common sequelae of this practice.

Table 2. Signs and Symptoms of CNS Depressant
Intoxication

Drowsiness	Ataxia
Slurred speech	Hypotonia
Motor incoordination	Hyporeflexia
Confusion/agitation	Memory impairment
Disorientation	Respiratory depression
Nystagmus	Inappropriate affect
Tremor	Rage reactions

2.4. Patterns of Abuse

2.4.1. Acute Intoxication and Overdose

2.4.1a. Etiology. Not infrequently, depressed patients may make a suicide attempt by overdosing on CNS depressants that they received for the treatment of insomnia and/or anxiety. Occasionally, a patient may become confused after ingesting the therapeutic dose and then forget he has taken it. Ingestion of a second, third, or even fourth dose ("drug automatism") then leads to increased confusion and subsequent overdose.

2.4.1b. Clinical Manifestations. Mild to moderate intoxication with central nervous system depressants closely resembles alcoholic drunkenness, but patients do not have alcoholic breath. The severity of symptoms depends on the drug or combination of drugs used, the route of administration, and the presence or absence of other complicating conditions (e.g., head injury). As summarized in Table 2, patients usually present with drowsiness, slurred speech, motor incoordination, impaired memory, confused thinking, and disorientation. Physical examination may reveal both horizontal and vertical nystagmus, tremor, and ataxia. In addition, patients may exhibit entreme irritability, agitation, inappropriate affect, and paranoia, sometimes accompanied by rage reactions and destructive behavior. The latter is most common when depressant drugs are combined with alcohol.

Severe overdose with CNS depressants is accompanied by signs of cerebrocortical and medullary depression. Patients may be stuporous or comatose, with absent corneal, gag, and deep tendon reflexes. Plantar stimulation may produce no response or an extensor response. They may also have impaired cardiopulmonary function, with shallow, irregular breathing, hypoxia, respiratory acidosis, and, in the late stages, paralytic dilation of the pupils. In terminal cases, the patient may develop shock, hypothermia, lung complications (e.g., pulmonary edema, pneumonia), and renal failure.

2.4.1c. Management. The clinical picture described above, coupled with a suspected or confirmed history of sedative intake, depression, and recent psychiatric or medical treatment, suggests the diagnosis of sedative overdose.

Additional history from family or friends also can be quite useful. Chromatographic analysis of blood and urine samples will confirm a drug ingestion.

Adequate treatment of sedative overdose requires a well-trained staff in a hospital setting. Generally, if more than 10 times the full hypnotic dose of a drug has been ingested, overdose will be severe, particularly if combined with alcohol intake. When the patient arrives in the emergency room, treatment will be dictated by his current state of consciousness. In the awake patient who has ingested a drug in the past several hours, vomiting should be induced or gastric lavage instituted. Samples of the vomitus, blood, and urine should be sent for toxicologic analysis. If the patient has ingested a fat-soluble drug like glutethimide, 60 ml of castor oil may be given via nasogastric tube. If bowel sounds are present, a cathartic (e.g., 15 to 30 g of sodium sulfate) should be instilled into the tube to prevent gastric dilation and regurgitation. If the patient's condition remains stable, *he should be continuously observed, with the monitoring of respiratory and cardiovascular functioning and the level of consciousness, both of which may fluctuate widely as the drugs are episodically released from tissue stores.* Patients who remain fully conscious and free of cardiopulmonary complications may be released after 24 hours of observation.

Patients who present in a stuporous or comatose state, or who are initially awake but then lapse into coma, clearly need more intensive treatment. The goal is to support vital functions until the patient is able to metabolize and excrete the drug. Thus, management is directed primarily toward maintaining adequate cardiopulmonary and renal function. If the drug ingestion has occurred within the previous six hours, gastric lavage should be attempted, but only after an unobstructed airway is established by passing a cuffed endotracheal tube. When oxygenation is adequate, the clinician should initiate mechanical ventilation and administer oxygen. If shock supervenes, transfusions of whole blood, plasma, or plasma expanders should be used to elevate blood pressure and prevent circulatory collapse. The use of vasopressor drugs [e.g., norepinephrine (Levophed)] has been advocated in some situations.

When renal function is satisfactory, forced diuresis should be attempted; enough saline and dextrose in water (approximately 500 ml/hr) should be administered to produce a urine output of 8 to 10 ml per minute. With the longer-acting barbiturates, like phenobarbital, alkalinization of the urine with sodium bicarbonate enhances excretion. Some authors advocate the use of diuretics [e.g., furosemide (Lasix)] to promote urinary excretion. In cases of profound intoxication, hemodialysis is often effective when more conservative measures fail. For the more lipid soluble short-acting barbiturates and some of the non-barbiturate sedative-hypnotics (e.g., glutethimide), the use of a lipid dialysate or hemoperfusion through charcoal or resins (e.g., the lipid-absorptive AMBERLITE XAD-4) may promote drug elimination more effectively than traditional dialysis methods.

In general, survival following an overdose of a CNS depressant depends on the maintenance of adequate respiratory, cardiac, and renal function until drug concentrations drop below potentially lethal levels. On recovery, psychiatric consultation should be obtained and the patient's suicide potential assessed. Patients who purposefully overdose on CNS depressants tend to repeat this action, especially if the underlying problem (e.g., depression) is not effectively treated.

2.4.2. Withdrawal from CNS Depressants

Chronic administration of CNS depressants, even in the usual therapeutic doses, may produce tolerance and eventually physical dependence. Although tolerance develops rapidly to the therapeutic dose, tolerance to a potentially lethal dose develops at a somewhat slower rate. Thus, even chronic users of these substances may become quite intoxicated and even comatose when the dose is raised only slightly.

Physical dependence implies the presence of an abstinence syndrome on withdrawal. In severe cases, withdrawal may carry significant risk of mortality and should be carried out in a hospital setting.

2.4.2 a. Clinical Manifestations.

Onset of withdrawal symptoms depends on the duration of action of the particular drug. In the case of the short-acting barbiturates, abstinence symptoms may occur within 12 to 16 hours after the last dose. Withdrawal of a longer-acting drug like diazepam may not result in abstinence symptoms until 7 to 10 days after the last dose. Severity of symptoms depends on the degree of physical dependence and on individual variables that are poorly understood.

Early manifestations of abstinence include agitation, anxiety, anorexia, nausea, and vomiting. As withdrawal progresses, the patient may complain of weakness and develop tachycardia, abdominal cramps, postural hypotension, hyperactive deep tendon reflexes, and a gross resting tremor. Although total sleep time is reduced, the percentage of rapid eye movement (REM) sleep increases, and nightmares become more frequent.

With the exception of the longer-acting barbiturates, withdrawal symptoms characteristically peak two or three days after the last dose; generalized seizures may occur within this period, either singly or as status epilepticus. About 50% of patients who have seizures develop delirium. The latter is characterized by anxiety, disorientation, frightening dreams, and visual hallucinations. Agitation and hyperthermia can lead to exhaustion, followed by cardiovascular collapse. Delirium is not easily reversed, even by giving large doses of the abused drug. If death does not supervene, the patient, after a lengthy period of sleep, usually clears by the eighth day.

2.4.2b. Management of CNS Depressant Withdrawal.

The treatment of CNS depressant withdrawal is complicated by the fact that sedative abusers are often inaccurate historians. They may wish to obtain as much drug from the clinician as possible and/or may have impaired memory secondary to chronic drug use. For this reason, the *pentobarbital tolerance test* is a useful tool in the management of withdrawal states. The test takes advantage of the fact that cross-tolerance exists among the various CNS depressants. As illus-

Table 3. Detoxification from CNS Depressants Using the Pentobarbital Tolerance Test

Day 1:

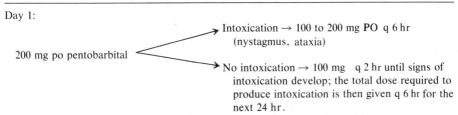

200 mg po pentobarbital

Intoxication → 100 to 200 mg PO q 6 hr (nystagmus, ataxia)

No intoxication → 100 mg q 2 hr until signs of intoxication develop; the total dose required to produce intoxication is then given q 6 hr for the next 24 hr.

Day 2: Give pentobarbital in the same dose as was given in the previous 24 hr.

Day 3 and beyond: Subtract 100 mg/day of pentobarbital from total dose given on previous day until detoxified. If signs of intoxication develop, eliminate a single dose and resume treatment 6 hr later. If signs of withdrawal develop, 100 to 200 mg pentobarbital PO or IM stat.

Phenobarbital substitution: 30 mg phenobarbital = 100 mg pentobarbital.

Advantages: more constant plasma level and significant anticonvulsant effects.

---

trated in Table 3, a patient showing signs of depressant withdrawal is given 200 mg of pentobarbital orally. One hour later, the clinician should examine the patient for signs of sedative intoxication, such as sedation, nystagmus, ataxia, and slurred speech. If mildly intoxicated by this dose, the patient has probably been taking less than the equivalent of 800 mg of pentobarbital a day. The clinician can stabilize these patients on a dose of 100 to 200 mg of pentobarbital every six hours, depending upon the degree of intoxication. If, after an initial test dose (200 mg), no signs of intoxication appear, the patient's tolerance is probably greater than that induced by prolonged daily use of 800 mg of pentobarbital. Consequently, additional increments of 100 mg of pentobarbital may be administered every two hours until signs of intoxication become evident, or until a total of 500 mg has been given. The clinician should then calculate the total dose required to produce intoxication and give this dose every six hours for the next 48 hours. If the patient becomes grossly intoxicated, the next six-hour dose may be omitted and the following day's dose reduced accordingly. Once stabilization has been achieved, the total daily dose of pentobarbital is reduced by 100 mg each day until withdrawal is completed. Patients should be free of tremulousness, insomnia and orthostatic hypotension. If these signs of abstinence recur during the tapering process, additional 100- to 200-mg doses of pentobarbital may be given. However, it is usually sufficient to stop the dosage reduction for one day and then cautiously resume tapering the drug.

One disadvantage of pentobarbital-mediated withdrawal is that patients sometimes require intoxicating doses to prevent the development of seizures and perhaps delirium. Thus, practical reasons exist for substituting a long-acting barbiturate, like *phenobarbital*, once stabilization on pentobarbital has been achieved. Use of the longer-acting phenobarbital produces a more constant plasma barbiturate level than can be obtained with the shorter-acting pentobarbital. Phenobarbital also provides a greater degree of anticonvulsant activity relative to its sedative effects, so that the patient need not be intoxicated to avoid the development of seizures. Finally, the lethal dose of phenobarbital is several times greater than the intoxicating dose, so that there is a greater margin of safety compared to pentobarbital. Thirty milligrams of phenobarbital can be substituted for every 100 mg of pentobarbital. The drug can be given in divided doses every eight hours. Once stabilization on phenobarbital has been achieved, the dose is lowered by 30 mg per day until total withdrawal is achieved. If the patient shows signs of barbiturate toxicity, one or more doses may be omitted. If signs of withdrawal are apparent, an additional 30 to 90 mg of phenobarbital can be given immediately IM and the total dose of pheno-barbital increased by 25%. Phenobarbital should not be administered in doses exceeding 500 mg per day.

Treatment with phenobarbital will suppress early symptoms of depressant withdrawal. Once delirium has developed, however, 24 to 72 hours of barbi-turate treatment may be required before it clears. Phenytoin (Dilantin) is of questionable efficacy in preventing withdrawal seizures in these patients. The antipsychotic drugs [e.g., chlorpromazine (Thorazine and others)], which them-selves lower seizure threshold, also should be avoided, although some have advocated their use in the treatment of delirium.

While some patients have been withdrawn from CNS depressants as out-patients, this is risky. Thirty mg of phenobarbital are substituted for each hyp-notic dose of the substance abused, and the total daily requirement of phen-obarbital is given in three divided doses. The total daily dose is then reduced by 30 mg per day until withdrawal is completed.

2.4.3. Mixed Opiate-Sedative Dependence

In the last decade, simultaneous abuse of more than one class of psy-choactive drug has become commonplace. Heroin addicts and patients on meth-adone maintenance may also abuse sedatives and alcohol. Although there is no cross-tolerance between opiates and CNS depressants, sedatives may par-tially alleviate the symptoms of opiate withdrawal. However, even large doses of methadone or heroin will not prevent sedative withdrawal.

When mixed opiate-sedative dependence is suspected, the clinician should first determine the degree of sedative dependence by using the pentobarbital tolerance test. Once this is done, the most prudent course is to maintain the patient on a dose of methadone sufficient to prevent symptoms of opiate with-drawal while gradually tapering the CNS depressants. Some have recom-mended tapering of both classes of drugs simultaneously, but this approach complicates the clinical picture.

3. Abuse of Stimulants/Amphetamines

3.1. Introduction

Currently, amphetamine and other CNS stimulants like methylphenidate are widely used in the *treatment of narcolepsy, Attention Deficit Disorder, and exogenous obesity*. Until the late 1960s, these drugs were frequently prescribed for the treatment of fatigue and depression as well. However, as their abuse potential became apparent, their prescription was placed under increased regulatory control, which, in turn, created a substantial illicit market. This has led to widespread drug substitution, so that most of what is sold "on the street" as amphetamine is often caffeine or other over-the-counter stimulants.

Many chronic amphetamine users first begin taking the drug in the context of treatment for obesity or depression. Truck drivers, students, and physicians may abuse the drugs to alleviate fatigue. With the development of tolerance, the user tends to raise the dose. Subsequently, attempts at withdrawal may produce abstinence symptoms and resumption of use.

Some amphetamine abusers use the drug intermittently, ingesting large doses in search of euphoria. Members of this group are often young, tend to abuse other drugs, and are more likely to use stimulants intravenously in the form of methamphetamine ("crystal"). With this pattern of use, the drugs may be injected many times each day in doses as high as one gram every three to four hours. Sprees of intoxication may last days or weeks and are usually followed by abrupt withdrawal ("crashing"), sometimes associated with concurrent use of barbiturates or opiates. After a period of exhaustion and sleep, amphetamine use is resumed.

3.2. Classification

A wide variety of drugs stimulate the central nervous system; a number of these have potential for serious abuse. Amphetamine and its related compounds are sympathomimetic agents: Their peripheral effects resemble that produced by stimulation of adrenergic (i.e., sympathetic) nerve endings. They also have central stimulatory effects, which contribute to their popularity as drugs of abuse. Dextroamphetamine (Dexedrine), the d-isomer of amphetamine, is three to four times as potent as the l-isomer. Other amphetamine derivatives include methamphetamine (Desoxyn), which is available in injectable form, methylphenidate (Ritalin), phenmetrazine (Preludin), and diethylpropion (Tenuate, Tepanil). This section will focus on amphetamines as examples of this class of agents.

3.3. Acute and Chronic Effects

In therapeutic doses, amphetamines produce wakefulness, mood elevation, increased mental alertness, a sense of confidence, and an increased ability to concentrate on simple tasks. Appetite is also diminished. Systolic and diastolic blood pressure are increased and heart rate is reflexly slowed. At higher doses, tremulousness, agitation, insomnia, headache, dizziness, confusion, and dysphoria occur.

With repetitive use, tolerance develops to some of the effects of the amphetamines, especially when high doses are administered frequently. The mechanism is unclear, but some have hypothesized replacement of norepinephrine stores with amphetamine metabolites, which act as "false transmitters." Tolerance develops rapidly to the mood-elevating and appetite-suppressant effects of these drugs. On the other hand, chronic low dose administration will continue to produce some stimulatory effects.

Upon sudden drug discontinuation after chronic amphetamine use, abstinence symptoms develop. These include lethargy, fatigue, and depression, along with a rebound increase in rapid eye movement (REM) sleep. These symptoms frequently set the stage for resumption of use, in what often develops into an alternating pattern of intoxication and withdrawal.

3.4. Patterns of Abuse

3.4.1. Acute Intoxication

3.4.1a. Clinical Manifestations. Serious toxic reactions from acute ingestion of amphetamine occur primarily in nontolerant (i.e., infrequent) users who consume relatively large doses (i.e., more than 60 mg/day) over a short period of time. The intoxication syndrome is characterized by restlessness, irritability, tremor, confusion, talkativeness, anxiety, and lability of mood. Peripheral effects include headache, chills, vomiting, dry mouth, and sweating. Blood pressure is variably affected and heartbeat may be irregular. In more severe cases auditory and/or visual hallucinations, seizures, and hyperpyrexia may occur.

Among intravenous methamphetamine users, prolonged episodes of intoxication ("speed runs") are accompanied by anorexia, weight loss, insomnia, and generalized deterioration in psychomotor abilities. Chronic users, while intoxicated, also exhibit a peculiar type of repetitive stereotyped behavior (e.g., taking things apart and putting them back together). Prolonged high dose use may result in hallucinations, parasitosis (i.e., picking at imaginary bugs), lability of mood, and paranoia. These individuals also are prone to episodes of unprovoked violence, especially when amphetamines are combined with barbiturates.

Tolerance to other toxic effects of amphetamine or methamphetamine varies. Some patients can become quite ill at doses of 30 mg, while chronic users may tolerate 1 g of dextroamphetamine or more. Even in chronic users, however, large doses of intravenous methamphetamine may be followed by chest pain, temporary paralysis, or simple inability to function. The conscious but "overamped" individual may experience racing thoughts coupled with euphoric mood and perhaps some degree of catatonia. Although deaths due to amphetamine overdose are relatively rare, hyperpyrexia, seizures, and shock are reported in fatal cases.

3.4.1b. Management. Treatment of acute amphetamine toxicity includes *reducing CNS irritability and autonomic nervous system hyperactivity, controlling psychotic symptoms, and promoting rapid excretion of the drug* and its metabolites. Fevers above 102° F should be treated vigorously. Seizures that occur with acute amphetamine toxicity may take the form of status epilepticus, which should be treated with diazepam 5 to 10 mg IV, injected at a rate not exceeding 5 mg per minute. This procedure may be repeated every 10 to 15 minutes as necessary to a total dose of 30 mg. Once the patient is no longer in acute distress, CNS irritability can be further reduced by avoiding excessive stimulation. The excretion of unchanged amphetamine can be enhanced by acidification of the urine. Provided there are no signs of liver or kidney failure, ammonium chloride 500 mg PO may be given every three to four hours.

Psychotic symptoms that accompany acute amphetamine toxicity are best treated by a dopamine blocking agent, like chlorpromazine or haloperidol. A test dose of chlorpromazine, 25 mg PO, may be followed by 50 mg qid until symptoms disappear, usually within 48 hours. Some patients may require larger doses. If severe agitation or aggressiveness is a problem, intramuscular administration of antipsychotic drugs should be considered. Patients receiving antipsychotics should be monitored for hypotension. In addition, illegally produced amphetamines sometimes are adulterated with anticholinergic substances, which can potentiate the anticholinergic effects of antipsychotic agents.

3.4.2. Amphetamine Withdrawal

Even without treatment, symptoms of acute amphetamine toxicity usually resolve within a week. The withdrawal period is characterized by fatigue, depression, hyperphagia and rebound increase in REM sleep. As recovery progresses, the clinician should treat the depression, which may be quite severe. The patient's potential for suicide must be evaluated. Treatment with heterocyclic antidepressants should be considered if the depression fails to lift within a few days. Although the efficacy of these drugs in reversing postamphetamine depression remains in doubt, some patients will experience depression and fatigue for several months and probably deserve a trial of antidepressant medication. In addition, patients with underlying mood disorders appear particularly vulnerable to the depression induced by amphetamine withdrawal.

3.4.3. Amphetamine-Induced Psychosis

Chronic high-dose amphetamine use may be accompanied by the development of a *toxic psychosis, which resembles paranoid schizophrenia.* In the early stages, patients are euphoric, loquacious, and overconfident in their abilities. As the syndrome progresses, suspiciousness, fear, and increased aggression are noted, along with delusions of persecution, ideas of reference, and auditory, visual, and tactile hallucinations. Bruxism, parasitosis, distorted time sense, changes in body image, and hyperactivity also are reported. Some patients exhibit compulsive, stereotyped behavior, which may appear purposeful but is characterized by doing and undoing a particular task. Unlike most toxic psychoses, confusion and disorientation are relatively absent.

In most cases of amphetamine psychosis, withdrawal of the drug is followed by slow, but complete, recovery within days to weeks. In some patients, however, psychotic symptoms may persist for years. Characteristically, there is hypermnesia for the psychotic episode, allowing the patient to describe retrospectively his condition in great detail.

Some have felt that the amphetamine psychosis occurs only in patients who are specifically predisposed to psychosis; however, the syndrome has been produced in normal volunteers given large doses of amphetamine over a five-day period. In practice, consistent use of large doses (over 100 mg per day) places the user at greater risk for the development of psychosis. Most patients who become psychotic have been taking the drug for weeks or months. Sudden increases in dosage, even in tolerant individuals, also may precipitate a psychotic episode.

As is the case with acute amphetamine intoxication, withdrawal of the drug and the use of antipsychotics (e.g., haloperidol, chlorpromazine) in doses sufficient to control symptoms is the treatment of choice for amphetamine psychosis. Once the psychosis clears (usually within several days), antipsychotic drugs should be stopped to permit clinical assessment in a drug-free state. If psychotic symptoms recur, antipsychotics can be reinstituted.

4. Abuse of CNS Stimulants/Cocaine

4.1. Introduction

The relatively high cost of illicitly acquired cocaine has contributed to its status as a drug of abuse by the middle and upper classes. The growing market for the drug, especially in urban areas, has also spawned an underground network of dealers who are often heavy users themselves. The drug is usually taken intranasally ("snorted"), although intravenous use is increasingly common. More recently, "freebasing," or smoking the alkaline precursor of cocaine, has come into vogue. Occasionally, cocaine is applied topically to the genitalia to enhance sexual excitement and delay orgasm.

The majority of cocaine users take the drug intermittently (e.g., once per week) and never experience significant physiologic or psychosocial problems. Some users, however, develop profound psychological dependence on cocaine and may experience serious emotional, social, and financial difficulties. These individuals may use the drug intensively over periods lasting days to weeks, during which time they sleep very little and remain almost continuously intoxicated.

4.2. Pharmacology

Cocaine is rapidly absorbed when administered intranasally, or by inhalation after smoking either coca paste or the alkalinized extract ("freebase"). Oral cocaine use is unusual in this country, but Andes Mountain Indians have chewed coca leaves (from which cocaine is extracted) for centuries. The usual street dose of cocaine is difficult to measure since both purity and the pattern of consumption varies widely. Fifteen to 25 mg is the usual intoxicating dose.

Following intranasal or intravenous (IV) administration, onset of action begins within two minutes. Peak effects occur at 10 to 20 minutes after intranasal use and 3 to 10 minutes after IV use. Freebase smoking results in almost immediate intoxication, but the effects last just a few minutes. With oral administration (i.e., chewing coca leaf), the rate of absorption is slower and the duration of action longer.

4.3. Acute and Chronic Effects

Perhaps no other drug has gained as much in popularity over the past decade as cocaine—a local anesthetic and CNS stimulant, whose actions resemble amphetamine but are of shorter duration and perhaps greater intensity (although research subjects who blindly compared the effects of the two drugs were unable to tell them apart).

Cocaine exerts a direct stimulatory effect on the cerebral cortex, producing excitation, restlessness, euphoria, and feelings of increased strength and mental ability. Its sympathomimetic effects include vasoconstriction, tachycardia, increased blood pressure and temperature, and dilated pupils.

In general, the subjective effects of cocaine are related to the plasma levels achieved, but the rate or rise of the plasma level also is important in determining the effects achieved. After a single dose, plasma levels fall rapidly as the drug is metabolized, both in the liver and by cholinesterase enzymes in plasma. The half-life of the drug is approximately 1 hour. The cocaine metabolite benzoylecgonine is excreted in the urine and can be detected by enzyme immunoassay up to 30 hours after the last dose.

While cocaine does not produce physical dependence in the classical sense, animal experiments suggest that the drug has powerful reinforcing properties. Clinical experience in man suggests that some users develop profound psychological dependence on cocaine and will pursue the drug experience to the exclusion of almost all other activities. In addition, hypersomnia, hyperphagia, and lassitude ("crash") seen after discontinuation of chronic use constitute a discrete withdrawal syndrome that may precipitate renewed use.

Although some chronic cocaine users may consume very large amounts of the drug, tolerance to the effects of cocaine has not been demonstrated. Indeed, some regular users may develop a "reverse tolerance" or sensitization to the drug's subjective and behavioral effects.

4.4. Patterns of Abuse

4.4.1. Acute Intoxication

Acute cocaine poisoning is most common among intravenous users, but freebasing and the smoking of coca paste also appear to be particularly hazardous modes of consumption. The symptoms are similar to those of acute amphetamine intoxication and often include intense anxiety, paranoia, and hallucinations. Elevated blood pressure, tachycardia, ventricular irritability, hyperthermia, and respiratory depression are symptomatic of more severe poisoning. Acute heart failure, stroke, and seizures also have been reported. Death from these complications is rare but can occur.

Initial treatment of acute cocaine poisoning should emphasize *general life-support measures*, including establishment of an airway, stabilization of the circulatory system, and reduction of severely elevated body temperature. Manifestations of sympathetic nervous system hyperactivity, such as hypertension, tachycardia, and tachypnea, may be treated with propranolol (Inderal, Inderide) 1 mg IV injected slowly q 1 minute for up to 8 minutes. Patients in hypertensive crisis who do not respond to this regimen may be given sodium nitroprusside (Nipride) or phentolamine (Regitine). Intravenous diazepam can be used in patients with repeated seizures. Once the patient is stabilized medically, chlorpromazine or haloperidol may be used to treat any psychotic symptoms that remain.

4.4.2. Sequelae of Chronic Cocaine Abuse

Infrequent cocaine use, even when sustained over a long period of time, usually does not lead to serious complications. Chronic heavy users, however, may develop perceptual disturbances, including auditory, visual, or tactile hallucinations (e.g., "cocaine bugs" crawling under the skin) as part of a paranoid psychosis similar to that seen in chronic amphetamine users. Heavy intranasal use may lead to chronic inflammation or ulceration of the nasal mucosa, and occasionally septal perforation. Smoking of freebase cocaine may impair pulmonary diffusing capacity. Patients with underlying affective disorder, e.g., recurrent depression, sometimes remain undiagnosed and untreated when the sequale of stimulant abuse cloud the clinical picture.

5. Abuse of Hallucinogens

5.1. Introduction

The hallucinogens are a group of structurally similar agents that produce perceptual distortions (primarily visual illusions and hallucinations) and enhance awareness of internal and external stimuli. Mundane events seem unusually important and the user experiences a tendency toward introspection and profound emotional lability. Because these drugs produce a state that mimics functional psychosis, some have referred to these substances as "psychedelic" (i.e., "mind-expanding") or "psychotomimetic." However, this similarity is superficial.

Though they were popular in the late 1960s, the prevalence of hallucinogen abuse has declined in recent years. The drugs have by no means disappeared, however, and the adverse consequences of their use are still apparent in emergency settings. Moreover, drugs sold on the street as hallucinogens often contain other agents (e.g., amphetamine, phencyclidine), so that patients who present with a "bad trip" presumably from mescaline may, in fact, be suffering from a PCP-induced psychosis.

5.2. Classification

The commonly abused hallucinogenic substances include the *indolealkylamines* like d-lysergic acid diethylamide (LSD), psilocybin, and dimethyltryptamine (DMT), which bear a structural resemblance to the neurotransmitter 5-hydroxytryptamine (serotonin); the *phenylethylamines* like mescaline; and the phenylisopropylamines like 2,5-dimethoxy-4-methylamphetamine (DOM, "STP"). The latter two types are structurally related to dopamine, norepinephrine, and the amphetamines.

The commonly abused hallucinogens and their important properties are summarized in Table 4. Since it is the best known from a pharmacologic and clinical standpoint and is the most commonly abused hallucinogen, we will focus primarily on LSD.

5.3. d-Lysergic Acid Diethylamide (LSD)

5.3.1. Pharmacology

LSD is a synthetic hallucinogen derived from an extract of the ergot fungus. It is the most potent hallucinogen, with intoxication resulting from doses as low as 50 micrograms. The drug is colorless, odorless, and tasteless. It is usually ingested as part of a pill or dissolved on a piece of paper. Occasionally, it is administered intravenously. Following oral administration, the drug is well absorbed from the gastrointestinal tract and distributed to body tissues. Only small amounts are detected in the brain, however. The plasma half-life of LSD is two to three hours. It is metabolized into nonhallucinogenic substances, primarily by conjugation in the liver.

5.3.2. Tolerance and Physical Dependence

With repeated administration, tolerance develops within two to four days to the behavioral effects of LSD. As a result, even chronic users do not take the drug more than twice a week, and the vast majority take it less frequently. Considerable cross-tolerance exists between LSD and the other hallucinogens. LSD users do not develop physical dependence, nor do they develop withdrawal symptoms after àbstinence. Only one fatality has been directly linked to an LSD overdose, although fatal accidents and suicides may occur during periods of intoxication.

5.3.3. Acute Intoxication

The effects of LSD begin 20 to 60 minutes after ingestion, depending on the amount ingested and the degree of tolerance developed by the user. Sym-

Table 4. Commonly Abused Hallucinogenic Drugs

Drug	Source	Psychedelic dose	Peak symptoms	Duration of action	Prominent somatic effects	Prominent psychological effects
d-lysergic acid diethylamide	Synthetic (from fungi)	50 mcg	2 to 3 hr	8 to 12 hr undulating activity as effect declines	Increased sympathetic nervous system activity: dilated pupils, increased BP, pulse, deep tendon reflexes, temperature, blood sugar, tremor	Hypervigilance, illusions, emotional lability, loss of body boundaries, time slowing, increased intensity of all sensations
Psilocybin	Mushroom	10 mg	90 min	4 to 6 hr	Like LSD, but milder	Like LSD, but less intense, more visual, more euphoria; paranoia
Dimethyltryptamine (DMT)	Synthetic	50 mg	5 to 20 min	30 to 60 min	Like LSD, but with more intense sympathomimetic symptoms	Like LSD, but usually more intense, in part because of sudden onset; must be smoked or injected; cannot be taken orally
Mescaline	Peyote cactus	200 mg	2 to 3 hr	8 to 12 hr	Nausea, vomiting; otherwise like LSD, perhaps more intense sympathomimetic effects	Like LSD but perhaps more sensory and perceptual changes; euphoria prominent
Dimethoxymethylamphetamine (DOM, "STP")	Synthetic	5 mg	3 to 5 hr	6 to 8 hr at doses below 5 mg; 16 to 24 hr at high doses (10 to 30 mg)	Minimal effects at low dose; autonomic effects prominent at doses above 5 mg	May resemble amphetamine combined with LSD, but long-lasting; high incidence of flashbacks, psychosis; chlorpromazine may aggravate symptoms

pathomimetic effects include tachycardia, increased blood pressure and body temperature, and pupillary dilation. Hyperreflexia, nausea, and muscle weakness also are observed. Peak effects occur between two and three hours after ingestion. Visual illusions, wavelike perceptual changes, macropsia or micropsia, and extreme emotional lability dominate this period. Perceptions in one sensory modality may affect or overflow into another (synesthesias) so that colors are "heard" and sounds "seen." Subjective time is slowed, and a generalized loss of body and ego boundaries is experienced. There also is a tendency toward increased fantasy production, diminished ego function, and feelings of depersonalization. In such a state, the lack of a supportive environment or companion can be detrimental, as the individual struggles to control his anxiety and prevent ego disintegration. As the effects of the drug begin to wane (i.e., 4 to 6 hours after ingestion), the patient experiences intermittent "waves of normalcy." After 8 to 12 hours, the intoxication syndrome is mostly cleared, although aftereffects, including a sense of psychic numbness, may last for days.

5.3.4. Adverse Reactions following Use of LSD or Other Hallucinogens

5.3.4a. Panic Reactions. As summarized in Table 5, the major hazards of hallucinogen use are psychological. The most common adverse reaction is a temporary episode of panic (a "bad trip"). The likelihood of panic is determined by the expectations or "set" of the individual taking the drug, the setting in which the drug is taken, the user's current level of psychological health, and the type and dose of the drug administered. Inexperienced users and those who are constricted, schizoid, or anxious, and who fear loss of control have difficulty coping with the disorganizing effects of these drugs. Taking the drug alone or in an unfamiliar or hostile setting also seems to predispose to panic.

Fortunately, most panic reactions are limited to the duration of action of the particular drug. Since there are no known methods for rapidly eliminating hallucinogenic substances from the body, the primary goal of treatment is to support the patient through this period (usually less than 24 hours), mostly by reassuring him that he is not "losing his mind" and that he will soon return to his normal state. The presence of calm, supportive friends can be very helpful. Such patients should not be left alone. When support and reassurance are ineffective and the patient is severely agitated, diazepam, 10 to 30 mg PO can be helpful. In most patients, psychotropic medication is not necessary.

5.3.4b. Toxic Delirium. Some hallucinogen users experience an acute toxic confusional state characterized by hallucinations, delusions, agitation, disorientation, and paranoia. In this state, assaults and inadvertent suicide attempts may take place (e.g., if the patient believes he can fly or stop a speeding train). No prior history of mental disorder, visual rather than auditory hallucinations, and the presence of some degree of observing ego suggest a diagnosis of toxic drug reaction, as opposed to schizophrenia.

Table 5. Adverse Reactions to Hallucinogens

Type	Duration	Predisposing factors	Treatment
Acute panic	2 to 24 hours	Obsessional character, large dose, inexperienced user	Support, reassurance, diazepam if necessary
Toxic delirium	2 to 24 hours	Large dose, idiosyncratic response	Support, reassurance, antipsychotics or diazepam if necessary
Drug-precipitated functional psychosis	Indefinite	Vulnerability to schizophrenia or affective disorder	Antipsychotics only after 48 hours
Flashbacks	Minutes to hours	Recent (< six months) use of a hallucinogen; use of marijuana or amphetamines	Reassurance; usually brief and not as intense as original experience

As in the case of any toxic delirium, the primary aim is to support the patient through the period of drug effect. In a majority of users, symptoms will subside gradually as the drug is metabolized. Diazepam may be effective in the treatment of associated anxiety, but it can also cloud the clinical picture and should be prescribed only when support and reassurance are ineffective. Phenothiazines must be given with caution, especially if atropine-type drugs may have been ingested. Haloperidol might be a better choice in such cases. At times, physical restraint also may be necessary to prevent the patient from harming himself or others. Untreated patients usually become mentally clear within 24 hours (as the drug is metabolized) with no obvious sequelae.

5.3.4c. Drug-Precipitated Functional Psychosis. Another untoward effect of hallucinogen use is psychosis that fails to clear after the drug is metabolized. This occurs primarily in patients with underlying affective disorder or schizophrenia, some of whom may use these drugs in the hope of achieving psychic reintegration or an anxiety-free state. Such patients often become more disorganized by the drug experience. Treatment may include judicious use of antipsychotic drugs and, when indicated, lithium and/or antidepressants. Following resolution of the acute psychotic episode, attention should be directed toward the precipitants for drug use.

5.3.4d. Recurrent Drug Experiences ("Flashbacks"). A fourth adverse consequence of hallucinogen use is the spontaneous recurrence of drug effects a few days to several months after the last drug experience. These "flashbacks," lasting a few seconds to several hours, can be precipitated by internal or external stress unrelated to drug use, or by use of marijuana or amphetamines. They are characterized by perceptual distortions, feelings of depersonalization, and emotional lability. Some patients respond to flashbacks with anxiety, depression, and paranoia; others enjoy them. Treatment consists of firm reassurance that the flashback will pass. In some cases, antianxiety agents like diazepam (10–20 mg PO) are helpful.

6. Phencyclidine (PCP) Abuse

6.1. Introduction

Phencyclidine (PCP, "angel dust," "hog," crystal joints, rocket fuel), a commonly used animal tranquilizer, has recently achieved considerable popularity among adolescent and young adult drug users. Phencyclidine abuse has become quite widespread in recent years, with approximately one of six young adults between ages 18 and 25 having used the drug knowingly, and more having taken the drug unwittingly in the form of adulterated marijuana or "LSD." Because of its behavioral toxicity, street samples of the drug have been shown to contain nearly 30 analogues of PCP; several are many times more potent per milligram than PCP. The drug poses a significant public health problem, with deaths resulting from drug-induced violence, suicide, and accidents.

6.2. Pharmacology

While classified as a dissociative anesthetic, PCP has stimulant, depressant, hallucinogenic, or analgesic effects, depending upon the dose and route of administration. Phencyclidine is usually administered by dissolving the drug onto marijuana or tobacco and then smoking the mixture. It can also be taken orally, intranasally, or intravenously. The drug is well absorbed via each of these routes, although absorption after oral ingestion may be slow. Phencyclidine is metabolized in the liver and stored in fatty tissues.

Behavioral tolerance occurs with chronic use, but physical dependence has not been reported. Although the serum half-life is generally about 45 minutes at low doses, the half-life may be as long as three days after an overdose; this is due to sequestration of PCP in brain and adipose tissue. Phencyclidine is a weak base with a PKa of about 8.5; thus, the drug is increasingly soluble in more acidic aqueous solutions. Acidification of the urine will, therefore, enhance excretion of PCP.

6.3. Acute Intoxication

In low doses (5 mg or less), PCP exerts a depressant effect on the central nervous system, resembling alcohol intoxication with muscular incoordination, generalized numbness of the extremities, and a "blank stare" appearance with mild ptosis of the lids. Ocular findings include vertical or horizontal nystagmus, miotic or normal-sized reactive pupils, and an absent corneal reflex. Impaired perception, mild analgesia, and various forms of motor disturbances are also seen. Higher doses (5 to 10 mg) produce nystagmus, slurred speech, ataxia, hyperreflexia, increased muscle tone, and catalepsy. Severe overdose (greater than 20 mg) may result in hypertensive crisis, muscular rigidity, seizures, respiratory depression, coma, and death.

The subjective effects of PCP include changes in body image, feelings of dissociation, perceptual distortions, auditory and visual hallucinations, and feelings of "nothingness." The behavioral state induced resembles the effects of sensory deprivation. Amnesia for the period of intoxication (usually four to six hours) is a frequent occurrence.

Many PCP users experience some degree of mood elevation, but feelings of anxiety are common as well. Indeed, most regular users report unwanted effects (most commonly perceptual disturbances, restlessness, disorientation, and anxiety) during each period of intoxication, while desired experiences (e.g., increased sensitivity to external stimuli, dissociation, stimulation, and elevated mood) occur only 60% of the time on the drug. This has led clinicians and researchers to wonder why so many people continue to take a drug that they find largely unpleasant. Major theories proposed have cited the reinforcing properties of the risks of a PCP experience and the fact that phencyclidine, if nothing else, alters consciousness profoundly. For many polydrug abusers (which most PCP users are), the degree of alteration in affective state is far more important than the type of alteration.

Patients acutely intoxicated with phencyclidine generally arrive at an emergency setting because they have aroused the concern of people around them. These patients are often confused and disoriented and may display bizarre posturing or catatonia. They may seem apprehensive and anxious or euphoric. Slurred speech is common, and the patients often appear to stare blankly into space. Increased bronchial and salivary secretions are common, as are systolic hypertension, horizontal or vertical nystagmus, and ataxia. The symptom picture of bizarre behavior with nystagmus, hypertension, and drooling strongly suggests a diagnosis of PCP intoxication.

Once the diagnosis is made, treatment efforts should be directed toward calming the patient, ensuring the patient's and the staff's safety, and treating any medical complications that arise. The patient should be placed in isolation in a "quiet room," which will decrease external stimulation; restraints may be necessary if the patient is combative or self-destructive. Diazepam (10 to 20 mg PO or 2.5 mg IV) may be useful in decreasing agitation and muscle hypertonicity. Since the patient may also have taken CNS depressants, diazepam should be used cautiously. To increase PCP excretion, the patient may be given cranberry juice or oral ascorbic acid (0.5 to 1.5 g). Nasogastric suctioning should only be carried out with extreme caution since PCP may predispose the patient to laryngospasm. Because of the risk of seizures, ipecac should not be used. Hypertensive crisis may be treated with diazoxide (Hyperstat, Proglycem), and status epilepticus, should it occur, is best treated with intravenous diazepam.

Most people improve within several hours after PCP ingestion. However, a patient should be observed until his sensorium has cleared, his vital signs are stable, and he is no longer combative or agitated.

6.4. PCP Overdose

PCP overdose is differentiated from simple intoxication primarily by the level of consciousness of the patient; the patient who has overdosed will be stuporous or comatose. Hypertension is frequently present and may be severe, respirations may be decreased, and seizures (sometimes leading to status epilepticus) are frequently seen. Horizontal and vertical nystagmus are always present, and muscle tone is increased.

Treatment consists of (1) maintenance of adequate oxygenation, (2) treatment of hypertensive crisis, if present, with diazoxide or hydralazine (Apresoline and others), and (3) use of intravenous diazepam if necessary for seizures. In severe overdose the half-life can be as long as 3 days, so that coma may last from several hours to 10 days.

Acidification of the urine facilitates drug excretion. This may be accomplished by administering ammonium chloride via nasogastric tube in a dose of 2.75 mEq/kg in 60 cc of saline solution every six hours, along with intravenous ascorbic acid (2 gm/500 cc IV fluid every six hours) until the urine pH drops below 5. For comatose patients, ammonium chloride should be given IV, 2.75 mEq/kg as a 1 to 2% solution in saline. When the urinary pH has reached 5, furosemide 20 to 50 mg IV should be given to promote further drug excretion. This may be repeated once if necessary.

6.5. PCP Psychosis

In some vulnerable individuals, PCP can produce psychotic symptoms that may persist for days or weeks after the last dose. Although this reaction occurs primarily in novice users, it may also occur in chronic users taking moderate to high doses regularly. It is also more likely to occur in patients with a history of prior schizophrenic episodes, even those who are being maintained on antipsychotic drugs.

Generally, the course of PCP psychosis may be divided into three phases, each lasting about five days. The initial phase of the psychosis, typically the most severe, is often characterized by *paranoid delusions, hyperactivity, anorexia, insomnia, agitation or catalepsy, and unpredictable assaultiveness.* During this time, patients are extremely sensitive to external stimuli. In the mixed phase of the psychosis, paranoia and restlessness remain, but the patient is usually calmer and intermittently in control of his behavior. In the absence of further drug use, the next one to two weeks are usually characterized by gradual reintegration and resolution of symptoms. However, in some patients psychotic symptoms may persist for months. Depression is also a common sequela of PCP psychosis.

The treatment of PCP psychosis is aimed at maintaining the physical safety of the patient and others, decreasing psychotic thinking with the use of antipsychotic drugs, and promoting rapid excretion of the drug through acidification of the urine. If drug ingestion has been relatively recent, gastric lavage may also be helpful. Injury prevention may be accomplished by prompt hospitalization and the use of a "quiet room" to reduce external sensory input. *Unlike hallucinogen users on "bad trips," patients intoxicated with PCP do not respond well to "talking down."* The use of antipsychotic drugs with significant anticholinergic effects (e.g., chlorpromazine) should be avoided since they may potentiate the anticholinergic effects of phencyclidine. *Haloperidol*, 5 mg IM given hourly as needed, may be useful, although response to treatment is often slow. Use of antipsychotics in conjunction with procedures designed to lower tissue levels of the drug may hasten recovery. Most patients are substantially better after two to three weeks of treatment—sooner if the drug can be rapidly eliminated from the body.

7. Marijuana Use and Abuse

7.1. Introduction

Marijuana, a plant used for recreational and medicinal purposes for centuries, is still widely popular today. The term *marijuana* refers to the dried leaves and flowers of the Indian hemp plant *Cannabis sativa*, which grows freely in warm climates and has psychoactive effects when smoked or ingested. Recent surveys suggest that between 40 and 45 million people over the age of 12 have tried marijuana at least once, including 60% of those between the ages of 18 and 25.

The majority of marijuana users (approximately 60%) may be classified as experimenters who give up the drug shortly after their initial experience. Another 35% use marijuana once or twice per week. The remaining 5% use the drug from several times per week to every day.

Most studies have demonstrated that casual users cannot be differentiated from nonusers on psychological tests or measures of psychomotor performance. On the other hand, heavy users (defined as those who smoke nearly every day) manifest an increased prevalence of all types of psychopathology. The use of other psychoactive substances, including alcohol, also is more frequent. On the other hand, there is no evidence that marijuana use *per se* leads directly to "harder" drugs. Clinical experience with chronic users suggests that some use the drug to treat predrug psychopathology. Most marijuana users who present to the ER have experienced an adverse reaction (see Table 6).

7.2. Pharmacology

Although marijuana has both stimulant and sedative properties and will produce hallucinations when taken in high enough doses, pharmacologically it appears to be in a class by itself. The plant is extremely complex, containing over 400 identifiable compounds. The principal psychoactive ingredient, however, appears to be delta-9-tetrahydrocannabinol (THC), which is found in highest concentration in the small upper leaves and flowering tops of the plant. Hashish, a dried, concentrated resinous exudate of the flowers, is several times more potent.

In this country, marijuana cigarettes ("joints") generally contain 0.5 to 1 g of marijuana leaf with an average THC content of 1 to 2% (i.e., 5 to 20 mg). During smoking, the degree of absorption varies, but the average experienced user will absorb approximately half the total dose into the bloodstream. Drug effects are noticeable almost immediately and reach peak intensity within 30 minutes. Speed of onset is partly determined by the concentration of THC in the preparation. After an hour, plasma levels begin to decline, and most of the subjective effects disappear by three hours after the last dose. Oral administration of marijuana is generally 20 to 30% as effective as smoking in delivering THC to the bloodstream. Onset of action also is slower (30 to 60 minutes after ingestion), but the subjective effects persist for a longer period of time (three to five hours). Predictably, the rate of absorption is influenced by the food content of the stomach. Following administration by either route, THC leaves the blood rapidly, as a result of both hepatic metabolism and efficient uptake by body tissues. THC is stored in fat depots, where it may remain for two to three weeks.

Daily use of marijuana may result in the development of tolerance, especially in those who consume more than five "joints" per day. This finding

Table 6. Adverse Reactions to Marijuana

Type	Predisposing factors	Symptoms	Treatment
Acute panic	Inexperienced users, hysterical or obsessional characters, oral administration	Anxiety, depression, no psychotic symptoms	Reassurance; occasionally anxiolytics; episode usually short-lived
Toxic delirium	Large dose, oral use	Confusion, disorientation, hallucinations, depersonalization, delusions	Most remit in 12 to 48 hours; antipsychotics if necessary
Flashbacks	Days or weeks after last dose, prior history of hallucinogenic use	Like hallucinogenic experience except brief	Reassurance; anxiolytics if necessary
Chronic psychosis	Prolonged heavy use of very potent marijuana or hashish; rare in U.S.	Paranoia, delusions, hallucinations, panic, bizarre behavior, occasionally violence	Antipsychotics
Amotivational syndrome	Prolonged heavy use; existence of syndrome is controversial	Apathy, decreased attention span, poor judgment, poor interpersonal relations	No known treatment

contrasts with earlier theories that experienced marijuana users exhibited "reverse tolerance," i.e., a greater sensitivity to the drug after repeated use. The latter phenomenon may be more a function of social learning than a drug effect. Mild physical dependence has also been demonstrated in heavy users. Withdrawal symptoms include restlessness, irritability, sleep disturbance, anorexia, sweating, tremor, nausea, vomiting, and diarrhea.

7.3. Acute Intoxication

7.3.1. Subjective Effects

As with other drugs, the clinical effects following a dose of marijuana depend on the strength of the preparation, route of administration, individual variables (e.g., metabolic rate, prior drug experience, and personal expectations), and the setting in which the drug is consumed.

Shortly after inhalation and absorption through the lungs, users experience a sense of well-being or euphoria, accompanied by feelings of friendliness and relaxation. Intoxicated persons also develop an altered time sense, or "temporal disintegration," a state in which the past, present, and future become fused. While awareness of their environment may be heightened, they may have less ability to communicate; their speech is often disconnected and tangential, and some smokers become remote and withdrawn. Thought processes are slowed, short-term memory is often impaired, and users have difficulty concentrating. Some feel that they have achieved special insights, others find mundane events more humorous or more poignant, and there is accompanying emotional lability.

7.3.2. Physiologic Changes

Two reliable signs of marijuana intoxication are increased heart rate and conjunctival injection. The rise in heart rate is directly related to the dose of THC. Decreases in salivation, intraocular pressure, and skin temperature also are found, and at high doses orthostatic hypotension can occur. Bronchodilation occurs acutely, but chronic marijuana smoking may result in obstructive pulmonary disease similar to that seen in tobacco smokers.

7.3.3. Cognitive and Psychomotor Effects

Various authors have studied the effect of marijuana on intellectual and psychomotor performance. Generally, naive and casual users given the drug in a laboratory setting demonstrate deterioration in both areas, probably because of memory disruption. Impairment is dose-related and dependent on the complexity of the task. More experienced users, however, are able to compensate for the acute intoxicating effects of THC. In most users, driving performance is impaired, with frequent misjudgment of speed and longer time required for braking.

7.4. Adverse Reactions following Marijuana Use

7.4.1. Acute Panic

Considering the extent of usage, the incidence of adverse reactions to marijuana use is quite low. The most common are summarized in Table 6. Panic can occur in inexperienced users; the likelihood is related to the dose of THC, the expectations of the user, and the setting in which the drug is taken. The tachycardia, disconnected thoughts, and paranoid ideation that often accompany marijuana use may precipitate panic attacks. A panic state may simulate acute psychosis, but careful examination reveals that the patient is not disoriented or hallucinating, and his ability to test reality is intact; he is aware that his condition is drug-related. In some patients, depression may be more prominent than anxiety.

The treatment of panic centers around firm reassurance in a nonthreatening environment. The patient is told that his symptoms have been caused by a strong dose of marijuana and that he will recover within several hours. Physical restraints, seclusion, or administration of antipsychotic drugs can exacerbate the problem. As drug effects subside, panic wanes, and the person, though shaken, regains control. The persistence of THC metabolites may cause some patients to feel intermittently intoxicated for several days.

7.4.2. Toxic Delirium

Following large doses of marijuana, taken either orally or by inhalation, users may experience psychic disorganization, accompanied by feelings of depersonalization and changes in perception and body image. Some patients are disoriented, with marked memory impairment. Confusion, derealization, paranoia, visual and auditory hallucinations, and dysphoria are also features of this toxic delirium. Individuals usually remain aware that these effects are drug-related. Toxic delirium is more likely after cannabis is ingested, perhaps due to the user's inability to titrate adequately the dose of THC. In most cases, the process is self-limited and lasts from a few hours to a few days; it resolves as plasma THC levels decline. Generally, no pharmacologic treatment is indicated, but patients should be carefully observed and prevented from doing harm to themselves or others.

7.4.3. Recurrent Reactions ("Flashbacks")

Although more characteristic of LSD, recurrent marijuana experiences, occurring days or weeks after the last dose, have been reported. Such phenomena are more common in individuals who have previously used hallucinogens. Flashbacks are rare in patients who last used the drug more than six months ago. When these reactions occur long after the last drug use, a psychiatric or neurologic disorder should be suspected, particularly if symptoms continue beyond several hours.

7.4.4. Sequelae of Chronic Use

7.4.4a. Cannabis Psychosis. In Western countries psychosis directly attributable to chronic cannabis use is rare. In Middle Eastern and Asian countries, however, chronic use of more potent marijuana or hashish (the concentrated resin) reportedly may result in a cannabis-induced psychosis. The clinical picture comprises paranoia, persecutory delusions, visual and auditory hallucinations, panic, bizarre behavior, and occasional aggressive outbursts. The role of preexisting psychopathology in these patients is unclear. Patients with this disorder usually respond quickly to treatment with antipsychotic drugs, although relapse is common upon resumption of cannabis use.

7.4.4b. Amotivational Syndrome. A number of authors have described an "amotivational syndrome," which develops gradually in chronic heavy marijuana users. It is characterized by decreased drive and ambition, a shortened attention span, poor judgment, a high degree of distractability, impaired communication skills, and diminished effectiveness in interpersonal situations. A tendency toward introversion and magical thinking also has been observed. The individual frequently feels incapacitated and makes few or no plans beyond the present day. Personal habits deteriorate, there is a progressive loss of insight, and feelings of depersonalization persist. Aggression is profoundly diminished, and, as a result, these patients appear apathetic and withdrawn rather than antisocial. The contribution of predrug psychopathology in this syndrome remains unclear. Indeed, some authors doubt the existence of the amotivational syndrome, since studies of chronic marijuana smokers in Jamaica, Costa Rica, and Greece found no difference in work output as the extent of use increased.

8. Inhalant Abuse

8.1. Introduction

Inhalants tend to be popular drugs of abuse among boys in their early teens, especially in poor and rural areas, where other, more expensive drugs of abuse are less available. Although the prevalence of inhalant abuse decreases with age, many users go on to abuse other drugs. Most commonly, the volatile gases are inhaled from a handkerchief or rag that has been soaked with the solvent material. Glue squirted into a paper gives off a vapor that can then be inhaled. Aerosol spray cans are a source of volatile hydrocarbons and nitrous oxide.

The inhalants constitute a heterogeneous group of volatile organic solvents that have profound toxic effects on the CNS. Some of the commonly inhaled substances and their major active ingredients include glues and paint thinners (toluene), lighter fluid (naphtha), aerosols (fluorinated hydrocarbons, nitrous oxide), cleaning solutions (trichlorethylene, carbon tetrachloride), and gasoline (benzene).

8.2. Acute Intoxication

High lipid solubility and rapid passage across the blood-brain barrier account for the rapidly intoxicating effects of the inhalants. Drug effects last up to 45 minutes, depending on the degree of exposure. The clinical picture resembles that of alcohol intoxication and includes euphoria, giddiness, and light-headedness. Irritation of the nasal mucosa, conjunctivitis, and unusual breath odor also suggest the diagnosis. Depending upon the solvent used, various toxic effects also may occur. These include induction of cardiac arrhythmias, hypoxia, seizures, and death. Tolerance to the effects of inhalants develops rather quickly, but no cross-tolerance occurs among the various solvents. Although physical dependence has not been documented, a syndrome resembling delirium tremens has been noted in some chronic users who stop using these agents abruptly. Abdominal pain, paresthesias, and headaches also can occur during drug-free periods. Strong psychological dependence often develops in inhalant abusers and accounts for much of the difficulty in treating these individuals.

8.3. Treatment Approaches

Chronic solvent abusers are notoriously difficult to treat due to the combined effects of low socioeconomic status, family problems, school failure, antisocial behavior, and brain damage. The aim of the emergency intervention should be to treat any medical problem and attempt to engage the patient in an ongoing treatment program. Therapeutic communities emphasizing work programs, remedial education, and other reality-based therapies may offer the best chance of success with these patients. Behavior modification programs may be useful in treating chronic relapsing behavior.

9. Summary

The epidemic spread of substance abuse is a phenomenon best understood through an eclectic perspective. The behavior of individuals who abuse one or more psychoactive substances is partially the result of developmental, sociocultural, and interpersonal factors. In some patients, genetic and/or biological factors may influence vulnerability as well. Although some have suggested that particular personality traits predispose to the development of drug abuse and dependence, some traits (e.g., passivity, manipulativeness, inability to tolerate frustration) may result from repetitive drug use and the drug-using life-style. Similarly, although the development of insight and the resolution of intrapsychic conflicts are clearly desirable goals, no hard data suggest that insight, by itself, leads to a decline in drug-using behavior.

A number of investigators have focused on the interaction between the effects of abused drugs and individual psychopathology. Thus, substance abusers have been viewed as self-medicating feelings of depression and tension while modifying internal drive states and avoiding the stark unpleasantness of the real world. However, clinical and laboratory studies of substance abusers have consistently found that although all these drugs serve as primary reinforcers in both animals and man, their chronic administration usually results in a host of unpleasant consequences. These may be subtle, like the effects of chronic marijuana use on ambition, or they may be dramatic, like the psychosis that often accompanies long-term PCP use.

Recently, there has been growing interest in the behavioral aspects of substance abuse disorders. Clearly, in some patients phenomena like conditioned abstinence contribute to drug-seeking behavior and relapse. Consequently, patients and their doctors must learn to anticipate the impact of environmental stimuli that may enhance craving and lead to renewed drug use. At the same time, the clinician should attempt to reshape attitudes and behavior through psychotherapy, group pressure, role modeling, and other techniques of social learning. The relative success of self-help organizations like Alcoholics Anonymous is clear testimony to the usefulness of providing concrete guidelines for behavioral change in a supportive setting.

Finally, biological approaches to substance abuse, although appealingly cost-effective, also have their pitfalls. In methadone maintenance programs, for example, some opiate addicts become alcoholics, and others spend their time diverting methadone to the street market. The narcotic antagonists, although pharmacologically effective, are not very popular with most opiate users. Disulfiram, an effective deterrent to impulsive drinking, is ineffective by itself in maintaining long-term abstinence.

In summary, substance abuse is an extremely complex and multidetermined behavior, and the treatment of substance abusers presents a bewildering array of theoretical and practical problems. Those who seek to alter such behavior need to recognize this and devise equally complex and multidisciplinary approaches to treatment. As in other areas of medicine, the doctor's adherence to dogma can be hazardous to the patient's health.

Bibliography

Opiates

Cushman P: The major medical sequelae of opioid addiction. *Drug Alcohol Dependence* 5:239–254, 1980.

Dole VP: Narcotic addiction, physical dependence and relapse. *N. Engl J Med* 286(18):988–992, 1972.

Gold, MS, Pottash ALC, Sweeney DR, Kleber HD, Redmond DE Jr: Rapid opiate detoxification: Clinical evidence of antidepressant and antipanic effects of opiates. *Am J Psychiatry* 136(7):982–986, 1979.

Goldstein A: Heroin addiction: Sequential treatment employing pharmacologic supports. *Arch Gen Psychiatry* 33:353–358, 1976.

Goldstein A: Heroin addiction and the role of methadone in its treatment. *Arch Gen Psychiatry* 26:291–297, 1972.

Jaffe JH: Drug addiction and drug abuse, in *The Pharmacological Basis of Therapeutics*. Goodman LS, Gilman A (eds): New York; Macmillan Co, 1980, chap 23, pp 535–584.

Jaffe JH, Martin WR: Opioid analgesics and antagonists, in *The Pharmacological Basis of Therapeutics*. Goodman LS, Gilman A (eds): New York; Macmillan Co, 1980, chap 22, pp 494–534.

Kleber HD, Slobetz F: Outpatient drug-free treatment, in *Handbook on Drug Abuse*. DuPont RL, Goldstein A, O'Donnell J (eds): Rockville, Md, National Institute on Drug Abuse, 1979, pp 31–38.

Ling W, Blaine JD: The use of LAAM in treatment, in *Handbook on Drug Abuse*. DuPont RL, Goldstein A, O'Donnell J (eds): Rockville, Md, National Institute on Drug Abuse, 1979, pp. 87–96.

Martin WR, Jasinski DR, Mansky PA: Naltrexone, an antagonist for the treatment of heroin dependence. *Arch Gen Psychiatry* 28:784–791, 1973.

Mello NK, Mendelson JH: Buprenorphine suppresses heroin use by heroin addicts. *Science* 207:657–659, 1980.

Meyer RE, Mirin SM: *The Heroin Stimulus: Implications for a Theory of Addiction*. New York; Plenum Medical Book Co, 1979.

Mirin SM, Meyer RE, Mendelson JH, Ellingboe J: Opiate use and sexual function. *Am J Psychiatry* 137(8):909–915, 1980.

Mirin SM, Meyer RE, McNamee HB: Psychopathology and mood during heroin use. *Arch Gen Psychiatry* 33:1503–1508, 1976.

National Research Council Committee on Clinical Evaluation of Narcotic Antagonists: Clinical evaluation of Naltrexone treatment of opiate-dependent individuals. *Arch Gen Psychiatry* 35:335–340, 1978.

Resnick RB, Schuyten-Resnick E, Washton AM: Treatment of opioid dependence with narcotic antagonists: A review and commentary, in DuPont RL, Goldstein, A, O'Donnell J (eds): *Handbook on Drug Abuse*. Rockville, Md, National Institute on Drug Abuse, 1979, pp 76–104.

Snyder SH: The opiate receptor and morphine-like peptides in the brain. *Am J Psychiatry* 135:645–652, 1978.

Stimmel B, Adamsons K: Narcotic dependency in pregnancy: Methadone maintenance compared to use of street drugs, *JAMA* 235:1121–1124, 1976.

U.S. Department of Health, Education, and Welfare: Public Health Service: Alcohol, Drug Abuse, and Mental Health Administration. Clinical management during pregnancy, in *Drug Dependence in Pregnancy: Clinical Management of Mother and Child*, National Institute on Drug Abuse, Services Research Monograph Series, Washington, US Government Printing Office, 1979, chap 3.

U.S. Department of Health, Education, and Welfare: Public Health Service: Alcohol, Drug Abuse, and Mental Health Administration. Management of labor, delivery, and the immediate postpartum period, in *Drug Dependence in Pregnancy: Clinical Management of Mother and Child*, National Institute on Drug Abuse, Services Research Monograph Series. Washington, US Government Printing Office, 1979, chap 4.

CNS Depressants

Cronin RJ, Klingler EL Jr, Avashti PS, Lubash GD: The treatment of nonbarbiturate sedative overdosage, in Browne PG (ed): *A Treatment Manual for Acute Drug Abuse Emergencies* Rockville, Md, National Institute on Drug Abuse, 1974, pp 58–62.

Dorpat TL: Drug automatism, barbiturate poisoning, and suicide behavior. *Arch Gen Psychiatry* 31:216–220, 1974.

Greenblatt DJ, Shader RI: Drug therapy: Benzodiazepines (First of two parts). *N Engl J Med*, 291(19):1011–1243, 1974.

Harvey SC: Hypnotics and sedatives, in Goodman LS, Gilman A (eds): *The Pharmacological Basis of Therapeutics*, New York; Macmillan Co, 1980, chap 17, pp 339–375.

Setter JG: Emergency treatment of acute barbiturate intoxication, in Browne PG (ed): *A Treatment Manual for Acute Drug Abuse Emergencies*, Rockville, Md, National Institute on Drug Abuse, 1974, pp 49–53.

Smith DE, Wesson DR, Seymour RB: The abuse of barbiturates and other sedative-hypnotics, in DuPont RL, Goldstein A, O'Donnell J (eds): *Handbook on Drug Abuse*. Rockville, Md, National Institute on Drug Abuse, 1979, pp 233–240.

Wesson DR, Smith DE: Managing the barbiturate withdrawal syndrome, in Browne PG (ed): *A Treatment Manual for Acute Drug Abuse Emergencies*. Rockville, Md, National Institute on Drug Abuse, 1974, pp 54–57.

Alcohol

Emrick CE: A review of psychologically oriented treatment of alcoholism II. The relative effectiveness of different treatment approaches and the effectiveness of treatment versus no treatment. *J Stud Alcohol* 36(1):88–108, 1975.

Fuller RK, Roth HP: Disulfiram for the treatment of alcoholism. *Ann Intern Med* 90:901–904, 1979.

Goodwin DW: Alcoholism and heredity. *Arch Gen Psychiatry* 36:57–61, 1979.

Hanson JW, Jones KL, Smith DW: Fetal alcohol syndrome: Experience with 41 patients. *JAMA* 235:1458–1460, 1976.

Mendelson JH, Mello NK: Biologic concomitants of alcoholism. *N Engl J Med* 301:912–921, 1979.

Mendelson JH, Mello NK: *The Diagnosis and Treatment of Alcoholism*. New York, McGraw-Hill, 1979.

Pattison EM, Nonabstinent drinking goals in the treatment of alcoholism: A clinical typology. *Arch Gen Psychiatry* 33:923–930, 1976.

Sollers EM, Kalant H: Alcohol intoxication and wihdrawal. *N Engl J Med* 94:757–762, 1976.

Stinson DJ, Smith WG, Amidjaya I, Kaplan JM: Systems of care and treatment outcomes for alcoholic patients. *Arch Gen Psychiatry* 36:535–539, 1979.

Victor M, Adams RD: Alcohol, in Isselbacher KJ, Adams RD, Braunwald E, Petersdorf RG, Wilson JD (eds): *Harrison's Principles of Internal Medicine*, ed 9. New York, McGraw-Hill, 1980, pp 969–977.

Weissman MM, Myers JK: Clinical depression in alcoholism. *Am J Psychiatry* 137(3):372–374, 1980.

CNS Stimulants

Byck R, Van Dyke C: What are the effects of cocaine in man? in Petersen RC, Stillman RC (eds): *Cocaine: 1977*. NIDA Research Monograph #13, Rockville, Md, 1977, pp 5–16.

Ellinwood EH, Jr: Amphetamines/Anorectics, in DuPont RL, Goldstein A, O'Donnell J (eds): Rockville, Md, National Institute on Drug Abuse, 1979, pp 221–231.

Ellinwood EH, Jr, Kilbey MM: Fundamental mechanisms underlying altered behavior following chronic administration of psychomotor stimulants. *Biol Psychiatry* 15(5): 749–757, 1980.

Grinspoon L, Bakalar JB: Cocaine, in DuPont, RL, Goldstein A, O'Donnell, J (eds): *Handbook on Drug Abuse*. Rockville, Md, National Institute on Drug Abuse, 1979, pp 241–248.

Grinspoon L, Hedblom P: *The Speed Culture: Amphetamine Use and Abuse in America*. Cambridge, Harvard University Press, 1975.

Petersen RC: Cocaine: An overview, in: Petersen RC, Stillman RC (eds): *Cocaine: 1977*. NIDA Research Monograph #13, Rockville, Md, 1977, pp 5–16.

Post, RM: Cocaine psychoses: A continuum model. *Am J Psychiatry* 132(3):225–231, 1975.

Tinklenberg JR: The treatment of acute amphetamine psychosis, in Browne PG (ed): *A Treatment Manual for Acute Drug Abuse Emergencies*. Rockville, Md, National Institute on Drug Abuse, 1975, pp 68–72.

Hallucinogens

Bowers MB Jr: Acute psychosis induced by psychotomimetic drug abuse. I. Clinical findings. *Arch Gen Psychiatry* 27:437–439, 1972.

Bowers MB Jr: Acute psychosis induced by psychotomimetic drug abuse. II. Neurochemical findings. *Arch Gen Psychiatry* 27:440–442, 1972.

Freedman DX: The use and abuse of LSD. *Arch Gen Psychiatry* 18:330–347, 1968.

Grinspoon L, Bakalar JB: *Psychedelic Drugs Reconsidered.* New York, Basic Books, 1979.

Tucker GJ, Quinlan D, Harrow M: Chronic hallucinogenic drug use and thought disturbance. *Arch Gen Psychiatry* 27:443–447, 1972.

Phencyclidine (PCP)

Fauman MA, Fauman BJ: The psychiatric aspects of chronic phencyclidine use: A study of chronic PCP users, in Petersen RC, Stillman RC (eds): *PCP: Phencyclidine Abuse: An Appraisal.* National Institute on Drug Abuse, Department of Health, Education, and Welfare Research Monograph #21, DHEW Publication No. 78–728. Washington, US Government Printing Office, 1978, pp 183–200.

Graeven DB: Patterns of phencyclidine use, in Petersen RC, Stillman RC (eds): *PCP: Phencyclidine Abuse: An Appraisal.* National Institute on Drug Abuse, Department of Health, Education, and Welfare Research Monograph #21, DHEW Publication No. 78–728. Washington, US Government Printing Office, 1978, pp 176–182.

Luisada PV: The phencyclidine psychosis: Phenomenology and treatment, in: Petersen RC, Stillman RC (eds): *PCP: Phencyclidine Abuse: An Appraisal,* National Institute on Drug Abuse, Department of Health, Education, and Welfare Research Monograph #21, DHEW Publication No. 78–728. Washington US Government Printing Office, 1978, pp 241–253.

Petersen RC, Stillman RC: Phencyclidine: An overview, in *Petersen RC, Stillman RC (eds): PCP: Phencyclidine Abuse: An Appraisal.* National Institute on Drug Abuse, Department of Health, Education, and Welfare Research Monograph #21, DHEW Publication No. 78–728. Washington, US Government Printing Office, 1978, pp 1–17.

Smith DE, Wesson DR, Buxton ME, Seymour R, Kramer HM: The diagnosis and treatment of the PCP abuse syndrome, in Petersen RC, Stillman RC (eds): *PCP: Phencyclidine Abuse: An Appraisal.* National Institute on Drug Abuse, Department of Health, Education, and Welfare Research Monograph #21, DHEW Publication No. 78–728. Washington, US Government Printing Office, 1978, pp 229–239.

Inhalants

Cohen S: Inhalants, in: DuPont RL, Goldstein A, O'Donnell J (eds): *Handbook on Drug Abuse,* Rockville, Md, National Institute on Drug Abuse, 1979, pp 213–220.

Glaser FB: Inhalation psychosis and related states, in Browne PG (ed): *A Treatment Manual for Acute Drug Abuse Emergencies.* Rockville, Md, National Institute on Drug Abuse, 1975, pp 95–104.

Marijuana

Bernstein JG: Marijuana—New potential, new problems. *Drug Ther.* 10:38–48, 1980.

Mendelson JH, Rossi AM, Meyer RE (eds): *The Use of Marihuana: A Psychological and Physiological Inquiry.* New York, Plenum Press, 1974.

Meyer RE: Psychiatric consequences of marijuana use: The state of the evidence, in Tinklenberg Jr (ed): *Marijuana and Health Hazards. Methodological Issues in Current Research.* New York, Academic Press, 1975, pp 133–152.

Mirin SM, Shapiro LM, Meyer RE, Pillard RC, Fisher S: Casual versus heavy use of marijuana: A redefinition of the marijuana problem. *Am J Psychiatry* 127(9):54–60, 1971.

Petersen RC (ed): *Marijuana Research Findings: 1980*. NIDA Research Monograph #31, Washington, US Government Printing Office, 1980.

Treffert DA: Marijuana use in schizophrenia: A clear hazard. *Am J Psychiatry* 135(10):1213–1220, 1978.

Weil AT: Adverse reactions to marihuana: Classification and suggested treatment. *N Engl J Med* 282(18):997–1000, 1970.

Emergency Presentations Related to Psychiatric Medication

Stephen C. Schoonover, M.D.
and Alan J. Gelenberg, M.D.

1. Introduction

Patients commonly use the emergency room because of various adverse effects from psychiatric medication. Among the most common are those related to the use of lithium, antipsychotic agents, and other psychiatric drugs with anticholinergic effects. This section describes the clinical manifestations and management of these drug effects. Agents used to treat medical disorders that also may cause behavioral effects are primarily described in the chapters on anxiety, depression, and acute psychoses.

2. Lithium Toxicity[1]

Lithium causes two types of toxic responses. The first, occurring at low serum levels, is characterized by fine hand tremor, gastric irritability, anorexia, vomiting, diarrhea, and thirst. These effects, coinciding with large fluctuations in serum lithium levels, usually abate over the first few weeks of therapy and do not require special treatment.

The second type of toxic response may result either from an acute overdose or from the chronic administration of an inappropriately high amount. Toxic reactions most often occur at serum levels in excess of 2.0 mEq/liter, although in some sensitive individuals they occur at lower levels. In these patients, gastrointestinal symptoms may initially appear, followed or accompanied by central nervous system depression, including somnolence, sluggishness, signs and symptoms of an organic brain syndrome, dysarthria, seizures, choreoathetoid movements, increased muscle tone, and increased deep tendon reflexes.

This chapter, reprinted here with permission, condenses material from Bassuk EL, Schoonover SC, Gelenberg AJ (eds): *The Practitioner's Guide to Psychoactive Drugs*, ed 2. New York, Plenum Publishing Corp, 1983.

S. C. Schoonover, M.D., and A. J. Gelenberg, M.D. • Harvard Medical Medical School, Boston, Massachusetts 02115.

Most often, more severe symptoms occur at serum lithium levels greater than 3.0 mEq/liter. Cardiovascular collapse marked by lowered blood pressure, irregular cardiac rhythm, decreased urine output, and conduction abnormalities (and EKG changes) may be life-threatening.

Acute intoxication causes significant central nervous system (CNS) depression. Patients develop pyramidal tract signs and impaired consciousness or coma. Individuals who chronically take too much medication gradually develop CNS impairment. Sluggishness and drowsiness may progress over a period of days. Often gastrointestinal symptoms, slurred speech, ataxia, and coarse tremor accompany these changes. If the initial signs of chronic intoxiciation are overlooked, a more florid CNS syndrome may develop, most often manifested by hyperpyrexia and stupor or coma. It may also include neurologic asymmetries, nystagmus, stiff neck, and hyperextension of the extremities

Lithium toxicity is generally managed by supportive measures. If the toxicity occurs as part of an acute medication regimen or minor overdose and kidney function is intact, careful observation usually suffices. Since lithium is excreted rapidly, the syndrome most often abates within a few days. However, in a large or chronic overdose, very large, total-body lithium stores may accumulate. In these cases, the patient often suffers persistent (several days or longer) life-threatening CNS depression and cardiovascular impairment

The key steps in the *management of serious toxic states* include the following:

- Evaluate rapidly (including clinical signs and symptoms, serum lithium levels, electrolytes and EKG), monitor vital signs and make an accurate diagnosis.
- Discontinue lithium.
- Support vital functions and monitor cardiac status.
- Limit absorption.
  - If alert, provide an emetic.
  - If obtunded, intubate and suction nasogastrically (prolonged suction may be helpful since lithium levels in gastric fluid may remain high for days.
- Prevent infection in comatose patients by body rotation and pulmonary toilet.
- In all cases, vigorously hydrate (ideally, 5 to 6 liters per day); monitor and balance the electrolytes.
- In moderately severe cases:
  - Implement osmotic diuresis with urea 20 g IV, 2 to 5 times per day, or mannitol 50 to 100 g IV per day.
  - Increase lithium clearance with aminophylline 0.5 g up to every six hours and alkalinize the urine with IV sodium lactate.
  - Ensure adequate intake of NaCl to promote excretion of lithium.
- Implement peritoneal or hemodialysis for severe toxicity, which is characterized by:

○ Serum levels between 2.0 and 4.0 mEq/liter, with severe clinical signs and symptoms (particularly decreasing urinary output and deepening CNS depression).

○ Serum lithium levels greater than 4.0 mEq/liter. Most patients completely recover from lithium toxicity; several may die; some develop permanent neurologic damage.

3. Extrapyramidal Effects[2]

Antipsychotic drugs may cause four types of extrapyramidal syndromes: acute dystonia, akathisia, Parkinson's syndrome, and, after longer-term use, tardive dyskinesia. This section describes each syndrome and its emergency treatment.

3.1. Acute Dystonic Reactions

Acute dystonic reactions, including acute dyskinesias (i.e., abnormal involuntary movements of various types) and oculogyric crises, typically occur during the early hours or days following the initiation of antipsychotic drug therapy or after a marked dosage increment. Involuntary muscle contractions are common, particularly about the mouth, jaw, face, and neck. The symptoms are episodic and recurrent, lasting from minutes to hours. There may be trismus ("lockjaw"), dystonia or dyskinesias of the tongue, opisthotonus (spasms of the neck that arch the head backward), or eye closure. In oculogyric crises, there is a dystonic reaction of the extraocular muscles, and gaze is fixed in one position.

Acute dystonic reactions are distressing, particularly to the patient, family member, or clinician who is unfamiliar with them. They may be uncomfortable, but they are rarely dangerous. In rare cases, however, there can be respiratory compromise, with potential for fatality.

The diagnosis of acute dystonic reaction is usually not difficult—if it is clear that a patient has recently begun taking an antipsychotic drug or has had a switch in the type of dosage or medication. At times, however, eliciting this information may be difficult; for example, patients who are taking prochlorperazine (Compazine) suppositories may say they are not taking any tranquilizer pills; some patients do not wish to acknowledge use of antipsychotic drugs, or have sought them for illicit use (described recently). Among the many neuropsychiatric syndromes that must be considered in the differential diagnosis of acute dystonic reactions are tetanus, seizures, and conversion reactions.

The highest-potency antipsychotic drugs have the greatest likelihood of producing acute dystonias, the low-potency agents much less, thioridazine (Mellaril) the least. Young people are at greater risk of developing this syndrome than the elderly, and males more frequently than females. When the acute dystonic reactions are frequent or severe in a patient, it may be worthwhile to assay the serum concentration of calcium, since rare cases of hypocalcemia can be detected.

The treatment of an acute dystonic reaction is straightforward, readily available, and usually dramatically successful. Parenteral treatment is preferred for the initiation of drug therapy, with intravenous being more rapid than intramuscular. The intravenous injection of contraactive medication provides both immediate relief and confirmation of the diagnosis. For this purpose, a number of classes of agents have been employed with considerable success. Some clinicians prefer to use a benzodiazepine intravenously, such as diazepam (Valium), up to 10 mg. This drug is safe and comfortable, and does not add additional anticholinergic effects. As with the injection of any other central depressant compound, equipment for support of the airway should be immediately available, should an emergency occur. Injection should be slow (5 mg of diazepam per minute), and care must be taken to avoid accidental intraarterial injection. Other clinicians prefer to administer an antihistamine drug, such as diphenhydramine (Benadryl), 50 mg. An injectable anticholinergic antiparkinson drug, such as benztropine (Cogentin), 1 mg, or biperiden (Akineton), 2 mg, also may be used.

Following immediate relief of acute dystonic signs, the clinician may wish to place the patient on an oral dose of one of these same drugs. The lowest effective dose should be used. If this successfully prevents any additional reactions, the contraactive medication can usually be tapered and discontinued within several weeks.

Would it be wise to coadminister an antiparkinson drug from the beginning of antipsychotic drug therapy in the hope of avoiding an acute dystonic reaction? To date, there is no definitive answer to this question. Some data, however, suggest that some patients may be partially protected through this "prophylactic" approach. Therefore, the physician may want to consider giving antiparkinson drugs to patients at highest risk (i.e., young males receiving high-potency antipsychotic agents), and for those in whom a reaction is likely to be clinically disruptive. For most others, it makes sense to avoid a drug that may be unnecessary, reserving treatment until signs of dystonia appear.

3.2. Akathisia

Akathisia is another extrapyramidal reaction associated with both antipsychotic drugs and postencephalitic Parkinson's syndrome. Akathisia is a symptom (i.e., subjective) defined as a compulsion to be in motion. Patients describe an inner restlessness, an intense desire to move about simply for the sake of moving. Persons who are virtually paralyzed by the akinesia of postencephalitic Parkinson's disorder have been known to ask other people to move their limbs, just to relieve this intense compulsion. Patients suffering from akathisia are often observed to pace aimlessly, fidget, and be markedly restless.

Akathisia can occur early in the course of drug treatment or it may not appear for several months. It, too, appears to be more prevalent with high-potency drugs. The natural course of akathisia is less clear than that of acute dystonic reactions: At times it appears to wane, yet some patients are troubled by it for a long time.

Treatment responses are variable in these patients. Nevertheless, akathisia is an important syndrome to recognize, as it may severely complicate a patient's response to antipsychotic drug therapy—and perhaps most important, it makes patients extremely unhappy. Patients may present to the emergency room complaining of anxiety, which must be distinguished from an akathisia. Approaches to treatment include lowering the dose of the antipsychotic drug, switching to a lower-potency agent, or adding a contraactive drug. The same drugs discussed for the treatment of acute dystonic reactions—anticholinergic antiparkinson agents, antihistamines, and benzodiazepines—also may be tried orally in cases of akathisia, although results are less universally successful.

3.3. Parkinson's Syndrome[3]

Parkinson's is characterized by a triad of signs: *tremor, rigidity, and akinesia (or bradykinesia)*. The tremor (by definition, a regular and rhythmic oscillation of a body part around a point) is in the neighborhood of four to eight cycles per second and is greater at rest than during activity. A Parkinsonian tremor often is observed in the hands, where the thumb rubbing against the pad of the index finger may produce a characteristic "pill rolling" appearance. The tremor also can involve the wrists, elbows, head, palate, or virtually any body part. In neuroleptic-induced Parkinson's syndrome, the tremor is typically bilateral; unilateral tremors should raise questions about the etiology. While tremor is very common and may be one of the earlier signs in naturally occurring Parkinson's disease, it is less common than rigidity and akinesia and may not appear until relatively late in the drug-related syndrome.

Rigidity is an increase in the normal resting tone of a body part. It is detectable only by palpation on physical examination. (In other words, a patient does not *look* rigid; he must *feel* rigid.) In testing for rigidity, the physician asks the patient to relax completely and allow body parts to be manipulated without moving them. The examiner then rotates the head on the neck, moves the major joints in the upper and lower extremities, and raises each extremity to note the rapidity with which it falls by gravity. An increased resistance to passive motion and a slow return from a raised position denotes the presence of rigidity. When tremor coexists with rigidity, the rigidity may take on the feel of a "cogwheel." In extreme forms of the condition, rigidity may mimic (or actually become) the waxy flexibility with sustained postures characteristic of catatonia.[3] In antipsychotic drug-induced Parkinson's syndrome, rigidity tends to be more common than tremor, but less common than the third sign of the triad—akinesia.

Akinesia is a disinclination to move in the absence of paralysis. Literally, akinesia means the absence of motion, while bradykinesia, truer to the clinical reality in most patients, implies a slowness of motion. The bradykinetic patient frequently shows a masklike facies, with diminished expressiveness and less frequent eye blinking.

The bradykinetic patient turns his body "en bloc." Instead of turning first with the eyes, then with the neck, followed in turn by shoulders, hips, and lower extremities, the Parkinsonian patient turns as if he were one solid block of wood—without joints. A typical stance includes a flexing of elbows and wrists, together with a stooped posture. The patient's gait is typically inclined forward, and he may walk with small, rapid steps (marche à petit pas). In the extreme forms, bradykinesia, as well as rigidity, may shade into catatonic immobility.[3]

In a less severe manifestation, the slowed movements of the Parkinsonian patient may appear primarily as apathy, boredom, and a "zombielike" appearance. If other signs of Parkinson's syndrome are not prominent, this social akinesia may be misdiagnosed as depression.[4] Together with the major triad of Parkinson's syndrome (tremor, rigidity, and bradykinesia), associated signs often include seborrhea and drooling.

Parkinson's syndrome usually occurs within weeks to months after the beginning of antipsychotic drug therapy. Although tolerance develops in many patients, the disorder may persist and require ongoing treatment in others. Women and the elderly are affected more commonly. Again, the high potency agents appear more likely to promote this disturbance. Probably a late-occurring variant of Parkinson's syndrome is the so-called rabbit syndrome, in which a rapid tremor of the mouth and jaw are reminiscent of the facial expression of a rabbit. The rabbit syndrome appears to respond pharmacologically like other forms of Parkinson's.

The treatment of Parkinson's syndrome reflects our understanding of the pathophysiology. One approach is to decrease the dose of the antipsychotic drug, presumably thereby decreasing the degree of dopamine blockade at the synaptic receptor. Alternatively, a less potent antipsychotic agent may be employed. As mentioned earlier, thioridazine has the lowest incidence of Parkinsonian reactions.

Table 1 lists available drugs that are useful for the treatment of drug-induced Parkinson's syndrome. The advantages of using one of these agents prophylactically in a patient receiving antipsychotic drug therapy have been debated, but the question remains unresolved. The alternative is to observe the patient for the development of extrapyramidal signs (including an awareness of the more subtle manifestations), and if and when they appear, to treat them vigorously. Because of additive untoward effects and toxicity, it may be simpler to use antiparkinson drugs only when necessary and to try to discontinue them (gradually) following several months of successful treatment. (Many patients, however, seem to require continued treatment.)

With the exception of amantadine, all the antiparkinson drugs listed in the table have anticholinergic and/or antihistaminic properties. Among these drugs, trihexyphenidyl has a relatively short half-life, while benztropine has a relatively long half-life. Amantadine is a dopamine agonist that has few anticholinergic effects. This feature may make it preferable in patients particularly

Table 1. Antiparkinson Agents[a]

Generic name	Trade name	Type of drug	Usual drug range (mg per day)	Injectable
Amantadine	Symmetrel	Dopamine agonist	100 to 300	No
Benztropine	Cogentin	Antihistamine and anticholinergic	1 to 6	Yes
Biperiden	Akineton	Anticholinergic	2 to 6	Yes
Diphenyhydramine	Benadryl	Antihistamine and anticholinergic	25 to 100	Yes
Ethopropazine	Parsidol	Antihistamine and anticholinergic	50	No
Orphenadrine	Disipal, Norflex	Antihistamine	300	No
Procyclidine	Kemadrin	Anticholinergic	6 to 20	No
Trihexyphenidyl	Artane, etc.	Anticholinergic	5 to 15	No

[a] Adapted from Wojcik.[5]

sensitive to anticholinergic ractions.[5] Amantadine, 100 mg bid to 100 mg tid, may be effective in some cases of drug-induced Parkinson's syndrome, particularly the more severe variety, when anticholinergic antiparkinson drugs have been ineffectual.[6] Amantadine has a relatively long half-life (approximately 24 hours). It is excreted in the urine unchanged with impaired renal function.

Antiparkinson drugs, as well as other chemicals with anticholinergic activity (e.g., belladonna-containing compounds), have been used for "recreational" purposes.[7] The anticholinergic activity provides a mood-elevating effect, creating a feeling of euphoria or a "high." Some afficionados of the drug culture actually use the drugs to create a toxic delirium, which they perceive as pleasurable. Many schizophrenic patients treated with antiparkinson drugs become more attached to these drugs than to their antipsychotic agents, possibly due to the relief of extrapyramidal symptoms or perhaps because of directly pleasurable effects. Trihexyphenidyl has been reported to be more commonly abused than other antiparkinson agents. If this is true, it could be related to the pharmacology of the drug or simply to its popularity and therefore availability.

3.4. Tardive Dyskinesia[2]

Tardive dyskinesia is characterized by abnormal, involuntary, choreoathetotic movements involving the tongue, lips, jaw, face, extremities, and, occasionally, the trunk. It typically involves orobuccolingual masticatory movements. These may include lip-smacking, chewing, puckering of the lips, protrusion of the tongue, and puffing of the cheeks. A common early sign is wormlike movements of the tongue. Other movements of the face can be observed, including grimacing, blinking, and frowning.

In the young, movements sometimes begin in the distal extremities and may consist of rapid, purposeless, quick, jerky movements distally—chorea ("dance")—or more sinuous, writhing movements proximally—athetosis. Occasionally, abnormal movements involve the trunk and pelvis. The signs of tardive dyskinesia can range in intensity from minimal to severe. Patients' awareness of the movements varies. Institutionalized chronic schizophrenic patients may deny even very severe movements, while a highly functioning patient with a mood disorder could be extremely troubled by the most minimal symptom. The movements may embarrass the patient and interfere with important activities, such as eating, talking, and dressing. In rare instances, tardive dyskinesia can impair breathing and swallowing.

The movements of tardive dyskinesia may appear during treatment when a patient is taking a constant dose of an antipsychotic—or they may initially appear when the dosage of the drug is lowered or stopped entirely. Conversely, if movements are present, increasing the dose of an antipsychotic drug can make the movements cease. This latter phenomenon has been referred to as "masking" of the movements and gives rise to the concept of "covert dyskinesia"—in other words, dyskinesia observed only when an antipsychotic drug has been discontinued.[8] On the other hand, when an antipsychotic drug is discontinued abruptly, a patient may show transient dyskinetic movements, which can disappear in a matter of days or weeks. This phenomenon has been known as withdrawal dyskinesia, and it might conceivably indicate that a patient is vulnerable to a persistent dyskinesia if the medication is reinstituted and continued.

Treatment approaches to tardive dyskinesia are based on our understanding (and beliefs) about the nature of antipsychotic drugs and tardive dyskinesia itself. First, of course, comes primary prevention. This can be accomplished in various ways: (1) Avoid unnecessary exposure of patients to antipsychotic drugs. In particular, the use of these agents to treat relatively benign conditions, or those that could respond equally well or better to other agents (e.g., anxiety, nonpsychotic depression), should be avoided whenever possible. (2) When it is necessary to employ antipsychotic drug therapy, use the lowest dose for the shortest period of time. Of course, most schizophrenic patients will require prolonged therapy with these agents, but the clinician should find the lowest effective maintenance dose. (3) Similarly, when treating patients with other chronic disorders, such as mental retardation and organic brain syndrome, the use of drugs should be minimized and constantly reevaluated.

Secondary prevention of a disorder means early detection. For tardive dyskinesia, this entails routine screening and monitoring patients for the presence of abnormal movements. The emergency clinician must consider the possibility of tardive dyskinesia in all patients with unusual movements and differentiate it from other extrapyramidal disorders. A standard neurologic examination can be employed for this purpose, or a clinician may want to use a specific examination procedure and rating scale, such as the Abnormal Involuntary Movement Scale, designed by the National Institute of Mental Health. However, all patients with suspected tardive dyskinesia should be referred to a consultant for further evaluation and treatment.

4. Anticholinergic Syndromes[9]

4.1. Description

Most psychoactive drugs have both peripheral and central anticholinergic effects. An anticholinergic syndrome can be caused by heterocyclic antidepressants, antipsychotics, some hypnotics, antihistamines, antiparkinson agents, and many over-the-counter preparations. Combinations of these drugs, such as an antipsychotic and an antiparkinson agent, may produce additive anticholinergic effects. Elderly patients and children seem particularly sensitive. Acute overdoses of the above-mentioned agents also frequently cause anticholinergic crises. In addition, plant alkaloids, such as ginseng weed and angel's trumpet, have become increasingly popular with adolescent drug abusers and commonly cause a toxic psychosis complicated by anticholinergic symptoms.

The anticholinergic syndrome may present with a mixture or a predominance of either peripheral or central symptoms. It should be suspected in patients who present with dry mouth, red face, dilated pupils, increased heart rate, widened pulse pressure, and increased temperature. In its florid state, the CNS picture consists of confusion, delirium with disorientation, agitation, visual and auditory hallucinations, anxiety, motor restlessness, pseudoseizures (myoclonic jerks and choreoathetoid movements with EEG seizure activity), and a thought disorder (e.g., delusions). The peripheral syndrome may be manifested by decreased bowel sounds and constipation, urinary retention, anhydrosis (decreased sweating), mydriasis (increased pupillary size), dry mouth, cycloplegia (decreased accommodation), increased body temperature, motor incoordination, flushing, and tachycardia. When these syndromes are caused by the heterocyclic antidepressants, there is also a high risk of life-threatening arrhythmias. Aliphatic and piperidine phenothiazines (especially thioridazine), and the tricyclics, amitriptyline (Elavil) and imipramine (Tofranil), are the most anticholinergic. A combination of the above drugs, or of these drugs with other anticholinergic agents, greatly increases the risk of an anticholinergic syndrome.

4.2. Anticholinesterase Therapy

Anticholinesterase therapy has proven very effective for the treatment of anticholinergic syndromes. All anticholinesterases counteract the peripheral manifestations of the syndrome. However, clinicians should use either physostigmine salicylate (Antilirium) or pyridostigmine bromide (Mestinon, Regonol) because they cross the blood-brain barrier and therefore counteract the central symptoms. Most clinical studies have focused on physostigmine, but equivalent doses of pyridostigmine also are effective. In general, the clinician should avoid using physostigmine in patients with unstable vital signs. In these cases, cardiac arrhythmias from cholinergic stimulation are common. Cholinergic effects can also produce seizures (particularly with rapid injection of physostigmine) and respiratory arrest in selected patients. Although practitioners have tried many different regimens, physostigmine salicylate 1 to 2 mg IM or IV will relieve symptoms dramatically. The clinician should infuse the drug very slowly (e.g., 1 mg over two minutes), monitor the cardiac status, and have means for respiratory support available. If no improvement occurs within 15 to 20 minutes, another dose of 1 to 2 mg should be given. Up to 4 mg may be administered over 10 to 15 minutes. The body degrades physostigmine almost completely within 1½ to 2 hours. Since the toxic agents may disappear more slowly, additional 1- to 2-mg doses at 30-minute intervals may be necessary, even if the initial treatment is successful. Physostigmine must be used cautiously, since it may produce hypotension, bradycardia, increased bronchial secretions, bronchoconstriction, and a lowered seizure threshold (particularly in a setting of cardiorespiratory compromise). Therefore, in such circumstances physostigmine must be administered only with careful monitoring.[10,11]

With heterocyclic antidepressant overdoses, various arrhythmias may result that have specific treatments. As described above, supraventricular arrhythmias from atropinelike effects should be treated with an anticholinesterase. Ventricular arrhythmias are best managed with lidocaine; heart block, with lidocaine or phenytoin. Clinicians should avoid using type I antiarrhythmics like procaineamide, quinidine (Quinidex, Quinora, and others), or disophyramide (Norpace) (since they may increase the impaired conduction caused by heterocyclics) and propranolol (since it may add significantly to depression of cardiac contactility). When severe arrhythmias persist, patients may require cardioversion or cardiac pacing. In addition, external cardiac massage and oxygenation should be continued for extended periods (i.e., two to three hours) in unresponsive, but previously healthy, patients even with complete asystole (since one patient recovered, possibly as a result of drug redistribution from continued perfusion).[12]

5. Conclusion

Patients who present to the emergency setting with symptoms and signs related to psychiatric drug use and abuse should be evaluated carefully and treated appropriately. The clinician should familarize himself with the wide range of adverse effects, their varied manifestations, and their acute management. Once the patient is stabilized, appropriate plans for follow-up should be arranged.

References

1. Schoonover SC: Bipolar affective disorders, in Bassuk EL, Schoonover, SC, Gelenberg AJ (eds): *The Practitioner's Guide to Psychoactive Drugs,* ed 2. Plenum Publishing Co, 1983, pp 33–35.
2. Gelenberg AJ: Psychoses, in Bassuk EL, Schoonover SC, Gelenberg AJ (eds): *The Practitioner's Guide to Psychoactive Drugs,* ed 2. Plenum Publishing Co, 1983, pp 64–79.
3. Gelenberg AJ, Mandel MR: Catatonic reactions to high potency neuroleptic drugs. *Arch Gen Psychiatry* 34:947–950, 1977.
4. Rifkin A, Quitkin F, Klein DF: Akinesia: A poorly recognized drug-induced extrapyramidal behavior disorder. *Arch Gen Psychiatry* 32:642–674, 1975.
5. Wojcik JD: Antiparkinson drug use. *Mass Gen Hosp Biol Ther Psychiatry Newsletter* 2:5–7, 1979.
6. Gelenberg AJ: Amantadine in the treatment of benztropine-refractory neuroleptic-induced movement disorders. *Curr Ther Res* 23:375–80, 1978.
7. Smith JM: Abuse of the antiparkinson drugs: A review of the literature. *J Clin Psychiatry* 41:351–354, 1980.
8. Gardos G, Cole JO, Tarsy D: Withdrawal syndromes associated with antipsychotic drugs. *Am J Psychiatry* 135:1321–1324, 1978.
9. Schoonover SC: Depression, in Bassuk EL, Schoonover SC, Gelenberg AJ (eds): *The Practitioner's Guide to Psychoactive Drugs,* ed 2. Plenum Publishing Co, 1983, pp 60–62.

10. Burks JS, Walker JE, Rumach BH, et al: Tricyclic antidepressant poisoning: Reversal of coma, choreoathetosis and myoclonus by physostigmine. *JAMA* 230:1405–1407, 1974.
11. Granacher RD, Baldessarini RJ: Physostigmine: Its use in acute anticholinergic syndrome with antidepressant and antiparkinson drugs. *Arch Gen Psychiatry* 32:375–379, 1975.
12. Orr DA, Bramble MG: Tricyclic antidepressant poisoning and external cardiac massage during asystole. *Br Med J* 283:1107–1108, 1981.

V

Patients and Clinical Syndromes 3
Behavioral, Cognitive, and Affective
Disturbances

Acute Psychoses

Arthur Barsky, III, M.D.

1. Overview

1.1. The General Medical Orientation

In caring for the acutely psychotic patient, the psychiatrist is similar to a general medical physician. He uses the traditional methods of clinical medicine: (1) data gathering (history, physical examination, laboratory investigation), (2) differential diagnosis, and (3) treatment. The acutely psychotic patient is presumed to be suffering a pathological process that has a specific treatment. The doctor's role tends to be more authoritarian than in many other areas of psychiatry—the psychiatrist must often take control of the situation, prescribing and proscribing rather than negotiating. Because judgment is impaired and decisions unrealistic, the acutely psychotic patient tends to play a relatively minor part in determining his emergency care. Although the psychiatrist values his alliance with the patient, with an acute psychotic there may be no real alliance established, or it may be subject to violation if good care must override patient wishes.

1.2. The Setting

Working with a psychotic patient in an emergency setting presents many difficulties. The patient is frequently unable or unwilling to give an adequate history. Clinical data may be ambiguous and confusing. At the same time, the pressures of the setting and the clinical situation dictate that the psychiatrist act quickly—time is at a premium. Thus, in spite of uncertain, ambiguous, and incomplete assessment data, managing the acute psychotic demands rapid, decisive, and definitive action.

1.3. Definition of Acute Psychosis

An acute psychosis is a rapidly developing pathological state in which an individual's thinking is disorganized, perceptions are distorted, feelings intense and unrealistic, and behaviors inappropriate. The patient's ability to perceive

Arthur Barsky, III, M.D. • Massachusetts General Hospital, Boston, Massachusetts 02114, and Harvard Medical School, Boston, Massachusetts 02115.

and deal with reality is grossly impaired. He cannot communicate with or relate to others normally, and cannot meet the ordinary demands of life. The state is classically characterized by disordered thinking (e.g., delusions) and impaired perception (e.g., hallucinations).

Although psychoses are labeled either organic or functional, it is entirely possible that the distinction results from incomplete knowledge. That is, organic psychosis refers to those disorders resulting from some *demonstrable* pathological lesion or pathophysiological process. Functional psychoses are those with no as yet demonstrable physical cause, and they include schizophrenia, mania, and depression.

2. Triage

Acute psychosis is a genuine medical emergency requiring immediate and complete attention. The first priority is to ensure the physical safety of the patient and others in the patient's environment. If the patient is at risk for losing control, then he must be secluded or restrained (see Chapter 2). Once physical safety is assured, the patient is triaged to that service or individual best able to perform the complicated evaluation. Since many physicians are trained only in emergency medicine, internal medicine, or neurology, the emergency psychiatrist should be called. Psychosis, like fever or abdominal pain, is a pathological state with many causes, some of which may be life-threatening. Other medical etiologies, while not acutely life-threatening, do cause irreversible damage if not promptly and definitively treated.

3. Assessment

3.1. Identifying Data

There are times when even the most basic demographic data cannot be obtained from the acutely psychotic individual. The confused, uncooperative, or totally disorganized patient may not be able to give his name, address, age, or names and telephone numbers of family or professionals already involved in his medical and psychiatric care. Under these conditions, clothes and possessions should be searched for identifying material such as address books, wallets, hotel receipts, bank books, and airline tickets. The patient's clothes or underwear may bear labels with his name or the laundry marks of a nursing home or state hospital at which the patient was a resident. Other health care personnel (e.g., ambulance drivers, desk clerks, security personnel) may know the patient from a prior visit to the hospital. Finally, state hospitals, shelters, and the police department should be contacted about persons reported missing.

3.2. Symptoms

3.2.1. Chief Complaint and Presentation

The acutely psychotic patient may or may not be able to specify a chief complaint. He may be uncooperative and mute, unable to acknowledge the psychiatrist's presence, much less to answer questions. He may be incomprehensible, reporting that he is the Son of God or answering each question by singing a song such as "It's Not for Me to Say." Thus, the evaluating psychiatrist may know nothing more than the immediate reason the patient was brought to the hospital. If the patient can articulate a chief complaint, it usually reveals the degree to which reality testing is preserved and some observing ego remains. Compare the chief complaint, "This is not the air force of the USSR," with "Voices are scaring me and telling me to run away."

3.2.2. Suicide

Suicide is a significant danger in all psychotic patients. If the patient also has a depressed mood, suicidal ideation, or history of self-destructive behavior, then the risk may be even higher. Psychotic patients are doubly at risk: (1) Self-destructive urges may be unchecked by internal controls and readily find expression in overt behavior, and (2) confused, deluded patients may take precipitate action that inadvertently results in their death—although they had not intended to die. For example, a paranoid and panicked man, hearing a knock at his door, might jump from his third-floor apartment window to escape his imagined pursuers. A careful suicide assessment is a mandatory part of the evaluation of every psychotic patient. The evaluation should include a consideration of the factors discussed in Chapter 7 on suicide. In addition, several specific characteristics of the psychotic state must be examined. Auditory hallucinations commanding the patient to act against himself are the most malignant sign and make hospitalization mandatory. A depressed mood or a diagnosis of psychotic depression is also an extremely grave sign.[1] Manic patients can be equally at risk because of their rapid mood shifts; depression may be just beneath the surface. The clinician should evaluate the degree to which psychosis has disrupted the patient's judgment so that he might inadvertently harm himself if the physical risks of his actions are misjudged. Patients with organic psychoses and deliria are also significant suicide risks.[2] For example, patients who have ingested phencyclidine are at greater risk because they are prone to violent, unpredictable, and bizarre actions.[3] (see Chapter 9).

3.2.3. Homicide and Violence

Assessment of violence is comparable to that of suicide. The acutely psychotic patient is at increased risk for committing violent or homicidal acts,[4] and a careful homicide assessment (see Chapter 6) is mandatory. Paranoid psychotics are particularly worrisome, becuase they may strike back at people whom they believe to wish them ill. These patients are most dangerous when their delusional system implicates one specific "villain" and when their psychoses are acute. Command hallucinations ordering the patient to commit violence put the patient in an extremely high-risk category. These patients almost always require hospitalization. Organic psychoses, deliria, and states of intoxication are also of concern—particularly when the latter involve alcohol, amphetamines, and phencyclidine.

3.2.4. Alcohol and Drug Use

Alcohol, illicit drugs of abuse, and prescribed psychotropic agents can, and commonly do, induce toxic psychoses and delirious states. Such clinical states can occur as a result of acute intoxication or long-term, chronic abuse. The hallucinogens, stimulants, agents with high anticholinergic potency, and alcohol are the most common offenders. They will be discussed in subsequent sections of this chapter (also, see Chapters 8 and 9).

3.2.5. Vegetative Symptoms

Acute psychosis disrupts many of the body's basic autonomic functions. The acute psychotic generally has profound insomnia (often with primitive nightmares), loss of appetite, disturbance of sexual function, and fatigue. These neurovegetative symptoms, in combination with increasing disruption of reality testing and personality disorganization, reflect the severity and acuteness of the psychosis but are not specific differential diagnostic points. The severely disorganized patient with somatic signs should be hospitalized more readily than the patient whose psychotic thinking and perceptual disturbances have not disrupted basic bodily functions or personal care.

3.3. History

3.3.1. Sources of History

It is important to obtain historical information from persons other than the patient. The psychotic patient's interpretation of events is important, but it is not sufficient to establish an "objective" picture of the crisis onset. Inaccurate and incomplete histories may be due to poor cognitive function or deliberate distortion.

> For example, a 38-year-old mother of two children entered the emergency room explaining that she had come to the hospital because she needed kidney surgery. Insisting that she see a urologist and not a psychiatrist, she gave a three-day history of insomnia and inability to work because of urinary tract symptoms. Although she appeared calm and cooperative, she failed to supply the truly relevant data. The patient's husband and sister, however, described the same three-day period during which the patient had awakened a neighbor in the middle of the night to accuse him of poisoning her, of trying to throw urine on her sister, and of disrobing in front of her terrified children.

Thus, it is essential to obtain history from all possible sources. These may include anyone who accompanied the patient to the emergency room; family, friends, neighbors, or roommates who can be contacted; and medical and psychiatric caretakers. It is not uncommon to spend more time on the telephone than interviewing the uncooperative, inaccessible, or disorganized patient.

3.3.2. Establishing the Temporal Course

When obtaining the history, the clinician should try to reconstruct the temporal course of the episode. He must establish how rapidly the acute illness evolved and ascertain the patient's prior clinical status and level of functioning. A longitudinal picture of the episode is necessary for several reasons: First, the differential diagnosis of an acute psychotic episode rests, in large part, upon the pattern and form of symptomatology over time; and second, to determine the goals and target symptoms of the emergency intervention, the clinician needs to obtain a clear picture of the patient's baseline state prior to the acute episode.

3.3.3. History of the Present Illness

The clinician should obtain a brief but accurate description of the presenting episode. This includes precipitating factors; the type, intensity, duration, and course of the psychotic symptoms; treatment (especially pharmacological); and response. It also should include a history of dangerous or impulsive behavior during this period, as well as pertinent drug, medication, and medical information.

3.3.4. Past History

It is most important to establish whether the patient has had previous psychotic experiences and what form they took, to what degree the patient has recovered between episodes, how the episodes were treated, and what treatment proved most effective.

The history should also include pertinent medical data and a review of systems—particularly if a medical etiology is suspected. Since the major functional psychoses may have a genetic component, a family history of psychosis can be useful for differential diagnosis.

3.4. Level of Functioning

The patient's level of functioning needs to be established for the period immediately preceding the acute episode as well as at the time of the emergency visit. Considerable disruption of functioning usually accompanies acute psychosis. Although the degree of impairment depends, in part, upon the nature and severity of the stresses, psychotic individuals are generally unable to function effectively at work, though some may "go through the motions." Similarly, most acute psychoses severely impair the individual's functioning within the social network of family, co-workers, neighbors, and friends.

In assessing functional level, the clinician should not ignore daily activities such as regular bathing, grooming, and eating, leaving the house, performing usual household tasks, and being left alone.

Functional level is particularly important in determining disposition after the emergency intervention. To the degree that the patient is "quietly crazy" and able to maintain some superficial level of appropriateness and predictability in his relationships and overt behavior, then an ambulatory disposition with close follow-up may be possible.

3.5. Social Network and Support Systems

The patient's social network is essential for home maintenance of the psychotic patient. They should be able to provide supervision and protection 24 hours per day, ensure that the patient takes his medication, and return the patient to the hospital if necessary. However, before entrusting the patient to home care, the psychiatrist should evaluate the family's relationship to the patient, whether their judgment is intact, and how enmeshed or intrusive they may be. Not uncommonly, the family proves unsuitable because of their need to deny that the patient is ill. Such families may be so frightened or appalled by the patient's disorder that they inappropriately minimize or ignore the illness. The clinician should also ascertain whether the patient trusts the members of his immediate social matrix in spite of his psychotic thinking.

3.6. Network and Systems Involvement

There may be a helping network ready to be mobilized for the psychotic patient who has had previous treatment. Professionals and agencies familiar with the patient can provide historical data and treatment suggestions. If hospitalization is to be avoided, then some system of outreach (e.g., crisis teams, professionals able to make home visits) or community-based ambulatory care (e.g., day treatment, walk-in facilities, neighborhood mental health centers) becomes very important. If these patients are to be managed on an ambulatory basis, then the entire network of care must be accessible, comprehensive, and continuous.

3.7. The Mental Status Examination (MSE)

The mental status examination is essential for diagnosing the acutely psychotic patient. It can be critical in differentiating organic from functional psychoses since, in general, significant impairment of cognitive functions suggests an organic etiology. Repeated administration of the MSE is also a quantifiable, objective measure of the disorder's course and of the impact of therapeutic intervention over time.

Appearance and behavior should be noted first. This includes general appearance, awareness and appreciation of surroundings, psychomotor activity, complex behaviors, and capacity to relate to the interviewer. General appearance may reflect the rapidity with which the psychosis has occurred. The well-dressed, carefully groomed psychotic may not have been psychotic in the very recent past. (Any illness that evolves over a few hours is likely to be organic.) If the patient is malodorous, dirty, and poorly dressed, it is likely that his condition evolved over days or weeks. Apparent lack of awareness of the environment may reflect the severity and disruption of the psychosis. The behavior of the acute psychotic may take almost any shape and form, but the particulars should be noted. Level of activity varies along a continuum from mute, catatonic, withdrawn immobility to hyperaroused, agitated, hypervigilant frenzy. In addition, the clinician should look for such classic behaviors as echopraxia and waxy flexibility, and evaluate impulsivity and unpredictability of the patient's actions. Orientation to the interviewer is important because it suggests opening maneuvers in establishing a therapeutic alliance.

Speech may well be affected during acute psychotic episodes, resulting in increased or decreased productions, blocking, or bizarre manners of speaking. True language disturbances (e.g., perseverations) might indicate an underlying organic disorder.

The patient's predominant emotion may be terror, despair, or elation. Emotion may be quite inappropriate to the thought content, may be poorly modulated, and is often very labile or unpredictable, with sudden upsurges of intense feeling. As opposed to the blunted and flat affect seen in chronic psychoses, the feeling tone during acute episodes is intense.

Perceptual disturbances are a cardinal feature of psychosis. Illusions are common in toxic psychoses and delirium; distortions of color, space, body, and time typically result from hallucinogen use. When the patient is hallucinating, the clinician needs to establish the sensory modalities involved as well as the content of the hallucinations. Visual hallucinations are more common in organic psychoses.

Thinking is disturbed in several characteristic ways. Thought flow, i.e., the evolution and interconnection of ideas, may be illogical and personalized. The patient may exhibit loose associations, word salad, clang associations, flight of ideas, etc. Thought content is also disturbed, with the formation of false beliefs (i.e., delusions) that are not susceptible to disproof and not socioculturally sanctioned. Possession of thought may also be disrupted in acute psychosis, with the patient experiencing thought control, insertion, withdrawal, and broadcasting. Tempo of thought is also often disordered. Mania has a characteristic acceleration of thinking, and depression is often accompanied by retardation.

Intellectual function is an important part of the mental status examination. It helps distinguish functional from organic psychoses; cognitive functions are generally preserved in functional conditions while intellectual impairment is much more likely to reflect an organic disorder. All cognitive function tests are rendered invalid if the patient cannot attend to the tests because of anxiety or distraction. Therefore, attention must be assessed before proceeding with cognitive function testing. Among the various tests of intellectual function, level of consciousness, orientation, memory, and general information are the most valid indicators of organic impairment.[5] The patient's judgment, insight, and arithmetic ability are also useful indicators. There are several standardized tests for cognitive function that are particularly easy to administer, can be repeated over time, and differentiate organic and functional conditions reliably. These include the Mini-Mental State Examination[6] and the Bender Gestalt Visual Motor Test.[7]

3.8. Physical Examination

Significant medical disease is surprisingly common among acute psychotics.[8] The medical illness may be causing the psychosis or may be concurrent. Physical examination is indicated in the emergency evaluation of these patients, entailing at least careful observation of vital signs or more complete physical and neurological examination, if necessary. The emergency psychiatrist should be capable of completing a basic physical examination, but may call upon other specialists when a more extended work-up is indicated.

Vital signs should routinely be obtained on every acutely psychotic patient. Although minor elevations of pulse or blood pressure may be nonspecific manifestations of stress and anxiety, more significant elevations may indicate withdrawal states or metabolic and endocrine disorders. Temperature elevations may be especially significant and may be the first indication of systemic or CNS infection. General observation of the patient may disclose signs of severe cardiac or respiratory compromise, adrenergic crisis (sweating, tremor, hyperarousal), anticholinergic toxicity (dry skin, flushing), or hepatic failure (asterixis). The head may reveal signs of trauma. Eyes should be examined for nystagmus (intoxication); pupil size, reactivity, and symmetry (substance intoxication or withdrawal, focal brain pathology); and extraocular movements (focal disease, Wernicke's encephalopathy). Eye grounds may reveal signs of increased intracranial pressure. The neck should be checked for suppleness (meningeal irritation). Deep tendon reflexes should be evaluated for asymmetry or hyperactivity. Pathological reflexes (Babinski, snout, glabellar) should be ruled out.

This physical screening will permit detection of the major, life-threatening causes of acute psychosis.[9] If, on the basis of the history, mental status, and physical examination outlined above, the clinician suspects serious medical illness, an extensive medical work-up should be ordered.

3.9. Laboratory Examination

The work-up of the acutely psychotic patient may include certain diagnostic laboratory tests. The most frequently used study is the toxicological assaying of blood or urine for psychotropics, poisons, stimulants, hallucinogens, narcotics, and hypnosedatives. The reliability, sensitivity, cost, and speed of these analyses are variable, and they may be difficult to obtain. When the screen is negative, the picture may not be much clearer; when it is positive, however, it can clarify an otherwise confusing clinical presentation.

When organic psychosis is suspected, the work-up should include
blood count, urine analysis, chest X ray, and electrocardiogram. Sod
tassium, calcium, glucose, BUN, thyroid, and liver function studies are
erally obtained. If neurological disease is suspected, lumbar puncture, el
troencephalogram, or CT scan may be helpful, depending upon the clinica
picture.

4. Differential Diagnosis

Etiological diagnosis is a crucial part of the approach to the acute psychotic. First, the clinician should distinguish between an organic and a functional psychosis. Further classification of functional psychosis may be difficult
given the single-point-in-time observation in the emergency setting. The emergency room psychiatrist's diagnosis may therefore be no more specific than
"acute psychotic episode," just as the emergency medical patient is admitted
with the general diagnosis "jaundice" or "respiratory failure." It may not be
possible to diagnose the specific psychiatric entity because historical detail is
unobtainable, the illness has not yet evolved longitudinally over time, or the
acute picture may not be specific to one classification.

4.1. Psychiatric Disorders Causing Acute Psychosis

4.1.1. Acute Schizophrenic Episode

Schizophrenia classically produces one or more acute psychotic episodes
during its course. The hallmark of these episodes is a disorder of perception,
thought control, and thought progression in the presence of a clear sensorium
and without manic or depressive symptoms. The patient is unable to control,
organize, or direct his thinking. His thoughts are illogical and idiosyncratic and
don't appear goal-directed. Delusions are prominent, frequently multiple, ab-
surd, or bizarre. They often involve persecution, bodily change, or experiences
of control or alienation. Hallucinations, most commonly auditory, are generally
prominent. Affect may be inappropriate, unpredictable, or contradictory, and
during the acute episode there is often panic, rage, or terror. Intellectual functions typically remain intact, although there may be transient periods of confusion or disorientation consistent with a particularly severe acute episode.

> For example, a 23-year-old factory worker was brought in by his girlfriend
> after two weeks of increasingly withdrawn and bizarre behavior. Three
> weeks previous to the EW visit, the man's boss had placed him on an
> undesirable shift. A week later he stopped going to work but was unable
> to account for his time. One evening the patient inexplicably punched out
> several windows in his neighborhood. He went marketing with his girlfriend
> and, instead of waiting for her in the parking lot, drove away and disap-
> peared. He returned a day later, having "lost" the car. He now slept little
> and refused to eat, mumbling that his food was not real. Finally, he angrily

r conspiring in a scheme in which the mayor had
his jaw and was controlling him via an army of
ls of their apartment. At this point his girlfriend
l. She described a somewhat similar episode 16
d a 10-week hospitalization. There had been no
The patient was dirty, unshaven, and malodo-
nd hypervigilant, but would suddenly break off
d stand immobile for several seconds. At other
drew from the interviewer, glancing around the
g to auditory hallucinations. His thoughts were
disorganized and difficult to follow. He repeated, for example, "Father and
mother, king and queen of evil, yelling and striking." Much of the content
was paranoid. At one point he claimed he was the mayor; at another he
implied that the interviewer was. Orientation, general information, and long-
and short-term memory were preserved.

4.1.2. *Major Depressive Episode with Psychotic Features*

Major depressions may have psychotic features. These patients look profoundly depressed and generally have severe psychomotor changes. They may
have incessant and urgent agitation, or profound anergia and total withdrawal.
They feel sad, hopeless, guilty, lonely, and helpless. The delusions and hallucinations of the acutely psychotic depressed patient are usually consistent
with the depressed affect. Delusions typically involve the patient's death, sinfulness, guilt, punishment, poverty, or physical disease. Hallucinations are
usually not as complex or bizarre as those in schizophrenia and may involve
voices condemning the patient or accusing him of errors or inadequacies. Intellectual functions are found to be preserved when the patient can be adequately tested, but testing may prove difficult because he is anergic, withdrawn,
and self-deprecating.

> For example, a 53-year-old, widowed mother of three with a previously
> negative psychiatric history was brought to the hospital after swallowing
> 20 aspirin and 12 digoxin. Over the preceding month, the patient had with-
> drawn from her family, had crying outbursts, relinquished household re-
> sponsibilities, and stopped a woman's club she had organized. She ate less,
> lost weight, and had profound insomnia about which she complained bit-
> terly. About a week prior to coming to the hospital, the patient confessed
> to her daughters a sexual indiscretion committed 36 years ago, and then
> began telling them she had developed cancer as just punishment for her
> promiscuity. She refused professional help and finally took the overdose
> that brought her to the emergency ward. At that time she sat quietly with
> red-rimmed, puffy eyes that were continuously downcast. She felt that her
> family was disgusted by her and that she was evil. Since she felt undeserving
> of treatment, she was negativistic and uncooperative with the interviewer.
> She did reveal that her dead husband condemned her, was calling her a
> traitor and a whore, and that his voice had commanded her to kill herself.

4.1.3. Acute Manic Episode

Initially, acute manics are elated, exuberant, grandiose, and overconfident. As time passes, they may become labile, then more disorganized and dysphoric; that is, hostile, paranoid, terrified, and frenzied. At this point, they may be explosive and assaultive.[10] Manic patients are characteristically hyperactive and have pressured speech, accelerated thoughts, and flights of ideas. The content of delusions and hallucinations is consistent with the overall manic state. Hallucinatory voices may praise or compliment the individual, or may be persecutory. Delusions may be grandiose and reveal a heightened sense of self-worth and ability, or they, too, may be persecutory. Intellectual functions are preserved, but attention span is diminished, distractability is increased, and the patient may not cooperate with the mental status examination.

> For example, a 24-year-old man from another city was brought by the police to the emergency room from a nearby airport. He had recently arrived and had been haranguing fellow air travelers about world politics. The patient denied anything was wrong, claiming to have been brought to the hospital only because he had "a big mouth." He saw no need to answer the psychiatrist's questions, although he did remove a Bible from his briefcase and lectured anyone in earshot about the absence of religion in current political decision-making. He felt his own intellect and vision offered people the opportunity to alter the situation. A telephone call to his family revealed that after losing his job one week ago, the patient had become increasingly active, outgoing, and hyperreligious. He began purchasing religious literature and giving it away to strangers. He was staying up almost all night, planning a cross-country campaign. During the course of his evaluation in the emergency room, he became increasingly labile and disorganized. He claimed to be the Son of God, would suddenly jump up, shout "on guard," and strike his head on the wall.

4.1.4. Schizoaffective Psychosis

The existence and definition of schizoaffective psychosis is controversial. The clinician encounters acutely psychotic patients who have both schizophrenic and affective symptoms. As mentioned above, with only a narrow cluster of observations and an inadequate history, the emergency clinician must often defer the question of definitive psychiatric diagnosis. Thus, questions about schizoaffective psychosis as a disease entity independent of schizophrenia and affective disorder need not be decided by the emergency psychiatrist.

4.1.5. Atypical and Brief Reactive Psychosis

Disagreement also exists about the definitions of the terms *brief*, *reactive*, and *atypical psychosis*. The basic point relevant for the emergency psychiatrist is that some acute psychotic episodes are milder and shorter and have more circumscribed effects than those described above. They produce fewer, "softer,'' and less flagrant symptoms; there is not the disorganization of the entire personality and the global impairment of reality testing seen in most schizophrenic and affective psychoses. Hallucinations are simple and nondescript; delusions are neither bizarre nor elaborate. The episodes are brief and occur in the context of obvious, massive stress. The psychotic thinking seems clearly related to the stressful situation or it may be precipitated by drug abuse. Often, ''soft'' psychotic signs are more prominent than clear-cut hallucinations or delusions: mild paranoia, overvalued ideas and ideas of reference, illusions, primitive or bizarre daydreams and dreams at night, depersonalization and derealization, and periods of perplexity. On mental status examination the clinician may observe inappropriate affect, parapraxes, and peculiar usage of certain words. It appears that at least some of these individuals are diagnosed as having borderline personality organization when not psychotic.

> For example, a 32-year-old woman came to the emergency room 36 hours after having been robbed on the street near her home. Three men had overpowered her, knocked her to the ground, stuffed a rag in her mouth, and torn off her jewelry. Soon after, while alone in her apartment, she heard a voice shout, ''Watch out!'' She became too terrified to leave her apartment and called an ambulance when she spotted a handkerchief on the floor that she believed was saturated with poison gas. In the emergency room, she said she thought she had been targeted for death by an international terrorist organization, but was not completely sure about it. Though the patient had never been overtly psychotic before, she had been sufficiently suspicious and critical of people so that she had left a series of jobs because her bosses were presumably neither supportive nor fair in their dealings with her. Two hours after taking 5 mg of oral haloperidol (Haldol), the patient had no further hallucinations but remained frightened and anxious. She remembered believing that the handkerchief was poisoned and that a conspiracy had been formed, but now felt this was no longer true.

4.2. Medical Disorders Causing Acute Psychosis (See Table 1)

4.2.1. Exogenous Substances

The use of stimulants (amphetamines, cocaine), alcohol, and hallucinogens (including marijuana) can produce a toxic psychosis that may be clinically indistinguishable from the functional psychoses discussed above (see Chapter 9). A single amphetamine overdose can cause a toxic delirium, while the repeated use of even moderate amounts can produce a chronic paranoid psychosis without any signs of organicity. The cessation of alcohol in the addicted individual can precipitate alcohol hallucinosis (i.e., no impairment of cognitive functioning) as well as the well-known withdrawal delirium. The ingestion of a single dose of a hallucinogen can cause an acute psychosis, and the prolonged use of these agents can produce a chronic psychosis that persists long after the individual has ceased using the drug. At the present time, the most common and most dangerous of the hallucinogens is phencyclidine (PCP or ''angel dust''). In addition to psychotic symptoms, it can produce severe agitation,

Table 1. Organic Causes of Psychosis[a]

1. Space-occupying lesions of the CNS
   Brain abscess (bacterial, fungal, TB, cysticercus)
   Metastatic carcinoma
   Primary cerebral tumors
   Subdural hematoma
2. Cerebral hypoxia
   Anemia
   Lowered cardiac output
   Pulmonary insufficiency
   Toxic—e.g., carbon monoxide
3. Neurologic disorders
   Alzheimer's disease
   Distant effects of carcinoma
   Huntington's chorea
   Normal pressure hydrocephalus
   Temporal lobe epilepsy
   Wilson's disease
4. Vascular disorders
   Aneurysms
   Collagen vascular disease
   Hypertensive encephalopathy
   Intracranial hemorrhage
   Lacunar state
5. Infections
   Brain abscess
   Encephalitis and postencephalitic states
   Malaria
   Meningitis (bacterial, fungal, TB)
   Subacute bacterial endocarditis
   Syphilis
   Toxoplasmosis
   Typhoid
6. Metabolic and endocrine disorders
   Adrenal disease (Addison's and Cushing's disease)
   Calcium-related disorders
   Diabetes mellitus
   Electrolyte imbalance
   Hepatic failure
   Homocystinuria
   Hypoglycemia and hyperglycemia
   Pituitary insufficiency
   Porphyria
   Thyroid disease (thyrotoxicosis and myxedema)
   Uremia
7. Nutritional deficiencies
   B12
   Niacin (pellagra)
   Thiamine (Wernicke-Korsakoff syndrome)
8. Drugs, medications, and toxic substances
   Alcohol (intoxication and withdrawal)
   Amphetamines
   Analgesics [Eq. pentazocine (Talwin), meperidine
   (Demerol)]

(Continued)

Table 1. (*Continued*)

---

8. Drugs, medications, and toxic substances (*Continued*)
   Anticholinergic agents
   Antiparkinson agents
   Barbiturates and other sedative-hypnotic agents
       (intoxication and withdrawal)
   Bromides and other heavy metals
   Carbon disulfide
   Cocaine
   Corticosteroids
   Cycloserine (Seromycin)
   Digitalis (Crystodigin)
   Disulfiram (Antabuse)
   Hallucinogens
   Isoniazid
   L-Dopa (Larodopa and others)
   Marijuana
   Propranolol
   Reserpine (Serpasil and others)

---

[a] Adpated from Schoonover.[11]

excitement, and sudden violent destructive outbursts. Psychotic symptoms include paranoid delusions and bizarre or violent delusions—that the patient is invulnerable or already dead, for example. Auditory and visual hallucinations may be present, and there are often prominent distortions of body and space.[3] There is the case of two young men, both under the influence of PCP, who set each other on fire attempting to prove that they would not burn since they were already dead. Another young man, a repeated user of PCP, jumped from an elevated train station believing he could fly. Unlike patients using hallucinogens, PCP users cannot be "talked down." Attempting to do so may exacerbate the psychosis and may in fact cause the patient to become violent. Instead, the patient should be isolated in a quiet room with minimal stimulation and carefully observed.

4.2.2. Metabolic and Endocrine Disorders

Electrolyte imbalance, uremia, and hepatic failure can produce confusional states with psychotic features. Endocrine disorders such as hyperparathyroidism, hypoglycemia (primary, or secondary to insulin administration), and thyroid and adrenal disease can likewise present with acute psychotic features.

4.2.3. Neurological Disorders

Brain diseases such as tumors (both primary and metastatic), strokes, concussion, subdural hematoma, and seizure disorders (especially temporal lobe epilepsy) must all be considered in the differential diagnosis of the acutely psychotic patient. It is not uncommon for encephalitis and meningitis to present initially with disturbance of cortical function before focal findings appear.

4.2.4. Other Systemic Illness

Any systemic process that acutely produces brain hypoxia or ischemia can result in psychotic symptoms. This includes pulmonary edema, pulmonary embolus, acute asthmatic attack, and sudden drops in cardiac output. Subacute bacterial endocarditis and hypertensive encephalopathy should be considered. Nutritional deficiency states also can produce a psychoticlike picture.

4.3. Differential Diagnostic Process

As mentioned above, the emergency psychiatrist must first decide whether the acutely psychotic patient has an organic or functional psychosis and then what the specific disease process is. This second step may not be completed in the emergency setting, especially when the psychosis does not appear to be organic. Definitive diagnosis may require hospitalization, the passage of time, and more intensive evaluation. No single symptom, historical feature, or mental status finding is sufficient to establish a particular diagnosis. (Even the classic picture of acute catatonia can be caused by many different psychiatric and medical disorders.[12]) The psychiatrist's impression is thus based on the overall picture composed of clinical history, family history, past psychiatric history, medical history, mental status, and physical findings.

Some historical features help distinguish between organic and functional psychoses. In general, one suspects an organic cause in older patients whose past psychiatric history is negative. Psychoses with very rapid onset (hours, or even minutes) tend to be caused by medical disorders, while functional psychoses usually evolve over days or weeks. A continually fluctuating picture, with symptom intensity waxing and waning, implies an organic etiology, especially if there is nocturnal exacerbation of symptoms.

An organic etiology should also be suspected when cognitive and intellectual functions are impaired. Hallucinations and delusions that are poorly formed, without detail, and rapidly shifting suggest an underlying medical cause. Conversely, psychotic content that is elaborate, bizarre, alien, and stable points toward a functional psychiatric disorder.

Visual, tactile, gustatory, and olfactory hallucinations suggest an organic condition, especially when auditory hallucinations are absent. Auditory hallucinations alone are more consistent with a functional etiology.

It is good clinical practice always to consider first the most common diagnoses, the most likely, and the most serious. The most serious causes of acute psychosis include meningitis and encephalitis, hypertensive crisis, intracranial hemorrhage, decreased oxygenation, hypoglycemia, and Wernicke's encephalopathy (see Table 1).

5. Management

5.1. Psychological

The acutely psychotic patient should be treated gently, but firmly. Communication should be simple and straightforward. The psychiatrist functions in the traditional mode of the impartial and professional physician who questions the patient, examines him, and then treats him. This does not mean, of course, that he omits trying to make empathic emotional contact with the patient, or that they do not talk about the patient's feelings. But the patient is not encouraged to ventilate his feelings. In the interest of not increasing the patient's anxiety, the interviewer should avoid interpretive comments.

The physician should convey to the patient that he is now in a safe, secure setting and will be protected. In addition, he can define clear guidelines for patient behavior, that is, what will be tolerated and what will lead to seclusion or restraint. The interviewer should explain what he will be doing to the patient and why. This can be done in a quiet, matter-of-fact way, without excessive elaboration: "I want to ask you some questions to see how clearly you are thinking. After that, we will do a physical examination to find out what is causing your difficulty."

The interviewer should always try to help the patient reality-test. Misperceptions and questions about the doctor or the procedure should receive direct and simple answers rather than further questions. It may be necessary to assure the patient explicitly that, in fact, "I cannot read your mind." When the physician must respond to delusional material, he should acknowledge that while he can understand how the patient might feel it to be true, he (the doctor) does not believe it is. For example, "Although I can understand why you think I am a CIA agent, I am not. I am a doctor and I would like to find out exactly what is bothering you so that I can help." It is not useful, however, to try to argue the patient out of his delusional beliefs. Similarly, the psychiatrist can acknowledge the patient's hallucinations, and the patient's emotional experience of them, but he should not imply that they are real, nor should he challenge their reality.

The approach to the withdrawn, mute, uncommunicative, and uncooperative patient is to try to make the patient comfortable enough so that he can talk meaningfully. The psychiatrist should convey his expectation that the patient can discuss his problems, and make it clear he wants to be helpful. The interviewer should try to address the patient's inner experience, whether it be paranoid fear, mountainous rage, or depressive despair. If the interviewer can address this accurately and the patient can acknowledge it, then the groundwork is laid for further interaction. The psychiatrist's initial impressions may be based upon the patient's behavior, appearance, or facial expression. He may begin by simply noting that the patient obviously doesn't feel like talking. If he has ancillary history from someone else, the doctor should tell the patient exactly what he has been told and then ask the patient for his views. Some mute patients will write answers to questions, or will nod yes or no in response.

With excited, agitated, and aroused patients, the interviewer must be careful not to seem intrusive to the patient. He needs to be firm, clear, "doctorly." Wearing a white coat, remaining at some distance (both physically and psychologically), and stating clearly that he is a doctor prepared to help the patient feel better will all reduce patient anxiety. Rather than making empathic comments as one might with a withdrawn patient, the psychiatrist can ask questions as he does in taking a medical history.[13] If the psychiatrist is afraid of the hyperaroused patient, he should take steps to feel safe before proceeding with the interview.

The disorganized patient may not be able to provide a coherent history no matter what interviewing techniques are employed. The interviewer should convey the expectation that the patient pull himself together and "act like an adult." Regression may be prevented by asking the patient to sit up in a chair, shake hands, adjust any clothing that may be in disarray, etc. Acute anxiety may contribute to the patient's disorganization and the interviewer should try to identify anything that might be heightening anxiety.

5.2. Physical

Acutely psychotic patients are confused, flooded with sensory input, and unable to focus their attention. As soon as possible, the patient should be placed in a private, moderately lighted, nonstimulating room containing no extraneous equipment. The room should be quiet and contain no dangerous objects or features that could be used by the patient to harm himself or others. These include live electric outlets, protruding light fixtures, sheets, equipment with sharp edges, cords, etc.

If the patient is a physical danger to himself, to the staff, or to other patients, then he will require security personnel, seclusion, and/or physical restraint. The least restrictive alternative should be employed first. Often the obvious presence of security personnel is all that is necessary to prevent violence. When the patient is made aware of their presence he is generally calmed and under better self-control, even in the case of the most severely disorganized and psychotic individuals. Adequate numbers are important; a massive show of force assures the patient that violence is out of the question.

Involuntary seclusion is a more restrictive form of physical management that can be used if the above measures are insufficient. The patient should be placed in a safe, private room. Patients must always be searched for matches, rope, and sharp or dangerous objects before being confined to such a room. If the secluded patient is still dangerous to caretakers when they enter the room or if he is actively self-destructive, physical restraints are necessary to protect him and to allow evaluation and treatment to proceed (see Chapter 2).

The final and most invasive restraint is pharmacological, used not as a specific treatment for psychosis but rather as a chemical inhibitor to prevent serious physical harm and to allow the staff to evaluate and treat the patient. For this purpose antipsychotics or benzodiazepines can be administered in repeated doses to sedate the patient sufficiently so that he may be examined by staff (see Chapter 2).

5.3. Pharmacological

Antipsychotic agents are safe and effective, and specifically reverse psychotic symptoms. If possible, they should be withheld until a complete history can be obtained, the patient has been observed, and any indicated medical work-up has been initiated. If necessary for restraint, however, they should be administered immediately.

If there is a medical cause for psychosis, then the primary treatment is directed at that medical disorder. If rapid management of psychotic behavior is also needed, then antipsychotics may be administered cautiously and in relatively low dosages (see below). If the clinician is unsure of the specific organic etiology, 100 mg of thiamine and 50 cc of 50% dextrose in water may be administered immediately in case the patient is hypoglycemic or has Wernicke's encephalopathy.

Once the diagnosis of an acute functional psychosis has been established, antipsychotic treatment should be initiated as soon as possible. If immediate hospitalization is planned, then the administration of antipsychotics may be delayed until the patient reaches the hospital. In general, however, antipsychotics should be started in the emergency setting when hospitalization is to be avoided.

In most cases of functional psychosis, treatment may be initiated with a high-potency antipsychotic agent, such as trifluoperazine (Stelazine), fluphenazine (Prolixin), or haloperidol (Haldol). There is relatively little danger of serious postural hypotension or arrhythmias. The weak sedating action is beneficial, allowing the psychotic thinking to be reversed without making the patient somnolent. The agent may be given in repeated doses, titrating the amount given against the target psychotic symptoms: hallucinations, delusions, and formal thought disorder. The agent may be given intramuscularly, or by mouth if the patient refuses the intramuscular route. The intramuscular route is preferable because it produces a more rapid effect—sharper onset of action—and the incremental effects of additional doses can be observed. Haloperidol, for example, may be administered with a 5-mg intramuscular injection, followed with 5 to 10 mg more every 30 to 60 minutes, depending upon patient's age and weight and the severity of the psychosis.[14] Administration is continued until the psychosis diminishes, the patient becomes somnolent, or the total dose reaches 40 to 50 mg. If the psychosis has not improved sufficiently, hospitalization is probably necessary and medication can be continued in that setting.[14] The patient should be observed for sedation, hypotension, and extrapyramidal effects (see Chapters 2 and 4).

If the patient goes home from the emergency setting, he should begin taking an oral dose of approximately one to two times the total amount he received in the emergency ward. This total dose may be spread over 24 hours in two to four divided doses. Extrapyramidal reactions, most often dystonia, tend to develop over the next few days. The patient should always be told about the possibility of extrapyramidal reactions. Because they occur frequently, a case could be made against the prophylactic prescription of an antiparkinson agent such as benztropine mesylate (Cogentin), 1 to 2 mg twice a day[15] (see Chapter 10).

For the patient with an organic psychosis, treatment is aimed at the underlying disorder. Treatment with antipsychotics is undertaken only when behavioral control is absolutely necessary. In general, haloperidol is effective for the treatment of organic psychoses because it is safe and has minimal medical effects. The doses used should be much lower than for functional psychoses. Starting doses are generally in the range of 0.5 mg to 2.0 mg. *Caution*: When treating psychoses due to exogenous substances, particularly anticholinergic toxicity, the anticholinergic properties of the antipsychotic agent can exacerbate the patient's condition. LSD psychosis is probably best managed with a benzodiazepine,[16] while most clinicians prefer haloperidol in the treatment of PCP psychosis.[17]

The patient should be told the name of the agent he is receiving and why it is being given. If the patient refuses medication, the physician should discuss the patient's concerns. If the patient continues to refuse medication that is necessary to prevent significant physical harm, then it should be administered, provided that the psychiatrist is aware of the legal issues involved in forcibly medicating a patient in an emergency (see Chapter 3).

6. Patient–Evaluator Interaction

6.1. General Reactions to the Psychotic Patient

Acutely psychotic patients provoke profound reactions in their caretakers. Anxiety and a feeling of threat underlie many staff reactions and may impair staff performance. They may experience lapses in judgment and think less clearly than they ordinarily do. Desk clerks forget to obtain identifying information; the triage officer sends the critically ill medical patient with a psychotic symptom to the psychiatry service. For example, a psychotic, weepy young man was triaged to psychiatry, although he had a compound fracture of the femur and severe physical pain. Similarly, a bizarre-appearing psychotic woman was triaged directly to psychiatry after jumping from a bridge into a river in the middle of the winter. The patient had not been checked for hypothermia and, when first seen by the psychiatrist, had a rectal temperature of 91°. Nurses unaccountably forget to obtain the vital signs of the acute psychotic. Medical physicians omit the most basic medical history in working up the patient. In another example, psychiatry was called to consult on the case of a 34-year-old hospital operating room technician who had suddenly become paranoid and combative on the job. Medical and neurological services had already worked up the patient with negative results. The psychiatrist was the first to learn from the patient that he was an insulin-dependent diabetic. His blood sugar was found to be 43 mg%.

The best approach to these problems is continuing in-service education. Such a program needs to be built into the routine emergency ward functioning. Discussions about such patients help "detoxify" them, make them less alien, and provide staff with a conceptual frame work for bizarre and frightening behavior. All of this diminishes staff anxiety and fear, thus improving patient care.

6.2. Specific Reactions of the Emergency Psychiatrist

Working with acute psychotics is extraordinarily difficult and requires rapid action. The psychiatrist working in this setting of ambiguity and uncertainty must learn to think clearly, work efficiently, and act decisively.

The first step is to recognize the inherent limitations of the setting. The emergency psychiatrist can be neither omniscient nor omnipotent. He should relieve himself of the pressure that derives from his own well-intentioned, but unrealistic, expectations.

The second step is to follow a standardized routine with all acutely psychotic patients. He should adhere to an overall frame work that will help him gather data, think logically and systematically, and maintain accurate clinical judgment. It may be helpful to think of the data-gathering process in sequence: psychiatric history, medical history, mental status observations, and then physical and laboratory examination. Next, the clinician should consider a complete differential diagnosis as a way to ensure that no important disease entities are missed. Management can be broken down into physical, psychological, and pharmacological interventions. Developing a systematic approach to the care of the psychotic patient will help ensure organization, thoroughness, and logic in a situation that often has a disorganizing effect upon the clinician.

Finally, the psychiatrist should remember that he must ultimately depend on his own clinical judgment and not on the family, other emergency personnel, consulting physicians, or even the patient himself. People have definite opinions about the management and disposition of the acutely psychotic individual. These opinions often conflict, so the psychiatrist should remember that he cannot placate, please, or agree with everyone involved.

6.3. Patient's Attitude toward the Psychiatrist

The acute psychotic perceives the external world as confusing, threatening, and intrusive. His own inner world of feeling is tumultous, unpredictable, and terrifying. Past, present, and future have no continuity; nothing about the recent past seems to predict anything about the immediate future. Given this experience, it is not surprising that the psychotic can form only a very tenuous and fragile therapeutic relationship. The psychiatrist cannot be perceived "objectively," and his intentions and abilities cannot be trusted. Some acute psychotics have sufficient observing ego to know they need help and to accept it. But many do not.

7. Treatment Planning

7.1. Requests

The requests of acutely psychotic patients are primitive, at one extreme on the spectrum of patient requests.[18] They request help for and with the following: (1) Reality testing—to help them to feel more sane, "check out" reality, and "keep in touch" with it. (2) Control—the patient feels overwhelmed and out of control, and fears he will lose his mind or hurt someone. He hopes the psychiatrist will stop his thoughts or feelings before they overpower him. (3) Nurturance—the patient feels empty, drained, and alone. He wants the psychiatrist to care, be involved, be warm and giving so that he in turn can feel replenished and comforted.[18]

Defining the patient's requests helps calm the patient and stabilize the situation. Conversely, should the psychiatrist misjudge the patient's requests, his intervention can make the patient more withdrawn, agitated, or disorganized.[18] Understanding the request and responding to it are a crucial part of the interaction with an acutely psychotic patient.

Acutely psychotic patients may or may not explicitly request hospitalization. Those who do are generally seeking to protect themselves and others from their violent impulses, and/or to find a safe port from the maelstrom of suffering and confusion in which they are caught. If the acute psychotic requests hospitalization, every effort should be made to accede. The patient is saying he doubts his control.

7.2. The Decision to Hospitalize

Hospitalization is one of the most critical treatment planning decisions. Many acute psychotic patients require hospitalization, but this is not invariable,[19] and there are significant advantages to returning a patient home. An ambulatory disposition requires, first, that there is no significant suicide or homicide risk. Second, there should be no serious or evolving medical disorder. Third, the patient must have a social matrix capable of watching, protecting, and treating him 24 hours per day for the duration of the acute psychotic episode. Fourth, the conditions that precipitated the episode should have been altered so that they no longer continue to act upon the patient after discharge. And fifth, the emergency intervention must have diminished the psychotic signs in order for the patient to be discharged back into the community. This means that antipsychotics have significantly tempered the psychotic symptoms without oversedating the patient, and that emotional contact was made with the patient. The clinician should be convinced that the patient will respect follow-up commitments. These conditions are stringent, but they are not infrequently met.[19] If they are, ambulatory follow-up offers some major advantages over hospitalization.

7.3. Availability and Nature of Resources

After emergency work-up and initial stabilization, the disposition of the acute psychotic depends, in part, on available resources. The least restrictive alternatives include disposition to the community, such as to the patient's own home or to an appropriate family member or friend. This requires close follow-up capability. Is there a facility where the patient can be seen daily and which is available for emergencies 24 hours a day? Is there the capacity for community outreach that would allow follow-up visits in the home? And most critically, are there family or friends able and willing to be involved in this way?

The next least restrictive option is voluntary hospitalization. If the patient wants to be hospitalized and is not a major suicide or homicide risk, he can be hospitalized on an open unit in a general or psychiatric hospital. The staff of such a unit should be experienced in treating acute psychotics since these patients require intensive observation and skilled care.

The most restrictive alternative is involuntary commitment to a locked unit. Acute psychosis by itself does not necessarily justify involuntary commitment. If the legal criteria for involuntary commitment are met, and other clinical signs warrant that alternative, arrangements should be made (see Chapter 3).

7.4. Negotiation about Treatment Planning

The psychiatrist may find that some of the patient's requests can be granted, some are negotiable, and some are not. While it may be appropriate to negotiate and compromise with the acute psychotic about the methods and conditions of treatment, the psychiatrist may not be able to compromise about the definition of the problem or the basic goals of treatment. Because of the patient's impaired judgment, lack of insight, faulty reality testing, and inaccurate perception of the external world, the psychiatrist needs to be directive and authoritarian without ignoring the patient's perspective or his wish to be heard and understood.

Negotiating with the patient's family is often difficult. While the family's goals and wishes are important, their view of the situation is colored by their own personal values, beliefs, and needs. They may seize upon minor aspects of the situation and exaggerate their importance. Or they may deny or minimize the psychotic symptoms because they feel responsible and guilty. It is essential to know the family's views, weigh them, and explain what is being done and why, but it often is neither possible nor advisable to accede to their requests if they conflict with professional judgment.

7.5. Administrative Issues

7.5.1. Facilities

A holding unit or overnight ward to which these patients can be admitted for 48 to 72 hours is useful. Such a unit can be used when prolonged medical, neurological, or psychiatric work-up is indicated, or when the psychosis is due to intoxication or poisoning. A holding unit can be employed to avoid the formal and prolonged hospitalization of a traditional inpatient unit.

7.5.2. Legal Problems

The management of acute psychotics raises difficult legal questions. The general guideline for the clinician is to exercise common sense and good clinical judgment rather than worrying about specific legal constraints and dictates. In the event legal questions might arise, written records should be explicit and detailed; they should include all clinical data on the possible alternative treatments, and the reasons for the procedures chosen. In short, the written record should convey the information on which the psychiatrist based his clinical reasoning. For example, if a patient was forcibly restrained, the written note should record verbal or physical threats, kinds of restraints employed, duration of restraint, and reasons for not employing alternative methods (see Chapter 3).

7.5.3. Dispositional Problems

Dispositional problems are common with acute psychotic patients, especially when the patient is chronically impaired and has been deinstitutionalized, or when he is elderly, an adolescent, or a child. For the chronically psychotic, deinstitutionalized patient with a superimposed acute exacerbation, community resources for ambulatory treatment may not be adequate. The patient may be caught between a reluctant inpatient facility and an inadequate ambulatory disposition based on community services. The elderly acute psychotic also presents problems: He commonly has concurrent medical illness, which psychiatric hospitals feel ill-equipped to manage; he may require nursing home placement after hosptialization, either because he is without social supports or because he is demented and unable to care for himself. Hospitals are reluctant to admit these patients if responsible aftercare is a major problem. Finally, inpatient facilities for psychotic children and adolescents are generally poor alternatives to good ambulatory care.

These dispositional problems are real and serious. The best solution at present is ongoing, open dialogue between emergency services and public/private sector inpatient facilities. The willingness of emergency facilities to provide emergency medical and psychiatric backup to these hospitals can be helpful in forging closer working relationships.

References

1. Shneidman ES, Farberow NL (eds.): *Clues to Suicide.* New York, McGraw-Hill, 1957.
2. Reich P, Kelly MJ: Suicide attempts by hospitalized medical and surgical patients. *N Engl J Med* 294:298–301, 1976.
3. Peralson GD: Psychiatric and medical syndromes associated with phencyclidine (PCP) abuse. *Johns Hopkins Med J* 148:25–33, 1981.
4. Lion JR: *Evaluation and Management of the Violent Patient.* Springfield, Ill, Charles C Thomas, 1972.
5. Keller MB, Manschreck TC: The biologic mental status examination. Higher intellectual functioning, in Lazare, A (ed): *Outpatient Psychiatry: Diagnosis and Treatment.* Baltimore, Williams & Wilkins, 1979, pp 203–214.
6. Folstein MF, Folstein SE, McHugh PR: Mini-mental state—A practical method for grading the cognitive state of patients for the clinician. *J Psychiatr Res* 12:189–198, 1976.
7. Bender L: A visual-motor test and its clinical use. American Orthopsychiatric Association Research Monograph #3. New York, American Orthopsychiatric Association, 1938.

8. Hall RCW, Popkin MK, Devaul RA, et al: Physical illness presenting as psychiatric disease. *Arch Gen Psychiatry* 35:1315–1320, 1978.

9. Anderson WH: The physical examination in office practice. *Am J Psychiatry* 137:1188–1192, 1980.

10. Carlson GA, Goodwin FK: The stages of mania. *Arch Gen Psychiatry* 28:221–228, 1973.

11. Schoonover SC: The practice of pharmacotherapy, in Bassuk EL, Schoonover SC, Gelenberg AJ (eds): *The Practitioner's Guide to Psychoactive Drugs*, ed 2. New York, Plenum Publishing Corp, 1983.

12. Gelenberg AJ: The catatonic syndrome. *Lancet* 1:1339–1341, 1976.

13. Havens LL: Taking a history from a difficult patient. *Lancet* 1:138–140, 1978.

14. Anderson WH, Kuehnle JC, Catanzano DM: Rapid treatment of acute psychoses. *Am J Psychiatry* 133:1076–1078, 1976.

15. Stern TA, Anderson WH: Benztropine prophylaxis of dystonic reactions. *Psychopharmacology* 61:261–262, 1979.

16. Khantzian EJ, McKenna GJ: Acute toxic and withdrawal reactions associated with drug use and abuse. *Ann Intern Med* 90:361–372, 1979.

17. Showalter CV, Thornton WE: Clinical pharmacology of phencyclidine toxicity. *Am J Psychiatry* 134:1234–1238, 1977.

18. Lazare A, Eisenthal S: A negotiated approach to the clinical encounter. I. Attending to the patient's perspective, in Lazare A (ed): *Outpatient Psychiatry: Diagnosis and Treatment*. Baltimore, Williams & Wilkins, 1979.

19. Anderson WH, Kuehnle JC: Strategies for the treatment of acute psychosis. *JAMA* 229:1884–1889, 1974.

Presentation of Depression in an Emergency Setting

Ronnie Fuchs, M.D.

1. Introduction

Depression affects approximately 20% of the population. Because of the associated risk of suicide, repetitive self-destructive acts, chronic self-neglect, and severe mood disturbance, depression accounts for a large proportion of emergency visits.

The depressive syndrome is defined by a persistent mood disturbance, but it frequently also involves corresponding physical, behavioral, and cognitive symptoms. The features of the syndrome can be grouped as follows:

- Mood: The dominant locus of the disorder. Symptoms—sadness, discouragement, lack of interest, feelings of worthlessness, helplessness, dread about the future.
- Physical correlates—sleep, appetite and sexual disturbances, low energy level, reduced stamina.
- Behavioral correlates—agitation, retardation, self-destructive acts, increased interpersonal and/or substance dependence.
- Cognitive correlates—negative predictions about the future, unfavorable self-assessment, poor concentration, impaired intellectual functioning.

These clinical features of depression may reflect a variety of diagnostic disorders: major medical or toxic disorders, bipolar or unipolar affective disorders, schizophrenia, characterologic problems, and situational depression. While good emergency management must be founded on sound etiologic premises, it is the total aggregate of symptoms, their severity and their collective potential to threaten the life of the patient that must be evaluated first (see Chapter 7).

This chapter discusses the evaluation, management, and disposition of depressed patients in the emergency setting. Because certain treatment decisions may depend on the presence of various symptom clusters, this chapter presents an approach to assessment that emphasizes the evaluation of these

Ronnie Fuchs, M.D. • Beth Israel Hospital, Boston, Massachusetts 02215, and Harvard Medical School, Boston, Massachusetts 02115.

Table 1. Major Depressive Illness—Diagnostic Criteria[a]

---

1. Dysphoric mood characterized by the following: feeling blue, irritable, hopeless, depressed or sad
2. Several (at least four) of the following symptoms present almost continuously for at least two weeks:
   a. Sleep disturbance
   b. Eating disorder with significant weight loss or gain
   c. Psychomotor agitation or retardation
   d. Loss of interest or pleasure in usual activities
   e. Fatigue and loss of energy
   f. Feeling worthless and guilty
   g. Difficulty concentrating or paying attention
   h. Preoccupying thoughts of death or suicidal feelings
3. Not due to schizophrenia or an organic problem

---

[a] Adapted from *Diagnostic and Statistical Manual of Mental Disorders.*[5]

symptoms. Clinical examples are included to highlight assessment and treatment issues.

2. Assessment

During the first few minutes of the emergency evaluation of a depressed patient, the presence of medically urgent conditions including, but not limited to, self-destructive acts, substance ingestion, and threatened suicide should be determined (see Chapters 2 and 7). If medically urgent symptoms can safely be ruled out, the clinician should assess the depressive syndrome itself, bearing in mind that the diagnosis of depressive disorder can be applied only if the mood disturbance is primary and predominant, and not secondary to an organic, medical, or psychotic disorder.

Some of the symptoms constituting a depression may be evident in a broad range of emergency patients, but it is the presence of some associated features and not others that will determine the clinician's initial diagnostic steps. It is useful, therefore, to outline in some detail the criteria for diagnosing a major depressive syndrome (see Table 1 and Section 4). The essential clinical feature is a lowered mood with consequent loss of interest in all, or nearly all, routine activities. Depression may be accompanied by significant agitation, resulting in restlessness, nervousness, pacing, and excited talking, or significant lethargy, manifested by slow speech and movement, fatigue, and reduced energy. Sleep patterns are frequently disturbed, with difficulty falling asleep, staying asleep, and, in some cases, terminating sleep. Appetite disturbances are also commonly associated with depression. Lack of appetite with consequent weight loss is typical, but compulsive overeating and weight gain can also correlate with depressive episodes. Particularly in the area of mental function, associated clinical symptoms can overlap diagnostic boundaries; these should receive special attention. For example, difficulty concentrating, memory lapses, disorien-

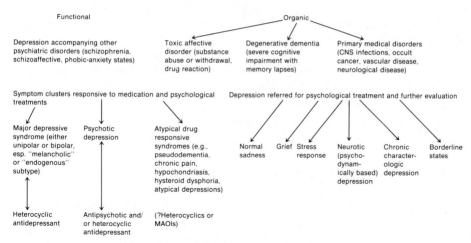

Figure 1. Assessment of depressive symptoms.

tation, and confusion can suggest an organic affective syndrome, schizophrenia or other psychotic disorder, major affective disorder, reactive depression, or pseudodementia secondary to major depression.

When the depressive syndrome does not itself present a moment-to-moment clinical emergency, steps should be taken to work through the following diagnostic tree: (1) Begin with an overall view of the patient by evaluating his internal assets, level of functioning, and external support network; (2) closely evaluate the specific complexion of the symptom cluster; determine the severity and persistence of each symptom; (3) differentiate crucial etiologic disjunctions, such as organic versus functional and primary versus secondary; and (4) consider the treatment implications. Are these syndromes responsive to medication and/or psychological treatments? Figure 1 is designed to help the clinician proceed step by step through critical assessment considerations.

The clinician should begin the evaluation by obtaining vital signs and completing a brief physical examination. A mental status examination (MSE) should be administered and a careful history taken. The history should include detailed information of possible precipitating events and of associated symptoms such as significant weight loss or gain, insomnia or hypersomnia, psychomotor agitation or lethargy, loss of interest or pleasure in life, loss of energy, feelings of worthlessness, guilt, difficulty in concentrating, memory loss or slowed thinking, wishes to be dead or suicidal impulses. To measure the disruptive effect of the current depressive episode, an impression of presymptom baseline mental functioning should be gathered, along with relevant facts from the past psychiatric and medical history. Patients should be carefully questioned about their use of prescribed and over-the-counter medication, alcohol, and other drugs subject to abuse. Other signs and symptoms, not usually identified with depression, may suggest the presence of an occult medical illness such as cancer of the pancreas. When a medical cause is suspected, simple laboratory tests such as blood counts and electrolytes can be obtained. Although vital signs should be taken on all emergency patients, a physical examination can also be performed. If the clinician continues to suspect a medical problem, the patient should be referred for a more complete work-up. If the patient is unable to give a complete history, family members or other persons in the patient's support network should be contacted. Similarly, current or previous therapists should be called for additional information.

3. Management and Disposition

Management goals within the first hour of emergency psychiatric care fall into three categories: (a) alleviating symptomatic distress by encouraging patients to express their feelings, to connect the feelings to significant life events or patterns of events, and to begin mobilizing internal and external counter-depressive resources; (b) formulating treatment plans; and (c) enlisting the patient's cooperation in effecting the transition from emergency care to post-emergency treatment.

Although it is not necessary to have made a definitive diagnosis during the first minutes of the emergency visit, it is essential to have refined the probable diagnosis by the end of the intervention so that disposition plans can be made to fit each patient's needs. Options for disposition are limited to hospitalization, referral for continuing (or follow-up) care (i.e., medication and/or psycho-therapeutic approaches), and no treatment.

3.1. Hospitalization

Many depressed patients require hospitalization either because of the severity of the depression and its associated symptoms or because the depression is secondary to another disorder, necessitating inpatient evaluation and/or treatment. Compelling suicidal intent, intense suffering, and chronic self-neglect or abuse are symptoms from which the patient needs protection. For these high-risk features of depression, a secure psychiatric unit offers several therapeutic advantages. Close observation and enforced, albeit structured, human contact can often help a patient survive an acute depressive and/or suicidal crisis. Milieu therapy provides a setting for the control of maladaptive patterns such as self-destructive rituals and the substitution of appropriate, depression-combating behaviors. For disorders with medically or psychiatrically urgent symptoms antecedent to the depressive syndrome, inpatient care may be the only option. Occult malignancies, such as carcinoma of the pancreas, are medical disorders of this type. The psychotic disorders may also require brief hospitalization, depending on the individual case.

It is advisable to inform the patient and his family of the need for hospitalization and then to assess the degree of cooperation that can be expected. Whenever possible, the clinician should encourage voluntary hospitalization, but if the patient is at greatly increased risk and refuses to cooperate, involuntary admission must be arranged (see Chapter 3).

3.2. Referral for Ongoing Care

Patients who do not require hospitalization, but who are likely to need medication, ongoing psychiatric treatment, or, at the very least, follow-up consultation, should be referred for outpatient psychotherapy. Depending on the (by now) well-refined diagnostic hypotheses, the patient's own wishes as well as those of his family, and the resources available to them, referral can be made to private therapists, psychiatric clinics, or community mental health centers. The type of therapy suitable for the patient should be based not only on the nature and severity of his symptoms but also on his psychological makeup and interpersonal style. Crisis intervention, behavior therapy, group and family therapy, marital counseling, even pastoral counseling are therapeutic modalities to be considered along with the more traditional formats.

Medication should be administered only when the patient has a drug-responsive symptom cluster such as a major depressive syndrome, psychotic depression, or various atypical syndromes (see Figure 1). Major tranquilizers can at times be used in the emergency setting for depressed patients with severe agitation. A drug such as haloperidol (Haldol) may provide immediate relief. If haloperidol (or a similar high-potency antipsychotic agent) is considered, the adverse effects (e.g., extrapyramidal reactions) should be explained to the patient and his response to the medication carefully monitored. Careful administration of medication in the emergency room increases the likelihood that the patient will follow ongoing treatment plans, including continued drug usage.

Antidepressant medication regimens, however, should not be started in the emergency room (see Chapter 4). There are several reasons for this policy: First, because the desired effect of antidepressant medications (mood elevation) is not evident clinically for 10 to 21 days after the medication is started, there is no particular advantage to their introduction in the emergency setting. Second, antidepressant medications are associated with various adverse effects requiring careful monitoring—the most serious of which are potentially lethal cardiac arrhythmias. And third, patients—especially those over 40 years old—should have a full medical evaluation (e.g., cardiovascular testing) before beginning medication. Antidepressants should be given in the context of an ongoing therapeutic relationship where adverse effects, clinical response, and the risk of deliberate or unwitting drug abuse can be monitored.

3.3. No Treatment

In the event that the emergency intervention successfully resolves the depressive crisis by allowing the patient to discuss and clarify his feelings and begin to grapple with the conditions precipitating his depression, the clinician may feel that no further treatment is warranted. In that case, the patient might be given the option of returning for a follow-up consultation and encouraged to seek help if the symptoms persist or recur. This outcome is most unlikely in patients with major depressive disorders.

3.4. Discussion

Hospitalization, medication, and referral for ongoing treatment are effective interventions only if they are actually implemented, and that depends on the patient's cooperation and motivation. The emergency room clinician must facilitate the patient's transition from emergency care to the next treatment setting by actively establishing rapport, explaining the rationale underlying treatment decisions, and helping the patient to clarify his own wishes and expectations. If it is necessary to ensure the transition, the clinician should contact the patient or his family and the proposed therapist or agency after the emergency visit is terminated.

4. Clinical Applications

4.1. Major Affective Disorders

Major affective disorders may present with a manic and/or depressive episode. To establish a diagnosis of bipolar illness, a depressed patient must be questioned about previous manic episodes. (For a full description of mania, see Chapter 11.) This section focuses on major depressive disorders.

Patients with major depressive disorders may experience a dysphoric mood and/or loss of interest or pleasure in almost all customary activities (see Table 1). This mood disorder is relatively persistent and is associated with other symptoms, such as appetite disturbance, change in weight, sleep disturbance (commonly early morning awakening), psychomotor retardation or agitation, decreased energy, feelings of guilt or worthlessness, difficulty concentrating or thinking, and thoughts of death or suicide. Other commonly associated features include anxiety, irritability, fear, brooding, tearfulness, excessive concern with physical health, panic attacks, and phobias. Hallucinations or delusions may be present and generally are depressive in content (e.g., persecutory delusions about sinfulness, delusions of cancer or poverty).

To establish a diagnosis of major depressive disorder, the patient's symptoms must be consistent with DSM III criteria (see Table 1). These criteria generally correspond to disorders responding to biological treatments (e.g., antidepressant medication). Factors correlating most positively with drug responsiveness include anorexia and weight loss, "middle and terminal" (rather than early) insomnia, diurnal mood variation, psychomotor retardation or agitation, decreased levels of functioning, acute onset and autonomous cause, family history of depression and/or family history of response to an antidepressant, and previous response to drug therapy. Poor drug responders more frequently exhibit other psychiatric disturbances (particularly hysterical or externalizing styles), chronic symptoms, mood-incongruent psychotic features (particularly delusions), prominent hypochondriacal concerns and/or somatization, and previous drug trial failures. Once the emergency evaluation has determined that the patient does in fact have a major depressive disorder requiring medication, the next objective should be to evaluate the level of suicidal risk, involve the patient in treatment planning, and ensure appropriate follow-up. Medication should always be administered in the context of an ongoing therapeutic relationship.

> A 48-year-old man presented to the emergency room complaining of depression, and difficulty concentrating at work. He had become increasingly withdrawn from his family and had stopped playing golf on the weekends because he "didn't enjoy it anymore." His wife encouraged him to seek help. He had no history of previous psychiatric difficulties or recent life changes. Further questioning revealed that he had sustained a 15-pound weight loss in the last month, and experienced early morning awakening. He had been warned that his job was in jeopardy because of his apparent lack of interest, apathy, and reduced energy. The patient's father had been hospitalized for depression and had recovered completely with medication.
>
> The patient was a depressed-appearing middle-aged man with psychomotor retardation. He kept referring to feeling worthless, hopeless, and a failure to his family. He could see no way to improve his situation and felt that suicide might be his only remaining option.
>
> History and mental status examination further indicated a major depressive disorder. This probable diagnosis was based on the patient's evidently depressed mood, loss of appetite, sleep disturbance, inability to concentrate, loss of interest in previously pleasurable activities, feelings of worthlessness, and suicidal ideation. Moreover, the family history was positive for medicable depression. The clinician felt that the patient probably would respond to antidepressant medication and recover completely from this episode. After explanation of the probable cause of his difficulty, the patient seemed eager to begin treatment. Since he was not acutely suicidal, his support system was adequate, and he preferred outpatient treatment, he was referred to a psychiatrist for antidepressant medication and supportive psychotherapy. He was also scheduled to see his internist for a full medical evaluation prior to that visit.

4.2. Organic Affective Disorders

The clinician must always consider the possibility that depression may be due to a medical disturbance or to the use of various medications or drugs (see Table 2). When the disorder closely resembles either a manic or a major depressive episode, and its etiology is organic or medical, it should be labeled an organic affective disorder. Medical illnesses that may present as depression include diseases of the brain (e.g., degenerative, neoplastic); infectious diseases (e.g., influenza); electrolyte disturbances (e.g., hyponatremia, hypercalcemia); endocrine disorders (e.g., hypothyroidism, hypoadrenocorticalism); occult malignancies (e.g., carcinoma of the pancreas). In addition, many medications and drugs of abuse may cause a depressive syndrome (see Chapter 9).

Table 2. Organic Causes of Depression[a]

1. Neurologic disorders	4. Effects of tumors
Alzheimer's disease	Cancer of the bowel
Cerebral arteriosclerosis	Cancer of the pancreas
CNS degenerative disorders	Carcinomatosis
Huntington's chorea	Cerebral metastases and tumors
Multiple sclerosis	Oat cell carcinoma
Normal pressure hydrocephalus	5. Drugs, medications, and poisons
Parkinson's disease	Alcohol
Postconcussion syndrome	Amphetamine withdrawal
Subdural hematoma	Antipsychotics
2. Metabolic and endocrine disorders	Barbiturates
Addison's disease	Bromides
Cushing's disease	Carbon disulfide
Diabetes	Carbon monoxide
Hepatic disease	Cocaine
Hyperparathyroidism	Digitalis
Hyperthyroidism	Heavy metals
Hypokalemia	Lead poisoning
Hyponatremia	Methyl dopa
Hypopituitarism	Opiates
Pellagra	Oral contraceptives
Pernicious anemia	Other sedatives
Porphyria	Propranolol (Inderal and others)
Uremia	Reserpine
Wernicke-Korsakoff syndrome	Steroids
Wilson's disease	6. Miscellaneous disorders
3. Infectious diseases	Anemia
Brucellosis	Cardiac compromise
Encephalitis (viral)	Chronic pyelonephritis
Hepatitis	Epilepsy
Influenza	Lupus erythematosus
Mononucleosis	Pancreatitis
Postencephalitic states	Peptic ulcer
Subacute bacterial endocarditis	Postpartum state
Syphilis	Rheumatoid arthritis
Tuberculosis	
Viral pneumonia	

[a] Adapted from Schoonover.[13]

A 55-year-old woman, accompanied by her husband, presented to the emergency room complaining of depression, lethargy, and decreased appetite. In the past four months she had become increasingly unable to perform her usual household chores and experienced little interest in family and friends. She felt "like a failure" and reported that she had become so depressed she was unable to leave the house. Her husband expressed a great deal of concern about her "change in personality over the last few months." They both denied any marital difficulties.

Careful medical history indicated that 10 years ago she had been treated with thyroid pills. A careful review of symptoms revealed that the patient's hair and skin had become increasingly dry and that her hair was thinning.

Her voice had also changed, becoming hoarse and deep. Frequently, she felt stiff and her muscles ached. Her pulse was 45 and regular. Mental status examination confirmed the clinical picture of a lethargic, depressed woman with slowed speech and movements. Cognitive functioning was grossly normal, and there was no indication of psychosis. Her affect was depressed and she expressed concern over her apathy and lack of energy, but denied suicidal ideation. The patient was referred for further medical evaluation because the emergency clinician suspected that the depression might be secondary to hypothyroidism.

Both hypothyroidism and depression can present with psychomotor retardation, slowed speech, loss of energy, decreased appetite, impaired level of functioning, and loss of interest in usual activities, but physical signs and the patient's history pointed to hypothyroidism. When the symptoms of depression can be attributed to a medical disorder, the diagnosis of a major depressive disorder cannot be made.

4.3. Pseudodementia in the Elderly

Some elderly patients present with symptoms and signs that can be clearly attributed to a major depressive disorder, bereavement, or a chronic characterologic problem, while others present a more confusing picture. Recent memory loss, confusion, and distractibility secondary to diminished attention span suggest a true dementia resulting from structural changes in the brain. However, these symptoms may also occur in depressed elderly patients. When secondary to depression, this condition is called pseudodementia and resolves when the depression is appropriately treated (see Chapter 19).

A psychiatric interview alone may not distinguish dementia from pseudodementia. On MSE, the patient with pseudodementia will seem confused and forgetful and may have difficulty with simple tests of attention and memory such as serial sevens and digit span. There may be disorientation to time and place. Loss of interest or pleasure in ordinary activities may appear as apathy, and difficulty in concentrating as inattentiveness. Unlike the patient with dementia, performance on the MSE may be inconsistent and erratic.

Clues to differentiating dementia from depression in the elderly often must come from family members or others close to the patient. A previous history of a major depressive disorder may suggest pseudodementia. Loss of appetite, with decreased weight and difficulty sleeping, also suggests depression. The course and onset of the confusion should be carefully delineated; a long, gradual, but steady decline in intellectual functioning points to a dementing process. A more acute onset, with rapidly progressing symptoms, is more suggestive of pseudodementia secondary to a major depressive syndrome. Sometimes, the diagnosis can be made with certainty only after a careful neurological evaluation (e.g., CAT scan) and neuropsychological testing.

The patient with pseudodementia sometimes requires hospitalization, particularly when the diagnosis is difficult to make. It is sometimes more efficient to do a complete neurologic work-up in the hospital. Also, confusion and memory loss often make it impossible for the patient to function independently at home. If the patient is seriously malnourished, he may require medical observation and treatment. If there is increased suicidal risk, a hospital setting helps to ensure the patient's safety. In addition, the major treatments for depression (antidepressant medication and electroconvulsive therapy) carry serious risks for the elderly. Elderly patients taking antidepressants are more susceptible to fatal cardiac arrhythmias, and they must be carefully evaluated and followed.

> An 82-year-old woman was brought to the emergency room by a neighbor because she was found wandering in the halls of her apartment building. She appeared lost and was unable to give a complete history. Mental status examination revealed a disheveled and cachectic-looking woman who was disoriented to time and place. She was unable to perform simple memory tests and was easily distracted. She seemed apathetic and listless, repeating that she just wanted to return home. The neighbor reported that four months ago the woman had seemed her usual self, chatting amiably in the hall with her friends. A relative described a depressive episode 15 years earlier. At that time, the patient had recovered completely after a course of ECT in a psychiatric hospital.
> Because the patient was unable to care for herself and needed a complete medical and neurologic examination, she was hospitalized. On the basis of the relatively rapid onset of symptoms and the presence of an earlier depressive episode responsive to ECT, the evaluator suspected that she might have pseudodementia secondary to a major depressive syndrome. After a course of antidepressant medication, she improved dramatically.

4.4. Other Major Psychiatric Disorders

Patients with other major psychiatric disorders, especially the psychoses, may experience intermittent depression requiring emergency intervention. Schizophrenic patients frequently become markedly depressed. During the acute psychotic phase they feel out of control, hopeless, alienated, and frightened by hallucinations or delusions. These experiences in themselves can foster feelings of worthlessness and helplessness. Moreover, command hallucinations telling the patient to kill himself place him at extremely high risk for suicide. Persecutory delusions may cause withdrawal. Depressed, acutely psychotic patients often need to be hospitalized, therefore, to institute appropriate treatment and to ensure their safety.

Schizophrenic patients may also become depressed following an acute psychotic episode. They frequently complain of loss of interest in pastimes and pleasurable activities, and report being unable to enjoy anything (anhedonia). They are unable to motivate themselves and are easily overwhelmed.

During a single emergency visit it may be difficult to differentiate some forms of schizophrenia from a major affective disorder. In both disorders the patient may appear extremely withdrawn, apathetic, depressed, and motorically retarded. The diagnosis of a major depressive episode is more likely if there is family history of an affective disorder, good premorbid adjustment, and previous episode(s) of an affective disturbance from which there was complete recovery. Emergency treatment is the same for both disorders. If the patient is extremely withdrawn and mute, and unable to care for himself, hospitalization is almost always indicated.

Other psychiatric disorders that may present with the complaint of depression include schizoaffective illness, cyclothymic disorders, obsessive compulsive disorder, or alcohol dependence. The intervention required will depend upon the severity of the depressive symptomatology, the patient's level of functioning, availability of the support network, and the presence of suicidal ideation.

4.5. Chronic Characterologic and Neurotic Disturbances

Many patients exhibit symptoms of depression that represent a chronic, repetitive way of relating to their environment. Depressive symptoms may be part of their character style or a habitual response to unconscious themes. Other patients may experience fantasized or real disappointment as a crisis, and may end up using the emergency setting repeatedly.

The essential feature of a depressive neurosis (or dysthymic disorder) is a chronically disturbed mood characterized by dysphoria and/or loss of interest or pleasure in usual activities and pastimes. The depressed mood is either relatively continuous or alternates with a short period of normal mood, but it is not persistent or severe enough to warrant a diagnosis of major depressive disorder. Social and occupational functioning are usually not significantly impaired. Although DSM III criteria for major depression are not specifically met, the individual may become overwhelmed and require psychiatric intervention at times of stress. The depressive features of this disorder are often viewed as secondary to an underlying character or personality disorder.

Some individuals with borderline personality disorder are chronic repeaters in the emergency room, presenting with depression and self-destructive ideation or actions. Self-abusive behavior may be repetitive but not immediately life-threatening (as with repeated superficial wrist-slashing). It can serve to discharge overwhelming affect, such as frustration, anger, or ennui, over which borderline patients feel they have no control. Their relationships are often unstable and intense, behavior similarly unpredictable and impulsive. These patients experience marked mood swings and exhibit intense, internally fueled anger. Although depressions secondary to personality disorders do not generally benefit from antidepressant medication, if a major depressive disorder develops in a patient of this sort, medication should be considered.

Patients in chronic crisis often tax clinicians and psychiatric systems. As angry, demanding, help-rejecting repeaters, they may actually abuse the legitimate function of emergency services and provoke negative countertransference feelings in emergency care providers. Feelings of frustration notwithstanding, the clinician must approach each emergency as if it were the first. Characterologically disturbed individuals should be screened for suicidal risk and referred as necessary for treatment ranging from crisis-oriented outpatient psychotherapy to involuntary psychiatric hospitalization.

A 26-year-old woman presented to the emergency room with her boyfriend after having taken five diazepam (Valium) tablets in a suicide attempt. The woman had made many low-lethal attempts in the past from minor overdoses to wrist-slashing. She had been in outpatient psychotherapy for the past two years and her therapist was currently on vacation. The woman had an unstable work and interpersonal history. Although she claimed that she had been depressed "all her life," there were no apparent vegetative signs. During a fight with her boyfriend, she impulsively took five pills, telling him that she wanted to die.

The patient appeared mildly depressed. When questioned about her therapist's vacation, she became tearful and angry. She denied further suicidal plans; the pills had been taken to "scare her boyfriend a little." The intent and lethality of the suicide attempt were evidently low. The evaluator urged her to express her feelings about the therapist and boyfriend more openly, and told her to call if there were continued distress.

4.6. Depression in Response to a Situational Disturbance

Most people feel sad in response to disappointments or loss and generally do not require psychiatric help. In certain individuals, however, the loss may be of such magnitude or have such a heavy psychological meaning that they require psychotherapy or pharmacotherapy. A precipitating event, usually real, can be discerned from the history. Individuals with this type of depression often have no prior psychiatric history and were functioning normally before the loss.

Bereavement conforms to the model for a typical depressive response to situational turbulence. Bereavement is a normal reaction to the death of a loved one. It is accompanied by loss of appetite and weight, insomnia, and lowered energy level. Guilt often centers around things that should not have been done or could have been done to forestall or prevent the death. The survivor may also feel he should have died instead or that he would now be better off dead.

According to Lindemann, the pathognomonic signs of acute grief during the impact phase of the crisis response include (1) somatic distress, (2) preoccupation with the image of the deceased, (3) guilt, (4) hostile reactions, and (5) interruption of routine patterns of functioning. The duration and course of the grief process depend upon the person's moving beyond the attachment to the deceased, readjusting to the remaining social system, and forming new relationships. This requires active mourning for the lost person. To grieve properly, people must acknowledge and tolerate a wide array of sad and painful affects. Resolving the crisis and integrating the issues related to the loss often takes as long as one to two years.

The depressed, grieving individual who presents to an emergency clinician clearly needs help. He sometimes requires only support and reassurance, an opportunity to ventilate and share his feelings, and, occasionally, a short-term medication (e.g., benzodiazepines) to relieve insomnia or anxiety. The depression, however, can progress to the point where the patient becomes morbidly preoccupied, feels worthless, has marked and persistent difficulty functioning, and develops active suicidal ideation. Such patients may be at high risk for self-injury, and appropriate measures must be taken to protect them.

Morbid (pathological) grief reactions are suspected when there is (1) delayed reaction to the loss, (2) distorted reactions, such as hyperactivity without acknowledgement of the loss, (3) acquisition of symptoms belonging to the last illness of the deceased, (4) alteration in relationships to friends and relatives, (5) furious hostility against specific persons, (6) persistent loss of usual patterns of social interaction, and (7) activities that are detrimental to the patient's own social and economic existence. If the intensity and nature of the symptoms and/or their temporal sequence are different from a typical grief reaction, the clinician should suspect pathology requiring additional treatment.

> A 65-year-old man was brought to the ER by his son. The man refused to talk with the psychiatrist, saying he just wanted to be left alone to die. History obtained from the son revealed that the man's wife had died suddenly five months earlier from a myocardial infarction. The man had not spoken of her death, nor had he cried at the funeral or afterwards. Since the death, he had been living with his son and daughter-in-law, but worried that he would become a burden. He had lost 20 pounds and was talking about buying a gun to "end all my misery." The patient had no psychiatric history. Prior to his wife's death he had been a successful businessman. The patient's son was concerned because his father was now refusing to work, had difficulty getting out of bed, and seemed headed for suicide. The intensity and duration of depressive symptoms (5 months) indicated pathological grieving; that is, the patient was still experiencing symptoms characteristic of the acute or impact phase of the loss. Because of the high suicidal risk and severely impaired functioning, hospitalization was recommended.

5. Summary

This chapter describes the emergency care of the depressed patient and focuses on the need to make symptom-specific decisions at two critical phases of the intervention: in the first few minutes, when the patient's life either is or could be at risk, and at the end of the visit, when the clinician must decide if the patient needs hospitalization, medication, and/or outpatient treatment. The fact that effective intervention and disposition demand solid etiologic grounding should not be ignored, but it cannot be emphasized too strongly that diagnostic acuity is no substitute for empathic management.

Selected Reading

1. Akiskal HS, McKinney WI Jr: Overview of recent research in depression; integration of ten conceptual models into a comprehensive clinical frame. *Arch Gen Psychiatry* 32:285–305, 1975.
2. Baldessarini RJ: The basis for amine hypotheses in affective disorders, a critical evaluation. *Arch Gen Psychiatry* 32:1087–1093, 1975.

3. Beck AT, Rush AJ, Shaw B, et al: *Cognitive Therapy of Depression*. New York, Guilford Press, 1979, pp 1–34.
4. Bibring E: The mechanism of depression, in Greenacre P (ed): *Affective Disorders*. New York, International Universities Press, 1965, pp 13–48.
5. *Diagnostic and Statistical Manual of Mental Disorders*, ed 3 (DSM III). Washington, American Psychiatric Association, 1980.
6. Gelenberg A: When is depression an emergency? *Drug Ther* 7:41–49, 1982.
7. Klerman G: Affective disorders, in Nicholi A: *The Harvard Guide to Modern Psychiatry*. Cambridge, Harvard University Press, 1978.
8. Kovacs M: The efficacy of cognitive and behavior therapies for depression. *Am J Psychiatry* 137:1495–1501, 1980.
9. Lindemann E: Symptomatology and management of acute grief. *Am J Psychiatry* 101:141–148, 1944.
10. Maas JW: Biogenic amines and depression: Biochemical and pharmacological separation of two types of depression. *Arch Gen Psychiatry* 32:1357–1367, 1975.
11. Schildkraut J: Catecholamine hypothesis of affective disorder. *Am J Psychiatry* 122:509–522, 1965.
12. Schoonover SC: Depression, in Bassuk EL, Schoonover SC, Gelenberg AJ (eds): *The Practitioner's Guide to Psychoactive Drugs*, ed 2. New York, Plenum Publishing Corp, 1983.
13. Schoonover SC: The practice of pharmacotherapy, in Bassuk EL, Schoonover SC, Gelenberg AJ (ed): *The Practitioner's Guide to Psychoactive Drugs*, ed 2. New York, Plenum Publishing Corp, 1983.
14. Weissman MM: The psychological treatment of depression. *Arch Gen Psychiatry* 36:1261–1268, 1979.
15. Weissman MM, Klerman GL, Prusoff GA, et al: Depressed outpatients results one year after treatment with drug and/or interpersonal psychotherapy. *Arch Gen Psychiatry* 38:51–55, 1981.
16. Weissman MM, Prusoff BA, DiMascio A, et al: The efficacy of drugs and psychotherapy in the treatment of acute depressive episodes. *Am J Psychiatry* 136:555–558, 1979.

Emergency Care of Anxious Patients

Roberta S. Isberg, M.D.

1. Introduction

Anxiety may be a normal response to stressful events or the symptom of an underlying disorder. Anxiety is both an emotional and a physical experience. Emotions range from apprehension to panic, with fears of losing control, going crazy, or dying. Physical symptoms include sweating, flushing, dizziness, fainting, racing heart, chest pain, hyperventilation, urinary frequency, diarrhea, nausea, and vomiting. The person's experience of anxiety is determined by his constitution, psychology, affective style, and severity of external stressors.

Emergency room (ER) patients may present with anxiety as a primary disturbance (e.g., panic disorder) or as a symptom of other medical or psychiatric illnesses. Presentations include:

1. Anxiety accompanying medical illness or organic psychiatric disorders.
2. Anxiety secondary to functional psychiatric disturbance such as schizophrenia, affective disorder, personality disorder, or dissociative state.
3. Anxiety as a primary psychiatric illness, such as panic disorder, phobia, or generalized anxiety disorder.
4. Anxiety as a response to stress, such as posttraumatic stress disorder and adjustment disorder.

Anxious patients generally seek emergency treatment when their internal capacity to bear anxiety and their external sources of support have been exhausted. To manage these patients effectively, the emergency clinician should keep in mind the following:

1. The immediate task is to provide a "safe harbor" for the patient. Establishing a calm relationship will facilitate the task of assessment and help to begin the process of treatment.
2. Assessment includes obtaining a careful description of the emotional and physical manifestations of anxiety and a history of events preceding the symptoms, and defining the characteristic coping mechanisms of the patient.[1] On the basis of these data the clinician can make a differential diagnosis and, possibly, a psychodynamic formulation.

Roberta S. Isberg, M.D. • Beth Israel Hospital, Boston, Massachusetts 02215, and Harvard Medical School, Boston, Massachusetts 02115.

3. Treatment of the immediate problem and referral for further therapy (when needed) complete the tasks of the interview.

2. Assessment

Assessment should follow a clear course beginning with observation of the appearance and behavior of the patient. The target complaint should be defined. The following guidelines apply: Patients complaining primarily of physical symptoms require medical evaluation. Anxious patients who appear confused or cognitively impaired must be evaluated for an organic disorder. Patients with bizarre or delusional symptoms may be suffering from other psychiatric disturbances.

Patients with a primary anxiety state are usually able to describe their problem coherently. As part of the relevant historical data, the interviewer should ascertain whether the current episode is the first of its kind or part of a recurrent pattern, whether it occurred spontaneously or in response to specific circumstances. The interviewer should encourage the patient to express his concerns. He may be anxious about his physical health: afraid that he is having a heart attack or dying. He may fear that he is losing his mind or be threatened by external circumstances beyond his control. He may have inordinate fears about things that appear trivial to others but have special personal meaning. He may describe conflicting feelings, or confess to having impulses or wishes that he finds shameful or repugnant.

To rule out other major disorders, the interviewer should routinely screen anxious patients in the following manner[2]: (1) measuring and recording vital signs; (2) completing a review of symptoms and evaluating any prominent or unusual symptoms with appropriate tests; (3) rapidly assessing mental status to identify possible psychosis, serious depression, or organic brain syndrome; and (4) obtaining a history.

Vital Signs. Pulse, blood pressure and respiratory rate should be measured and recorded. Anxious patients commonly have a sinus tachycardia to 120, but rarely exceeding 130–140 beats per minute.[2] A pulse of 140 or greater is more suggestive of supraventricular tachycardia and requires further evaluation, including an EKG. Blood pressure may be temporarily elevated in acute anxiety states. A drop in blood pressure in the presence of an elevated pulse indicates an abnormal hemodynamic state, such as hypovolemia or shock, and requires immediate medical treatment. An elevated respiratory rate may be a sign of anxiety-induced hyperventilation. However, a history of cardiac or respiratory illness, or accompanying symptoms such as chest pain or wheezing, demand further medical examination. While minimally elevated temperature may be associated with anxiety, significant increases are due to other causes.

Systems Review. Anxiety can be either the cause or the result of cardiovascular, pulmonary, neurological, and/or gastrointestinal complaints. When a patient has specific complaints referrable to the cardiovascular or pulmonary system, a screening chest examination is indicated. A patient over 35 with complaints suggestive of cardiac disease should have a physical exam and EKG. Symptoms suggestive of neurologic disease should be pursued with a routine neurologic examination and further tests when indicated.

When the suspected medical disorder does not seem life-threatening or particularly urgent, the evaluation need not be completed in the ER, and the patient should be referred for outpatient work-up. Patients over 30 with recent onset of anxiety should at some time in the course of their evaluation be seen by an internist for a physical examination and indicated laboratory studies; this may include routine metabolic and hematologic screening, as well as thyroid function tests.

Mental Status. The routine mental status examination (MSE) measures the "vital signs" of the patient's consciousness, including level of awareness, attention, visual and auditory perception, speech, orientation, memory, and other cognitive functions. Abnormalities in these functions suggest the presence of an organic brain syndrome.

History. Each patient should be asked specifically for a medical, psychiatric, and drug use history. Unless specifically questioned about such problems, many patients will inadvertently forget, or purposely avoid divulging important information.

2.1. Assessment of Physical Complaints of Anxious Patients

2.1.1. Guidelines for Evaluating Physical Complaints

Many medical disorders present with physical symptoms of anxiety such as air hunger, chest tightness, or palpitations. Other disorders can give rise to emotional symptoms of anxiety. See Table 1 in the Appendix for a detailed list of these disorders. The clinician should be familiar with these disorders and their work-up.

2.1.2. Hyperventilation Syndrome

Hyperventilation syndrome is an anxiety-induced physiologic disturbance that causes physical distress, provoking even greater anxiety. Patients with hyperventilation syndrome may fear they are having a heart attack, asthma attack, or catastrophic illness. Rapid treatment of hyperventilation reassures the patient about his physical health.

The patient with hyperventilation usually presents with a feeling that he cannot catch his breath or get enough air. He may complain of lightheadedness, dizziness, and tightness or pain in his chest. In more advanced stages, blurred vision, paresthesias in the extremities and perioral region, and carpopedal spasm may occur. The patient may even lose consciousness, thereby automatically aborting the attack. A rapid respiratory rate and elevated pulse will be present, and the patient may appear pale and sweaty. Often, the patient himself is not aware of breathing rapidly and will therefore attribute his anxiety to other somatic causes.[1]

The physical symptoms are caused by the fall in PCO_2 and resulting respiratory alkalosis that occurs when any healthy individual overbreathes. Arterial blood gas measurements during acute hyperventilation reveal a decrease in PCO_2, an increase in PO_2, and an increase in pH. The respiratory alkalosis can lead to tetany with carpopedal spasm. Symptoms of faintness and blurred vision may result from diminished cerebral blood flow caused by the constriction of cerebral blood vessels in response to lowered PCO_2.[3] All these uncomfortable physical sensations can be reversed if the PCO_2 is restored to normal. Resumption of a normal rate of respiration automatically raises PCO_2 levels.

It sometimes helps to demonstrate that the patient can still hold his breath even during an attack when he feels he is suffocating.[3] This may help to abort the attack. The attack can also be terminated by breathing in and out of a paper bag or by inhaling a 5% CO_2 mixture.

Once the attack is terminated, the patient should be informed about the mechanism of the attack and ways of controlling it: As he became anxious, he began to overbreathe without being aware of it and developed symptoms as his body reacted to the overbreathing.[1]

Usually the initial management of such patients is provided by the medical rather than the psychiatric service of an emergency room. Before a referral to psychiatry is made, it should be remembered that there are other physiologic causes of hyperventilation. These include central nervous system lesions, metabolic acidosis (as is seen in the Kussmaul breathing of uncontrolled diabetes mellitus and chronic renal failure), salicylate poisoning, acute or chronic hypoxia (as at high altitude), or hepatic coma. All these conditions are easily distinguished from anxiety-induced hyperventilation by the presence of other physical signs and by abnormal findings in arterial blood gases.

2.2. Anxiety as a Manifestation of Other Psychiatric Disorders

Just as anxiety can be a symptom of many medical illnesses, it can also reflect various psychiatric illnesses other than a primary anxiety disorder. Since different forms of treatment are indicated for these other psychiatric disorders, it is important to recognize the underlying illness. Anxiety can be a symptom of psychotic, affective, or personality disorders. The related problems of conversion hysteria, somatization disorder, and hypochondriasis, malingering, and dissociative reactions are also discussed in the differential diagnosis of anxiety disorders.

2.2.1. Psychosis

The psychotic patient often appears anxious and frightened. The mental status examination reveals delusions, hallucinations, loose associations, illogical thinking, or other signs of a thought disorder. Patients with anxiety disorder often *fear* that they are going crazy but maintain the ability to distinguish reality from fantasy. In general, they realize that their fears have an exaggerated quality. In contrast, psychotic patients confuse their mental constructions with reality (see Chapter 11).

2.2.2. Affective Disorders

Anxiety may be the presenting symptom of an agitated depression or early mania. When other signs of depression are present—depressed mood, change in appetite, insomnia, self-reproach, and suicidal thoughts (see Chapter 12)— a major depressive disorder should be suspected as the primary psychiatric illness.

Early in the course of a manic episode, feelings of irritability and hyperactivity may be interpreted by the patient and his family as anxiety. "Racing thoughts" are common to both anxiety attacks and mania. Loss of reality testing or severe mood disturbance, grandiose ideas, buying sprees, sexual indiscretions, and uncontrolled and reckless ventures are characteristic of mania but are rarely seen in patients with primary anxiety disorders.

2.2.3. Personality Disorders

Assessment of the anxious patient should include an evaluation of the patient's usual style of coping with stress. Sometimes this reveals rigid personality traits causing significant functional impairment or distress[4] (p. 305). If these maladaptive traits are enduring personal characteristics and not a product of unusually stressful circumstances, the diagnosis of personality disorder should be considered.

The presence of a personality disorder does not exclude the possibility of other coexisting psychiatric illness. Patients with personality disorders may have panic attacks that are amenable to medication or they may be victims of situational trauma and suffer posttraumatic stress symptoms. Some patients who were thought to have dependent or histrionic personality disorders may actually have a primary panic disorder, which has led to the development of certain dependent or hysterical traits.

2.2.4. Dissociative Disorders

Persons with extreme anxiety often experience themselves (depersonalization) or the world (derealization) as unreal. Depersonalization, the most common presentation of a dissociative state, occurs in 30 to 70% of young adults[4] (p. 259). When such an alteration in consciousness becomes the predominant symptom, or when it gives rise to significant amnesia, fugue state, or multiple personality, the primary diagnosis of dissociative disorder should be made. It may be difficult to distinguish these states from drug-induced phenomena or the early stages of psychosis, but they can usually be differentiated by taking a careful history, doing a mental status and a physical examination, and obtaining a toxic screen. In patients with primary dissociation, reality testing remains generally unimpaired. Possible neurologic causes for the altered state should be carefully explored.

The interviewer should try to interrupt the altered state of consciousness. If usual interviewing techniques fail, hypnosis or drugs can sometimes be useful. Under hypnosis, restoration of normal language and reconstruction of the precipitating event may be possible.[5] Some clinicians use the sodium amytal interview after ruling out head trauma, medical illness, or drug ingestion. It should be used only by clinicians familiar with its risks. To distinguish between psychosis and a dissociative state, IM haloperidol (Haldol) can be used. If the patient is clearly not psychotic, a benzodiazepine can be administered. With either haloperidol or benzodiazepine, the patient may become sedated or even fall asleep, and awake in a normal state of consciousness.

2.2.5. Somatoform Disorders

Many patients experience a great deal of anxiety in association with real or imagined medical disorders. Other patients experience little or no anxiety but develop a physical symptom as a substitute for emotional awareness.

2.5.2a. Conversion Reactions. In conversion reactions a loss or alteration of physical functioning results from psychologic conflict. Two different mechanisms are commonly suggested to explain the formation of the symptom[4] (p. 244). In one, the individual achieves a "primary gain" by keeping an internal conflict out of awareness: For example, an unconscious conflict about "taking a stand" on a particular issue may be expressed as difficulty standing or poor balance. In the other mechanism, the individual achieves "secondary gain" by avoiding a particular activity or by getting extra support from the environment: A policeman, transferred to a dangerous beat, may develop fainting attacks that force his transfer back to a desk job. A common feature of both mechanisms is the use of repression as a defense against painful affects.

Although such patients have been described as having *la belle indifférence*, many of them are extremely frightened and demanding.[1] These patients are often seen by hospital personnel as "not really sick"; it is sometimes hard for the clinician to believe that the symptoms are not under voluntary control.

The history may contain clues to the mechanism of symptom formation. A history of previous episodes, or similar episodes in family members, may also be found. It should be borne in mind that many patients with indisputable organic disease also have coexistent "hysterical" symptoms. The initial physical disease may form the basis for subsequent psychogenic symptoms. These patients are able to imitate (consciously or unconsciously) "the symptoms that they know best."[6] It is important that the evaluator recognize the coexistence of organic and psychogenic disorders.

Hypnosis performed by an appropriately trained person sometimes can be useful in the immediate management of hysterical symptoms. Other patients respond to reassuring medical attention and sympathetic interviewing alone. Some patients, unable and unwilling to recognize the psychologic roots of their distress, should be referred back to their primary physicians for symptom management. Still others may benefit from psychotherapy. It is not uncommon, however, for patients who achieve relief of the troublesome physical symptom to lose interest in further psychiatric intervention. Because many different types of patients—neurotic, borderline, and character-disordered—can develop conversion symptoms, the type of intervention should depend on the patient's underlying pathology.

2.2.5b. Somatization Disorder. Somatization disorder, previously referred to as Briquet's syndrome or hysteria, is a chronic disorder characterized by recurrent and multiple somatic complaints. The patient repeatedly seeks medical attention, but no physical cause for the symptoms is discovered[4] (p. 241). Because these patients commonly complain of chronic anxiety, they may be referred to a psychiatrist. While psychiatric consultation may help the physician manage such a patient, psychotherapy itself may be of little benefit. Optimal management is usually accomplished by a primary care physician whose consistent and understanding approach to the patient's physical distress can contain his anxiety.

2.2.5c. Hypochondriasis. Hypochondriasis is characterized by preoccupying fears about having a particular disease. The somatic delusions of a psychotic patient and the anxiety of panic disorder must be differentiated from hypochondriasis: Patients with somatic delusions usually have other features of psychosis, and patients with primary panic disorders usually feel reassured about their state of health once the panic attacks are under control. The patient who clings tenaciously to his fear of physical illness, despite all contrary medical evidence, is the hypochondriac.

Patients who express psychologic issues through their preoccupation with a given organ system or illness vary greatly in their ability to use psychologic insight to understand their fears. Management by a primary care physician alone may be indicated over psychotherapy.

2.2.6. Malingering and Drug-Seeking Behavior

Patients who report a subjective sense of anxiety that far exceeds their apparent distress, patients who request a particular drug that is not commonly used as an antianxiety agent, and those with a history more consistent with drug abuse than with anxiety may be using the ER to obtain drugs. Anxiety is a typical disguise for this covert agenda. Before any prescription is written (or refilled), the ER clinician should consult the patient's primary therapist (if there is one) or write enough for only 24 hours pending follow-up consultation.

2.3. Anxiety as a Primary Psychiatric Disorder

Primary anxiety disorders can be divided into two categories: (1) when anxiety occurs without an identifiable cause or as an abnormal response to external reality and (2) when anxiety occurs in response to stressful life events. This section describes the first category of patients with anxiety as a primary emotional disorder.

Primary anxiety disorders include panic disorder, agoraphobia with or without panic attacks, simple or social phobias, obsessive-compulsive disorder, and generalized anxiety disorder. Posttraumatic stress disorder and adjustment reactions are described in Section 2.4. Separation anxiety, school phobia, and other childhood disorders are discussed in Chapter 18.

Many people suffer from agoraphobia or panic attacks for years without seeking help. The visit to the emergency room often reflects a breakdown in the patient's usual manner of compensating for this disorder: for example, the agoraphobic patient whose family can no longer provide constant companionship or the phobic patient who experiences increased demands at work.

2.3.1. Panic Disorder

According to Klein, the onset of the first panic attack may occur during a routine activity such as walking down the street, eating a meal, or even sleeping.[7] Suddenly, the patient is overtaken by a sense of terror that gives rise to heart-pounding and shortness of breath. Strange thoughts race through his head. He fears he is having a heart attack or that he is going to die. Sweating, faintness, numbness, and tingling sensations may occur. A sense of unreality prevails. The attack usually lasts for 10 to 30 minutes but sometimes continues for hours.[7]

Although the patient may not seek professional help after the first attack, repeated episodes eventually lead him to an internist or to the emergency room—since the symptoms suggest that he has a physical illness. No physical basis for his symptoms is found.

The patient, however, may be convinced that there is something wrong with him that the doctors have been unable to find. He feels constantly tense and apprehensive, always anticipating another attack. He begins to avoid situations in which an attack might occur: restaurants, subways, highways. Eventually he may be unable to leave the house. A minor tranquilizer may provide temporary relief but doesn't prevent the attacks.

The patient may come to the emergency room. During an attack, he displays signs of physical distress—tachycardia, tachypnea, sweating, tremor, dilated pupils, and hyperactive reflexes. An electrocardiogram taken at this time usually reveals sinus tachycardia. Following the episode, these signs disappear, although an elevated heart rate may persist. Between attacks, chronic anxiety, muscle tension, abdominal distress, and headaches are typical. When the medical work-ups reveal no physical disorder, the patient may be referred to a psychiatrist. Recognition and validation of the existence of the disorder is the first therapeutic step in the management of such patients.

The patient with panic disorder, or agoraphobia with panic attacks, usually experiences two different kinds of anxiety: the acute panic attack, and the chronic dread, or "anticipatory anxiety," that the next attack could occur at any time.[8] Although the disorder usually begins with an unexpected panic attack, repeated attacks soon breed a general sense of apprehension. The onset of "anticipatory anxiety" marks the second stage in the three-stage process (described by Donald F. Klein) that leads to the development of panic disorder and avoidant behavior.[7]

Following the standard stimulus-generalization model, the patient begins to associate certain situations with the attack even when they are not causally related.[8] The patient then avoids them in an ineffective attempt to prevent another panic attack. This marks the development of a phobia, the third stage of the disorder. Obviously, patients vary greatly in the degree to which these fears change their lives. Some people continue to function, while others even refuse to leave their homes unless accompanied by a trusted companion.

Many patients use minor tranquilizers, barbiturates, or alcohol to calm their anxiety. While these substances do decrease the general level of anticipatory anxiety, they do not prevent the occurrence of further panic attacks, and may result in dependence on the drug.

Recognizing panic as a discrete disorder, distinct from other complaints of anxiety, is necessary for specific treatment. Tricyclic antidepressants and MAO inhibitors can inhibit panic attacks and make dramatic recoveries possible. Treatment of panic disorder is discussed in Section 3.2.

2.3.2. Agoraphobia, Social Phobia, and Simple Phobia

Agoraphobia can develop in response to recurrent panic attacks or can exist without concurrent panic attacks. When a patient has agoraphobia with panic attacks, proper evaluation and psychopharmacologic treatment are indicated. After the panic attacks have been inhibited with medication, avoidance behavior can be treated specifically with behavior therapy. Sometimes these symptoms occur against a background of psychological problems that need to be treated in insight-oriented psychotherapy.

For agoraphobia without panic attacks, the etiology is less clear. Character assessment and psychodynamic explorations may reveal information useful for treatment and referral decisions.

The stimulus situation for phobic patients should be specified. Common simple phobias are claustrophobia (fear of closed spaces), acrophobia (fear of heights), and fear of spiders, snakes or other animals[4] (p. 229). Social situations, such as speaking or eating in public, are stimuli for "social phobias." In contrast to panic disorder, however, phobic symptoms do not occur randomly or spontaneously, but only in association with the stimulus situation. Because such patients can control their symptoms by avoiding phobic stimuli, they rarely use the emergency room. A visit by such a patient signals a disruption of usual coping strategies, reflecting some change in responsibilities or avail-

support. Medication may not be as effective as behavior ~~;~~rapy, or other forms of psychotherapy.

~~e~~-Compulsive Disorder

~~ith~~ obsessive-compulsive disorder may experience extreme anxiety ~~n~~ ~~...~~ ~~empt~~ to resist their obsessions and compulsions. Certain patients with this disorder experience anxiety attacks and may respond to treatment with MAOIs.[9,10] These patients rarely present for emergency treatment. When they do, it is usually because of an extreme exacerbation of a chronic problem: Patients with ritualized behaviors may be unable to attend to basic physical needs, such as eating and sleeping. In other cases, the need for emergency treatment may reflect a new crisis imposed on the background of a chronic problem.

2.3.4. Generalized Anxiety Disorder

Some patients complain of a diffuse, but persistent, feeling of dread not apparently elicited by an external stimulus. They have symptoms of autonomic hyperactivity such as sweating, palpitations, and dry mouth. They are distracted and preoccupied by the vague sense that something awful is about to happen. When the signs of organic disease, panic disorder, psychosis, or affective disorder are absent, and the anxiety is not a characteristic of an underlying personality disorder, the clinician should consider the diagnosis of generalized anxiety disorder.

This diagnosis covers a heterogeneous group of patients who share the common symptoms of persistent anxiety. Among them are patients who, in other classification systems, would be said to have neurotic anxiety. In such patients an exploratory interview will usually reveal evidence of internal conflict or of unconscious causes of anxiety. These patients should be referred for further psychological evaluation or directly for psychotherapy. Unlike panic disorder, which is a distinct syndrome responsive to specific pharmacologic intervention, generalized anxiety disorder has no common etiology and no specific course of treatment. In DSM III it is a diagnosis based on exclusion, the result of our current inability to distinguish among various causes and types of anxiety.

Patients with persistent anxiety usually do not seek emergency treatment unless intervening events have precipitated a crisis. The interviewer should explore the events leading to the emergency room visit, the course of the anxiety disorder, and the patient's manner of dealing with stress.

2.4. Anxiety as a Psychological Response

Anxiety is an expected response to stressful life events. In posttraumatic stress syndrome the traumatic event is extraordinary, outside the range of usual human experience: rape, military combat, flood, concentration camp. Such an event would evoke significant symptoms of distress in almost everyone[4] (p. 236). In adjustment disorder the event or life-stage is disruptive, but not extraordinary; i.e., not everyone would develop psychiatric symptoms in response to such a stress. Examples include transitional life-stages, loss of a loved one, marital conflict, business setbacks, and physical illness. This section presents a model developed by Mardi Harowitz for understanding the stress response syndrome.[12–14]

2.4.1. Posttraumatic Stress Disorder

In response to traumatic events, individuals develop a common pattern and progression of symptoms. Initially, the individual may react intensely or feel stunned and dazed. This may be followed by a period of relative denial and numbing.[12] Accident victims, victims of violence, and family members of patients who die suddenly may arrive in the emergency room during the initial phases of emotional response (see Part VI). Sometime after the initial impact, the individual may experience recurrent episodes of intrusive flashbacks, strong emotion, or compulsive behavior, or may suffer denial, numbing, and efforts to ward off the disruptive implications of the trauma.[12] These two symptomatic processes—reexperiencing of the trauma and numbing of responsiveness—are essential features of the posttraumatic stress disorder[4] (p. 238) and are associated more specifically with symptoms of anxiety than with other symptoms of emotional distress.[13]

The psychological task is to reestablish a state of relative homeostasis.[12] The individual needs to revise previous impressions about the world and himself; old feelings of invulnerability must yield to the new reality of personal injury or loss. Both the repetitive experiences and the numbing response serve important functions. Reexperiencing the trauma facilitates reexamination of the event and ultimately integration. Avoidance and numbing control the intrusive experience and keep the disruptive feelings from becoming overwhelming. Carried to completion, these processes lead to working through of the experience. When either of these two processes becomes exaggerated or uncontrolled, however, the reparative function is interrupted. The reexperiencing of the trauma may become overwhelming, so vivid that the person behaves as though actually experiencing the trauma at that moment. Alternatively, reduced emotional responsiveness and withdrawal from involvement may become severe, with inability to feel, love, or care for others.

Should the intrusive reexperiencing of the trauma become uncontrolled and overwhelming, the person may seek emergency treatment. The history indicates a posttraumatic stress disorder. The stress may be recent, or it may be long past, as in delayed or chronic forms of the disorder. A current experience may give rise to sequelae from a past trauma: Following a car accident, a combat veteran may reexperience the horror of wartime.

2.4.2. Adjustment Disorder (or Adjustment Reaction)

Significant life changes such as divorce, illness, business crises, or developmental transitions—leaving home, getting married, or retiring—would normally stimulate some degree of anxiety. Excessive anxiety elicited by these events brings patients to the emergency room. Such anxiety is often a response to feelings aroused by the event rather than a response to the event itself. Anger in response to a business loss is not necessarily frightening, but the impulse to unleash one's rage against particular individuals, with the consequent loss of love and respect from others, is anxiety-provoking indeed. These imagined sequelae may be conscious, but unspeakable, for the patient, or they may be just barely accessible to consciousness, revealed only by intrusive images or dreams.

The following case demonstrates the kind of anxiety that can arise out of intrapsychic conflict. In this example, a developmental transition causes a college student to confront her adult sexuality.

> A 19-year-old college student was brought to the emergency room by her roommates because she had refused to leave her room after dark for the past week. After becoming seriously interested in her boyfriend, she had developed a preoccupying fear of being raped in the streets at night. Because of her fear of going out, she became unable to visit her boyfriend, who lived in his own apartment. Now he could only visit her in the suite she shared with three other roommates. When the boyfriend stopped by to visit one evening—when her roommates were away—the patient suddenly had her first anxiety attack.
>
> On the surface, the patient had "no good reason" for being so afraid of being raped. It was the history of events leading up to the formation of the symptoms that suggested possible intrapsychic causes for anxiety. Alone in her boyfriend's apartment, she felt threatened by the possibility of acting on her wishes for sexual involvement. A rigidly moralistic upbringing and an enduring need for support from her parents made acting on her sexual impulses seem particularly dangerous. Her fear of going out at night served two purposes. In her own mind, it resolved the conflict between sexual desire and parental prohibition by projecting all the sexual desire onto the imagined rapists; more practically, it made it impossible for her to enter the "danger zone" of her boyfriend's apartment. Safely surrounded by her three roommates, she was sure that she would not act on her impulses. When these external controls were unexpectedly removed on the evening her boyfriend stopped by, the patient experienced a panic attack.
>
> The emergency room interview was helpful in revealing to the patient the underlying source of her anxiety. Initially, she was unwilling to believe that her fear of being raped was irrational and argued that she had no other cause for anxiety. But as she discussed her feelings about her developing relationship, it became clear that this was an even more urgent source of anxiety. In hearing herself tell the story, the patient was able to connect her irrational fears of being raped with her more understandable fears of losing control of her sexual impulses. This had a calming effect on the patient. Furthermore, it helped to convince her that she could use more help in sorting out her feelings about sexuality.

Anxiety about sexual impulses, sexual identity, or sexual preference can be seen in patients of all ages and all diagnostic categories. It is important to

understand each patient in terms of his particular conflict, rathe[...]
that the patient suffers from "oedipal guilt," "castration an[...]
sexual panic," or other familiar complexes. For example, a m[...]
express anxiety about homosexual fantasies, while his underlyin[...]
involve dependency or power rather than sexual gratification. O[...]
ments on this symbolic use of sexuality for nonsexual purposes[...] who
express anxiety over homosexuality. Men experiencing conflict over dependency, defeat, or aggression may symbolize their concerns in terms of genital
organs in their dreams and fantasies. This may precipitate a fear of having
homosexual desires, leading, in some individuals, to a state of panic involving
loss of self-esteem.[16] Woods[16] points out that such men may use violence to
ward off this "pseudohomosexual anxiety" through a demonstration of power
and strength. He comments on the importance of helping the patient to identify
his underlying nonsexual conflicts, and of dealing with the shame and humiliation that the patient has experienced in association with his homosexual ideation.

Many patients are unable to identify internal sources of anxiety during the
emergency ward interview. Even when the interviewer can guess at these conflicts, the patient may fail to see any connection. The evaluator should be
cautious not to impose a mistaken or premature interpretation on the patient.
Nevertheless, the suggestion that unrecognized sources of anxiety lurk behind
the symptom can help patients begin to understand their distress. Sometimes
a single interview is all the help that a patient will want. Other patients will
use the interview as an introduction to further psychotherapy.

3. Treatment

3.1. Introduction

The anxious patient comes to the ER because he feels overwhelmed. Affects that are intolerable for a person to handle alone are often more bearable
in the context of a relationship with a concerned, but unintrusive, individual,
i.e., the ER clinician. There are two treatment issues to be considered: medication and supportive interviewing.

Despite the calmest and most reassuring approach on the part of the interviewer, some anxious patients are beyond comfort. The patient should be
informed that he must continue to tolerate a certain amount of painful anxiety
and that the beneficial effects of treatment occur gradually.

Most anxious patients come to the ER with a relative or close friend. While
an attempt should be made to interview the patient alone, the companion should
also be interviewed and consulted about treatment planning. Successful treatment may depend on the cooperation of the companion.

3.2. Treatment of Primary Anxiety Disorders

For panic disorder, the ER clinician should first acknowledge that the panic
attacks *do* consist of a feeling of real terror, even when there is no apparent

cause for fear. Sometimes there are precipitating events—either situational or intrapsychic—but there is often no identifiable cause. The patient can be assured that his anticipatory anxiety about recurrent panic attacks is also understandable, given the real threat of repeated panic attacks. Hospitalization should be avoided unless there is a concern about suicide or life-threatening self-neglect.

While tranquilizers have long been known to decrease generalized anxiety, it is only within the last 20 years that other medications have been shown to be effective in inhibiting the recurrence of panic attacks. In 1959, while studying the effects of imipramine, Donald Klein discovered that this medication reduced the frequency of panic attacks.[7] Since then, other antidepressants, including desipramine (Norpramin, Pertofrane) and nortriptyline (Aventyl, Pamelor), have been shown effective. More recently, the MAOIs, particularly phenelzine sulfate (Nardil), have been shown to be even more effective in some patients with panic disorder.[17] Because of dietary restrictions with MAOIs, many clinicians prefer to use imipramine (Tofranil) rather than phenelzine, as a first-line drug for panic disorder.

Until recently the benzodiazepines appeared to alleviate anticipatory anxiety but to have little effect on the recurrence of panic attacks.[18] An exception, however, is one of the newer benzodiazepines, alprazolam (Xanax), which appears to be effective in the treatment of panic disorder.[19] Because alprazolam, like the other benzodiazepines, has fewer uncomfortable side effects and takes effect more rapidly than the antidepressants, many clinicians now initiate drug treatment of panic disorder with alprazolam, in the hope that it will be the only medication required for prevention of panic attacks. The usual starting dose is 0.25 to 0.5 mg tid, which can be increased to a recommended maximum of 4 mg daily.[20] Alprazolam, like other benzodiazepines, can also be used in combination with antidepressant medication.

Both imipramine and phenelzine have a delayed onset of therapeutic effect of two to six weeks. Since the patient will continue to experience panic attacks during this time,[19] benzodiazepine can be taken simultaneously to alleviate the symptoms of anxiety. The benzodiazepine dose will depend on the patient's drug history and tolerance. Patients who are on no medication can be started on 2 to 5 mg of diazepam, or an equivalent dose of another benzodiazepine. (If alprazolam is used, as noted above, there may be no need for additional medication with an antidepressant.) For the management of chronic anticipatory anxiety, the benzodiazepine should be prescribed on a regular rather than a prn schedule.[8] Generally, the decision to start benzodiazepine treatment in the ER, before the patient is engaged in an ongoing treatment program, should depend on various factors such as (1) severity of anxiety, (2) patient's motivation and reliability, and (3) potential for abusing the medication.

Rather than beginning antidepressant treatment in the emergency room, the clinician should usually refer the patient to an outpatient program consisting of both medication and psychotherapy. The disorder is usually long standing, and the therapeutic effect of the antidepressant is delayed, so that starting medication is not an emergency issue. The *sense* of emergency is associated with the panic attack, rather than an indication of a true medical or psychiatric emergency.

In certain patients, the clinician could start a tricyclic antidepressant (TCA) or MAOI during an emergency room visit. One such case is the patient who has taken the medication before with good results, wants to resume treatment, and is motivated to follow through. Antidepressants can be started in the emergency room if the following conditions are met: (1) The diagnosis is certain; (2) the appropriate medical work-up has been completed; (3) the clinician and patient have reviewed the use and adverse effects of the medication; (4) a follow-up appointment can be provided in four to five days, with immediate entry into a more encompassing outpatient treatment program; and (5) a telephone number is available in case of an emergency.

Imipramine can be started at a dose of 25 mg at night and increased by 25 mg each day until 200 mg is reached, or unless adverse effects prevent further increase.[8] More gradual increases, of 25 mg every two or three days, may decrease the discomfort of side effects. A follow-up visit should be arranged for four to five days after starting the medication.

Because of the dietary and medication restrictions with phenelzine, the clinician generally should not prescribe this medication in an emergency room, where there is little time for proper patient education. A patient familiar with the drug from past successful use could restart it. The patient should also be given a written list of food and drug restrictions. These apply 24 hours *before* starting the medication and two weeks after stopping.[21]

Since phenelzine may produce greater improvement than imipramine in patients with panic disorder,[17] phenelzine could be the first drug tried with certain responsible and motivated patients. For the patient who has only a moderate response to an adequate trial of imipramine, a later trial of phenelzine (after several days' interruption between medications) may be indicated. While other MAOIs have also been used successfully in treating panic disorder, phenelzine has the lowest risk of causing hypertensive crisis when drug and food restrictions are violated.[21]

It is rare that medications other than benzodiazepines and TCAs would be useful in the emergency room management of a patient with panic disorder. While some patients are profoundly disorganized by their anxiety, there is almost no indication for using antipsychotics. They are not effective in reducing the frequency of panic attacks or in alleviating anticipatory anxiety.

Propranolol (Inderal, Indexide) and other beta blockers are also being used to treat anxiety. While propranolol is more effective than placebo in the treatment of anxiety, there is no conclusive evidence of its effectiveness relative to the benzodiazepines, TCAs, and MAOIs.[22] Therefore, it should not be used in the initial treatment of typical panic disorder. However, in patients with anxiety *and* other medical conditions—such as mitral valve prolapse syndrome—propranolol may be the drug of choice (see Section 3.2 and Appendix for a more complete discussion of MVPS and panic disorder).

It is always a good idea to consult the regular physician or therapist before prescribing more or new medication. Most patients should be referred back to their regular doctor if they need refills or medication adjustment. If the therapist is not available or if the patient is suffering adverse effects, recommendations can be made to the patient for a brief period until the patient can again consult his regular doctor.

The role of TCAs and MAOIs in treating anxiety without panic is less clear. Generalized anxiety disorders, if medicated, should be treated with minor tranquilizers. Some patients feel that all they need is an occasional dose at times of unbearable anxiety. Many patients, however, can be most successfully treated by psychotherapy alone.

3.3. Treatment of Anxiety in Response to Stress

When the patient's anxiety is related to a stressful experience, the interviewer should obtain a detailed account of the events leading to the onset of anxiety and should assess the patient's usual coping mechanisms. Such information will help the interviewer to support the patient's adaptive defenses and to make interventions consistent with his capacity to tolerate affect. The patient's ability to use insight and interpretation in the emergency room can be used as an indicator of whether insight-oriented or supportive psychotherapy is appropriate. Psychotherapy is not necessarily the treatment of choice; some patients are able to use the support and clarification provided by a single interview to resume their usual activities. Among patients referred for psychotherapy, only a small number will follow through, so that the emergency room interview may remain the sole treatment, regardless of the interviewer's recommendations.

Many patients demand medication. While medication may play a helpful role in the management of anxiety, it should not be given until the patient and interviewer have had a chance to explore the circumstances leading to the anxiety attack. Some patients are reassured to learn that they are capable of tolerating the anxiety without medication. Others may experience the refusal of medication as rejection—so serious as to make it impossible for them to return for follow-up.[1] Such patients may be prescribed a low dose of minor tranquilizers (i.e., benzodiazepines). Often, such prescriptions are never filled by the patient but provide reassurance that help is available. The medication should be given with the message that it is of short-term benefit and that the long-term solution requires better understanding of the situation. Accordingly, a specific appointment for follow-up treatment is always important.

3.3.1. Treatment of Posttraumatic Stress Disorder

The patient who has suffered a serious trauma can become overwhelmed by intrusive memories and fears. The emergency room interview can help the patient to establish a more controlled way of allowing distressing feelings into awareness. The goal of the interview is not to deepen the affective experience or "to help get the feelings out." Rather, it is to help the patient organize and begin to integrate his experience.

The management of such a patient is illustrated by the case of a 20-year-old man who survived a train wreck in which his father was killed. Following an initial period of intense grief, shared by the entire family, the patient fears that he will become the victim of a fatal accident. Terrified of leaving his house, he is plagued by recurrent nightmares and gruesome images of the event. At times he awakens from a dream, convinced that the accident is actually happening, but that this time he is to die and his father is to survive. Although reluctant to seek psychiatric help, he is persuaded by his family to go to the ER. The goals of the emergency room interview are necessarily limited to being the transition to a suitable form of ongoing therapy.

In talking with the interviewer, this young man reveals that he has irrational fears of death, as well as rational thoughts about his own and his father's vulnerability. In an irrational way, he feels that anything that had happened to father will happen to him.

One task of brief psychotherapy with such a patient is to help him to become aware of his identification with his father. Such an examination will promote more realistic perceptions about himself and his father and will free him from the irrational assumption that he has to die as well. It can enable him to preserve his positive identification with his father, as well as the freedom to be different. Such a task is completed over the course of many psychotherapy sessions, but it can be started during the emergency room intervention.

In some patients with posttraumatic stress disorder the clinician's general approach to treatment should be modified. For example, post-Vietnam syndrome seen in combat veterans is characterized by intrusive combat-related thoughts and nightmares, numbed responsiveness, and specific symptoms such as drug dependence, sleep disturbance, depression, anxiety, and rage.[23] Many clinicians advocate group rather than individual psychotherapy for combat veterans, who can share their feelings to help one another recover from the trauma. Alcohol abuse and drug dependence, more common in combat veterans than in their nonveteran peers, need treatment simultaneously. Intoxication increases the psychic numbing and interferes with the process of integrating the traumatic experience.

When head trauma or other physical injury accompanies the traumatic event, medical evaluation is an essential part of management. The symptoms of postconcussive syndrome should be evaluated and treated and should not be attributed automatically to emotional disturbance. (See the Appendix and Section 5.4 for a more complete discussion of postconcussive syndrome.)

3.3.2. Treatment of Anxiety in Adjustment Disorder

For patients with adjustment disorder, the external stress may not appear catastrophic, but the underlying fears can be overwhelming. The patient should be helped to identify and understand the thoughts and feelings that give rise to anxiety. Examining these thoughts is the first step toward resolution.

A 30-year-old businessman, recently divorced from, but living in the same city as, his wife, came to the emergency room because of sleeplessness, inability to concentrate at work, and extreme anxiety. His first anxiety attack occurred after his boss had offered him a promotion to a job in a distant city. Thrilled to have been chosen for the position, he immediately accepted. After all, he no longer felt tied down by his marriage. Suddenly, it occurred to him that he could not leave his wife. Although divorced, he always assumed that she needed him. Following his decision to move out of town, he was plagued by nightmares in which his wife would be hurt or suddenly taken ill. These intense feelings were hard for him to understand, because the divorce had been "particularly amicable." "Hardly an angry word between us," he reported.

The patient's insistence upon feeling no hostility toward his former wife revealed his discomfort over the possibility that he might be angry with her. Further discussion revealed that the patient actually had felt hurt and angry. Bringing these hostile feelings into conscious awareness would free him to make a more informed choice about leaving. He could then acknowledge that he might really want to leave, but that unrecognized guilt feelings kept him from leaving. This is the work of longer-term therapy. The goals of the emergency room interview are limited to evaluation and establishment of a relationship that facilitates further exploration of the problem in psychotherapy.

4. Conclusion

This chapter emphasizes the necessity of recognizing the variety of medical and psychiatric problems that present with anxiety symptoms, and of treating the symptom within its appropriate medical or psychiatric context. It is important for the interviewer to communicate to anxious patients that feelings that seem so overwhelming can, in fact, be tolerated, understood, and treated. Because the emergency room encounter is time-limited, the chief task of the clinician is to facilitate a transition to the next stage in the appropriate treatment process.

Appendix

Physiologic Disorders Associated with Anxiety Symptoms (See Table 1)

Drug-Related Symptoms

Substance Abuse and Medication Effects. A careful history of prescription and non-prescription drug intake is essential to the evaluation of every anxious patient.

Drug Withdrawal Syndrome. Withdrawal from alcohol, benzodiazepines, barbiturates, opiates, and other sedative-hypnotics gives rise to anxiety.

Table 1. Physiologic Disorders Associated with Anxiety Symptoms

Drug-related disorders
    Stimulants: amphetamines, cocaine, "diet pills," ephedrine, aminophylline
    Hallucinogens: D-lysergic acid diethylamide (LSD), phencyclidine hydrochloride (PCP)
    Sedative-hypnotics: paradoxical effects of barbiturates
    Medication effects or toxicity: thyroid preparations, corticosteroids, antipsychotic medications,
        (akathisia), anticholinergic toxicity, antihistamines, over-the-counter cold pills, digitalis tox-
        icity
    Dietary: caffeinism, MSG, tyramine in foods with MAOIs, vitamin deficiency diseases
    Drug withdrawal syndromes: alcohol, barbiturates, opiates, benzodiazepines, meprobamate,
        other sedative-hypnotics
Endocrine disorders
    Hyperthyroidism, pheochromocytoma, drug-induced hypoglycemia, insulinoma, reactive hypo-
        glycemia, Cushing's syndrome, hypoparathyroidism, menopause, electrolyte disturbance
Cardiovascular disorders
    Hyperventilation syndrome, pulmonary embolism, pulmonary infection, pulmonary edema,
        asthma, pneumothorax, COPD, restrictive lung disease
Neurologic disorders
    Organic brain syndromes, seizure disorders, cerebrovascular insufficiency, subclavian steal syn-
        drome, head injury, postconcussive syndrome, tumor, infections, metabolic or toxic enceph-
        alitis, multiple sclerosis, vertigo, vasculitis, Wilson's disease, Huntington's chorea, postero-
        lateral sclerosis, polyneuritis, cerebral syphilis, migraine headache
Hematologic disorders
    Intermittent acute porphyria, anemia
Neoplastic (secreting tumors)
    Carcinoid tumor, pheochromocytoma, insulinoma[2]
Immunologic
    Autoimmune disease, anaphylaxis[2]
Infection
    Acute or chronic infections

Endocrine Disorders

Endocrine disorders are frequently associated with emotional disturbances. Since anxiety is a common feature of hyperthyroidism, careful questioning of anxious patients for other symptoms of thyroid dysfunction is indicated. Infrequently, patients have both endocrine disorders and primary panic
anxiety. Hyperthyroid patients who were treated adequately for hyperthyroidism continued to have panic attacks until a specific antianxiety treatment, imipramine, was begun.

Hyperthyroidism. Hyperthyroid patients frequently present with symptoms of chronic anxiety such as nervousness and palpitations. They also may
complain of heat intolerance, increased perspiration, frequent loose stools, and
increased appetite without weight gain; women report irregular menses. Physical findings include tachycardia, tremor, warm, moist skin, and weight loss.
In Graves's disease, the most common cause of hyperthyroidism, a diffusely
enlarged thyroid, a staring gaze, "lid lag," and pretibial myxedema can also
be found. Diagnosis of hyperthyroidism can be made by measuring the serum

thyroxine (T4), triiodothyronine (T$_3$), and T$_3$ resin uptake (RT3). Caution in interpreting results of abnormal thyroid function tests is warranted because of recent evidence that the free T$_4$ and free T$_3$ may be elevated in acute psychiatric disturbances with return to normal after two to three weeks of hospitalization.[24]

Patients with hypothyroidism who take replacement hormone can also become thyrotoxic from exogenous thyroid hormone. A history of recent changes in the dose of medication or physical status and the appropriate serum assay will reveal exogenous thyrotoxicity.

Pheochromocytoma. A rare, but surgically treatable, cause of anxiety is a pheochromocytoma—a catecholamine-secreting tumor, usually benign, which arises from the adrenal medulla. The secretion of norepinephrine and epinephrine can be paroxysmal or continuous, producing acute or chronic symptoms, respectively. In acute attacks, experienced by about 50%[25] of patients, headache, flushing, and elevations of blood pressure occur. Such episodes can be precipitated by postural change, pressure on the abdomen, sexual activity, smoking, eating, exercise, laughing, and emotional stress. Diagnostic tests include urine assays for free catecholamines, metanephrine, and vanillylmandelic acid. These test results will be falsely elevated in patients using MAOIs, chlorpromazine (Thorazine and others), or sympathomimetic amines.

Hypoglycemia. Hypoglycemia, an abnormally low serum glucose, produces acute anxiety accompanied by sweating, hunger, tremor, headache, and fatigue. In severe episodes, confusion, seizures, and coma can ensue. The diagnosis is easily made by obtaining a serum glucose during an episode.

Drug-induced hypoglycemia is by far the most common form of this disorder. Diabetic patients on insulin or oral agents frequently become hypoglycemic because changes in medication, diet, or general state of health. While most diabetics can readily identify the symptoms of hypoglycemia, new diabetics or experienced patients who have recently started a new drug, such as a beta-blocker, may fail to recognize them. As soon as blood is drawn for serum glucose, oral or intravenous dextrose must be rapidly administered. Hypoglycemia also may be seen in medically sophisticated patients who self-administer insulin to produce a factitious syndrome.

Insulinoma, a rare, insulin-secreting tumor of the pancreas, can produce hypoglycemia manifested by anxiety and other behavior changes.

Reactive hypoglycemia can result from digestive disorders (e.g., in patients with gastrectomies) or from endocrine disorders as in early diabetes, hypoadrenal states, or hypothyroidism.[25]

Idiopathic hypoglycemia is rare, despite its popularity as an explanation for many dysphoric states. "Low blood sugar" should not be cited as the cause of anxiety except when it has been documented either during an attack or following the provocative glucose load of a glucose tolerance test.

Cushing's Syndrome. Cushing's syndrome—the result of elevated corticosteroids—can be caused by endogenous hormones as in adrenal hyperplasia, or by treatment with exogenous steroids. The endogenous disorder can cause depression, mania, or paranoid psychosis, accompanied by anxiety.[25] Exogenous corticosteroids can also cause euphoria, depression, or psychosis. Associated features include increased body weight, hirsutism, hypertension, weakness, and amenorrhea.

Hypoparathyroidism. Hypoparathyroidism and the resulting hypocalcemia cause organic brain syndrome more commonly than anxiety.[25] Symptoms include muscular cramps, paresthesias in the extremities and perioral region, and carpopedal spasm. Similar symptoms occur transiently during hyperventilation and are not elicited by provocative tests, as in true hypocalcemic states. Because of inadvertent surgical damage to the parathyroid gland, patients who have had thyroidectomies are at risk for hypoparathyroidism.

Menopause. The symptoms of menopause, commonly described as "hot flashes," can be mistaken for anxiety symptoms. These symptoms can also occur as a result of surgical removal of the ovaries.

Other Metabolic Disorders. A number of illnesses and medications can cause electrolyte or metabolic abnormalities, such as hyponatremia or uremia. While anxiety is rarely a primary symptom, cognitive impairment and confusion may cause patients to appear agitated and feel anxious. In patients whose symptoms and history suggest metabolic disorders, a screen of electrolytes, glucose, creatinine, BUN, and calcium may reveal an organic etiology.

Cardiovascular Disorders

Patients with anxiety may complain of feeling weak in the chest, difficulty taking a deep enough breath, palpitations, and dizziness. It is often difficult to determine whether or not organic heart disease is contributing to the patient's complaints. The association between anxiety and cardiac symptoms has long been noted. In 1871 DaCosta described the syndrome of "the irritable heart"[26] in Civil War soldiers, and in 1919 Lewis descibed World War I soldiers with "soldier's heart," and their female counterparts with "effort syndrome."[27] This section emphasizes the more familiar cardiac emergencies—such as arrhythmias and ischemia—which are "not to be missed" in an emergency room evaluation. Once these life-threatening disorders have been ruled out, a more leisurely study of the patient's cardiac function can be arranged.

Cardiac Arrhythmias. Cardiac arrhythmias can produce palpitations, chest discomfort, dyspnea, dizziness, and syncope. These symptoms, except for syncope, are commonly part of an anxiety attack. Diagnosis during an acute episode is straightforward, since most arrhythmias will be noted when the pulse is taken. The clinician should always evaluate a pulse rate that is less than 60 or greater than 120, or an irregular rhythm by EKG and physical exam. An EKG may also be required when evaluating a patient on cardiotoxic medications or with known heart disease. While anxiety often causes sinus tachycardia in healthy patients, other arrhythmias should not be attributed to anxiety alone.

Diagnosis is more difficult if an acute attack is not directly observed. The history of a patient with recurrent supraventricular tachycardias may be impossible to distinguish from a history of panic attacks. In these patients, a Holter monitor should be used to record the patient's EKG for 24 hours. If the patient records a sensation of "anxiety" on the Holter log at the same time that an irregular rhythm occurs on the recording, it documents the connection between the patient's symptoms and the arrhythmia.

Mitral Valve Prolapse Syndrome (MVPS). Mitral valve prolapse is a common, highly variable, and usually benign condition in which a portion of the mitral valve billows into the left atrium with each contraction of the heart.[28] This condition—manifested by a "midsystolic click and murmur" on auscultation and by echocardiographic findings—can result from various abnormalities of the mitral valve. It can be completely asymptomatic or associated with serious dysfunction, including arrhythmia, atypical chest pain, and an increased risk of sudden cardiac death.

The symptoms of panic disorder are similar to those reported by many patients with mitral valve prolapse: palpitations, increased awareness of one's heart, dyspnea, fatigue, chest pain, and syncope.[29] It has been reported that as many as 50% of patients with panic disorder have mitral valve prolapse.[30] The meaning of this association is not clear. There is some evidence that this association reflects a selection bias of highly symptomatic individuals, rather than a true association between the two disorders; most studies do not include the large population of asymptomatic patients with MVPS. A recent study of family members of patients with MVPS revealed *no* increased prevalence of panic disorder in family members with or without MVPS.[29]

Since MVP is found in many patients with panic disorder, some experts recommend screening all patients with panic disorder for MVP. While extensive cardiac evaluation is not always indicated, a careful history and physical exam by an internist should be part of the optimal evaluation of a patient with panic disorder.

Since the course of MVP is usually benign, no special medical treatment is indicated for asymptomatic patients, except for medical follow-up. The finding of mitral valve prolapse is not a contraindication to treatment with TCA or MAOIs. Imipramine has been used quite successfully to obtain remission of symptoms in patients with panic disorder, who were also found to have MVP.[31]

Propranolol is frequently used to treat chest pain and arrythmias in patients with MVPS. For those patients with panic disorder and cardiac symptoms from MVP, propranolol may successfully treat the anxiety as well as the cardiac symptoms. Propranolol should not, however, be used together with an MAOI except in an unusual and closely monitored situation. Since MAOIs increase adrenergic activity at both alpha and beta receptors, blockade of beta receptors by propranolol could cause a dangerous increase in unopposed alpha adrenergic activity.

Another cardiovascular syndrome—the "hyperdynamic beta adrenergic circulatory state"—has been suggested as a cause of anxiety states.[32] It is described as a state of increased "cardiac awareness, increased heart rate responsiveness to various stimuli, and hyperkinetic circulation." The experimental induction of a "hysterical outburst" following infusion of isoproteronol, a beta agonist, promptly reversed by propranolol, a beta antagonist, in several such patients has been cited as evidence of such a syndrome.[32] Patients with this syndrome, and other patients in whom anxiety is experienced with prominent cardiovascular symptomatology, may be best treated with a beta blocker such as propranolol. At present, several studies suggest this, but none demonstrates the superiority of propranolol over other agents used to treat anxiety.

Cardiac Ischemia. A typical episode of anginal pain is easily distinguished from a panic attack. It is often described as heavy pressure, squeezing, or constriction in the chest. It is usually brought on by exertion, but it can also be precipitated by anger, excitement, or other emotional states. Atypical angina can be described as a vague chest discomfort or even as a feeling of anxiety. Patients who come to the emergency room with chest pain as the predominant complaint should be examined by an internist for evidence of myocardial ischemia or infarction. This is particularly true of patients over 40 with recent onset of symptoms. Panic disorder usually begins in people under 40, while angina and myocardial infarction usually appear in patients over 40. Angina is usually relieved by rest or by TNG. Panic attacks are not. A trial of TNG can be used by the internist to help distinguish angina from anxiety. An abnormal EKG during the time when the patient is symptomatic, which returns to normal afterwards, suggests cardiac ischemia. There are, however, some minor ST segment and T wave abnormalities that can be seen during anxiety attacks even in people without other evidence of cardiac disease. Unfortunately, history, physical examination, and EKG are often insufficient for diagnosing angina, and more definitive diagnosis must await further studies such as exercise tolerance testing or, ultimately, coronary angiography. However, for the patient who comes to the emergency room with chest pain and anxiety, a careful evaluation to rule out the presence of a life-threatening condition can be reassuring to both the patient and the interviewer.

Other Abnormal Hemodynamic States. Hypovolemia from dehydration or blood loss, as in gastrotestinal bleeding, can present with tachycardia, dizziness, and faintness. Cardiovascular collapse, or shock, as seen in cardiac pump failure, sepsis, and anaphylactic reactions, also causes tachycardia, sweating, and syncope.

Respiratory Disorders

Any patient who becomes aware of difficulty breathing will experience extreme anxiety. It is the task of the emergency room evaluator to distinguish primary anxiety, with hyperawareness of breathing (or hyperventilation syndrome), from primary respiratory illness, with resulting anxiety. The syndrome of anxiety-induced hyperventilation has been discussed in detail in Section 2.1.2. in this chapter. Here, we will consider other respiratory disorders.

Recurrent pulmonary emboli may present with repeated episodes of hyperventilation accompanied by anxiety. Since physical findings are often minimal, arterial blood gases may be necessary to distinguish pulmonary emboli from anxiety-related respiratory distress. In psychogenic hyperventilation, arterial blood gases will usually reveal an elevated PO_2, while in pulmonary embolism the PO_2 is usually decreased. In equivocal cases, use of ventilation perfusion lung scan or even pulmonary arteriography may be necessary to make the diagnosis with certainty. Asthma, respiratory infections, spontaneous pneumothorax, restrictive lung disease, pulmonary edema, and chronic obstructive pulmonary disease are usually easier to recognize because of their more distinctive physical findings. The exacerbation of asthma can, of course, be precipitated by emotional states. While medical intervention is of primary concern during an acute asthmatic episode, psychiatric consultation or ongoing intervention often helps in managing this illness.

Neurologic Disorders

Neurologic disease affecting either the central or the peripheral nervous system can be confused with anxiety disorders. Delirium or dementia can present with agitation and anxiety. Peripheral nervous system disease is sometimes mistakenly diagnosed as "hysteria" or conversion disorder.

Organic Brain Syndromes. Patients with organic brain syndromes, such as delirium or dementia, present with inability to concentrate, sensory misperception, disorientation, and other features often associated with emotional disturbance, such as anxiety, fear, or irritability. Patients with delirium are commonly agitated. Their anxiety may be a response to terrifying hallucinations or to the frightening loss of ability to think and perceive things clearly. A careful test of cognitive skills—orientation, short-term memory, calculations, writing, reading, drawing constructions, and following commands—will help to distinguish organic brain syndrome from primary anxiety states. Recognizing an organic brain syndrome is the first diagnostic step. Defining the etiology of the syndrome requires further medical or neurologic evaluation.

Seizure Disorders. Temporal lobe epilepsy (TLE) is the seizure disorder most commonly associated with psychiatric symptoms, but occipital, frontal, and parietal foci may cause similar symptoms, perhaps by secondary involvement of the temporal lobe.[33] Altered emotional states can be part of the aura of a generalized seizure or can be the sole manifestation of a partial complex seizure. Fear is a common emotional correlate of epilepsy—identified as the primary emotion experienced by over half of epileptic patients with ictal affect.[34] Actual panic attacks are much less common, occurring in only 1% of patients with temporal lobe epilepsy and in 4% of patients with occipital foci.[35] Patients with TLE usually have other symptoms, including ictal hallucinations, abdominal symptoms, and masticatory movements and interictal personality changes, which help distinguish them from patients with primary emotional disorders. A sleep EEG, particularly with nasopharyngeal leads, can identify the majority of patients with TLE. The difficult differentiation of hysterical seizures from epileptic seizures usually requires a more extensive evaluation than can be accomplished in the emergency room.

Cerebrovascular Insufficiency. Several forms of cerebrovascular insufficiency can cause intermittent or chronic anxiety. Transient ischemic attacks usually lasting 2 to 10 minutes are frequently accompanied by anxiety. While anxiety may predominate early in the disorder, other disturbances of sensorimotor function, speech, and cognition usually develop as the cerebrovascular disease progresses[36] (p. 22). The subclavian steal syndrome caused by partial occlusion of the subclavian or inominate arteries can also cause episodes of anxiety, dizziness, and intermittent confusion.[37] Relative cerebrovascular insufficiency may also occur in disorders such as chronic anemia, cardiac arrhythmias, and intermittent or sustained hypertension. Early symptoms often include anxiety.

Head Injury. Anxiety states are common sequelae of head injury.[38] In the postconcussive syndrome, which can last for several months following an injury, the patient may experience episodes of anxiety, dizziness, lability of mood, personality change, and headache.[39] When the circumstances of the injury are emotionally traumatic, it can be difficult to tell whether the ensuing symptoms result from physical or emotional trauma. The symptoms specific to postconcussive syndrome are reportedly made worse by changes in posture, exposure to heat or sunlight, alcohol ingestion, or strenuous exercise.[40] Subdural hematoma must also be considered in the differential diagnosis.

Infection. Anxiety states can follow encephalitis or can be a manifestation of subclinical encephalitis. History of a preceding upper respiratory infection associated with headache, fever, or photophobia are clues to the diagnosis, which can be confirmed by viral titers.

Multiple Sclerosis. The early, transient sensorimotor disturbances of multiple sclerosis are frequently misdiagnosed as hysterical conversion symptoms. Anxiety and other mood disturbances commonly precede the appearance of other, more easily recognized symptoms of the disorder.

Tumors. Tumors and other mass lesions of the central nervous system can present with various psychiatric disturbances, including anxiety. According to Penfield and Jasper,[38,39] anxiety is a predominant feature of tumors involving the third ventricle.

Other Neurologic Disorders. Wilson's disease, Huntington's chorea, cerebral syphilis, and any other dementing disorder may initially present with anxiety and later evolve into the more easily identified disorder. Toxic-metabolic and infectious encephalopathies can cause neuropsychiatric disturbance. Neurologic disorders causing vertigo, such as Meniere's, also have features in common with anxiety attacks. Systemic diseases that can affect CNS function, such as SLE, and other forms of cerebral vasculitis, can cause psychiatric disturbance. Migraine headaches can be heralded by a sense of vague premonition, visual symptoms of bright spots or homonymous field cuts, paresthesias, hemiparesis, transient aphasia, or confusion. These symptoms, in their early stage, can be accompanied by extreme anxiety, presenting the picture of a panic attack. The full development of characteristic symptoms distinguishes the migraine headache from panic attack. Polyneuritis, posterolateral sclerosis, and early myasthenia gravis can produce peripheral motor and sensory disturbances easily misdiagnosed as "conversion symptoms." Since such symptoms cause anxiety in psychologically healthy patients, the mere presence of anxiety does not rule out a diagnosis of neurologic disease. Hereditary tremor, and the tremors seen in other neurologic disease, should also be distinguished from anxiety tremor.

Hematologic Disorders

Neuropsychiatric symptoms can be precipitated by ingestion of barbiturates in intermittent acute porphyria. Anemia can present with fatigue, depression, anxiety, or other emotional distress.

Neoplastic

The secreting tumors, such as pheochromocytoma and insulinoma, sometimes cause anxiety symptoms. Carcinoid tumors, which secrete the biologically active agents serotonin, bradykinin, histamine, and ACTH, can cause flushing, intestinal hypermotility, and cardiac lesions, all of which might be misinterpreted as symptoms of anxiety.

Immunologic Disorders

The autoimmune diseases, such as systemic lupus erythematosus, can cause neuropsychiatric disturbances. Symptoms of an anaphylactic reaction include tachycardia, sweating, faintness, and dyspnea, which, in their early stages, might be mistaken for anxiety.

Infection

Acute or chronic infection can give rise to mood disturbance, irritability, and restlessness, which are occasionally experienced or labeled as anxiety.

References

1. Glick RA: Anxiety and related states, in Glick RA, Meyerson AT, Robbins E, et al (ed): *Psychiatric Emergencies*. New York, Grune and Stratton, 1976, pp 121–134.
2. Rosenbaum JF: Anxiety, in Lazare A (ed): *Outpatient Psychiatry: Diagnosis and Treatment*. Baltimore, Williams & Wilkins, 1979, pp 252–256.
3. West JB: Disorders of regulation of respiration, in Isselbacher KJ, Adams RD, Braunwald E, et al (eds): *Principles of Internal Medicine*. New York, McGraw-Hill Book Co, 1980, pp 1271–1276.
4. *Diagnostic and Statistical Manual of Mental Disorders* ed 3 (DSM III). Washington, American Psychiatric Association, 1980.
5. Frankel FH: The use of hypnosis in crisis intervention. *Int J Clin Exp Hypn* 22:188–200, 1974.
6. Caplan LR, Nadelson T: Multiple sclerosis and hysteria: Lessons learned from their association. *JAMA* 243:2418–2421, 1980.
7. Klein DF: Anxiety reconceptualized, in Klein DF, Rabkin JG (eds): *Anxiety: New Research and Changing Concepts*. New York, Raven Press, 1981, pp 235–263.
8. Muskin PR, Fyer AJ: Treatment of panic disorder. *J Clin Pharmacol* 1:81–90, 1981.
9. Jenike MA: Rapid response of severe obsessive-compulsive disorder to tranylcypromine. *Am J Psychiatry* 138:1249–1250, 1981.
10. Isberg RS: A comparison of phenelzine and imipramine in an obsessive-compulsive patient. *Am J Psychiatry* 138:1250–1251, 1981.
11. Thoren P, Asberg M, Cronhom B, et al: Clomipramine treatment of obsessive-compulsive disorder. *Arch Gen Psychiatry* 37:1281–1285, 1980.
12. Horowitz MJ: Psychoanalytic theory, in Kutash IL, Schlesinger LB, et al (eds): *Handbook on Stress and Anxiety*. San Francisco, Jossey-Bass Publ, 1980, pp 364–391.
13. Horowitz MJ, Wilner M, Klatreider N, et al: Signs and symptoms of posttraumatic stress disorder. *Arch Gen Psychiatry* 37:85–92, 1980.
14. Krupnick JL, Horowitz MJ: Stress response syndromes: Recurrent themes. *Arch Gen Psychiatry* 38:428–435, 1981.
15. Ovesey L: *Homosexuality and Pseudohomosexuality*. New York, Science House, 1969.
16. Woods SM: Violence: Psychotherapy of pseudohomosexual panic. *Arch Gen Psychiat* 27:255–258, 1972.
17. Sheehan DV, Ballenger J, Jacobsen G: Treatment of endogenous anxiety with phobic, hysterical, and hypochondriacal symptoms. *Arch Gen Psychiatry* 37:51–59, 1980.
18. Gelenberg AJ: Treating panic attacks. *Mass Gen Hosp Newsletter: Biol Ther Psychiatry* 5:1–2, 1982.
19. Klein DF, in Lipton MA (ed): *Psychopharmacology: A Generation of Progress*. New York, Raven Press, 1978, p 1402.
20. Alprazolam, in *Med Letter* 24:41, 1982.
21. Sheehan DV, Claycomb JB, Kouretas N: Monoamine oxidase inhibitors: Prescription and patient management. *Int J Psychiatry Med* 10:99–121, 1980–81.
22. Noyes R, Rathol R, Clancy J, et al: Antianxiety effects of propranolol: A review of clinical studies, in Klein DF, Rabkin J (eds): *Anxiety: New Research and Changing Concepts*. New York, Raven Press, 1981, pp 81–93.
23. Friedman MJ: Post-Vietnam syndrome: Recognition and management. *Psychosomatics* 22:931–943, 1981.
24. Morley JE: Thyroid function screening in new psychiatric admissions. *Arch Intern Med* 142:591–593, 1982.
25. Dietch JT: Diagnosis of organic anxiety disorders. *Psychosomatics* 22:661–669, 1981.
26. DaCosta JM: On irritable heart: A clinical study of a form of functional cardiac disorder and its consequences. *Am J Med Sci* 61:2–52, 1871.
27. Lewis T: *Diseases of the Heart*. New York, Macmillan, 1933, pp 158–164.
28. Shrivastava S, Guthrie RB, and Edwards JE: Prolapse of the mitral valve. *Mod Concepts Cardiovasc Dis* 46:57–61, 1977.

29. Hartman M, Kramer R, Brown T, et al: Panic disorder in patients with mitral valve prolapse. *Am J Psychiatry* 139:669–670, 1982.
30. Gorman JM, Fyer AF, Gliklich J, et al: Effect of sodium lactate on patients with panic disorder and mitral valve prolapse. *Am J Psychiatry* 138:247–249, 1981.
31. Gorman JM, Fyer AF, Glicklich J, et al: Mitral valve prolapse and panic disorder: Effect of imipramine. in Klein DF, Rabkin J (eds): *Anxiety: New Research and Changing Concepts.* New York, Raven Press, 1981, pp 317–340.
32. Frolich ED, Tarazi RC, Dustan HP: Hyperdynamic beta-adrenergic state. *Arch Intern Med* 123:1–7, 1969.
33. Schneider RC, Crosby EC, Bagchi BK, et al: Temporal or occipital lobe hallucinations triggered from frontal lobe lesions. *Neurology* 11:172–179, 1961.
34. Weil AA: Ictal emotions occuring in temporal lobe dysfunction. *Arch Neurol* 1:101–111, 1959.
35. Currie S, Heathfield KWG, Henson RA, et al: Clinical course and prognosis of temporal lobe epilepsy: A survey of 666 patients. *Brain* 94:173–190, 1971.
36. Hall RCW (ed): *Psychiatric Presentations of Medical Illness.* New York, Spectrum Publications, 1980.
37. Santschi DR, Frahm CJ, Pascale LR: The subclavian steal syndrome: Clinical and angiographic considerations in 74 cases in adults. *J Thorac Cardiovasc Surg* 51:103–112, 1966.
38. Merskey H, Woodforde JM: Psychiatric sequelae of minor head injury. *Brain* 95:521–528, 1972.
39. Miller H, Ster G: The long-term prognosis of severe head injury. *Lancet* 1:225–228, 1965.
40. Penfield W, Jasper H: Functional localization in the cerebral cortex, in Penfield S, Jasper H (eds): *Epilepsy and the Functional Anatomy of the Human Brain.* Boston, Little, Brown and Co, 1954, pp 41–155.

VI

Patients and Clinical Syndromes 4
Victims of Situational Crises

1. Introduction

Unlike psychiatric emergencies that are caused by factors indigenous to the patient, such as medical and intrapsychic conditions, a dichotomous category exists that can be attributed to events or causes external to the patient. These situations transcend ordinary daily experiences and expectations. They destroy an individual's sense of personal inviolability and frustrate normally effective techniques for integrating experiences into existing cognitive and emotional schemes. Such events, or patterns of events, produce overwhelming reactions both at the time of their occurrence and subsequently; the intensity and type of emotional reaction depends not only on the nature of the event but on the strengths and inherent flexibility of the victim's internal psychological organization. It is commonly agreed that situations such as natural disasters, war, or accidents and those of personal victimization such as rape or domestic violence do produce psychological crisis and that, depending on the individual's interpretation of the event, situations such as marital separation, loss of a loved one, chronic illness, or surgery can also precipitate an emotional crisis.

2. General Response to Crisis: Three Phases

Although the type and content of psychological reactions to crisis are highly variable, a general pattern can be delineated. This pattern is presented in Table 1.

3. The Tasks

Emergency personnel become involved with persons experiencing situational crises at two specific times. Only the first, the impact phase, correlates temporally with the occurrence of the event. The second point can occur during any of the latter two stages. For reasons specific to the victim's personality, past history, and psychological status, he fails to regain a pretrauma level of emotional stability.

The chief tasks for emergency personnel during or immediately following a crisis are to provide aid, alleviate immediate distress, and evaluate each victim's potential for developing serious psychological sequalae. The symp-

Table 1. General Emotional Responses to Crisis[a]

Phase	Symptoms	Temporal course
Acute reaction during the impact phase of the crisis	The symptoms include shock, disbelief, disorientation, panic, extreme grief, anger, or other intense emotional states. There may be somatic symptoms as well. The individual experiences a complete disruption of normal functioning on both a practical and cognitive level.	Begins immediately following the trauma; may last from 1 to 3 months.
Adjustment reaction during the recoil phase of the crisis	As symptoms of the first stage begin to subside, the individual resumes normal activity and actively attempts to put the crisis into perspective.	May overlap with the first stage, but follows the termination of the acute reaction; may last 3 to 6 months.
Integration and long-term resolution of the crisis	The individual attempts to resolve the crisis by working through the emotional issues and integrating them.	Overlaps with the second stage; may last 1 to 2 years.

[a] If the event is not sudden and unanticipated, a fourth stage (first in the temporal sequence) can be identified—the anticipatory phase. It involves the assessment of, emotional response to, and behaviors deemed necessary for the impending crisis.

toms manifested during the acute phase are not necessarily reliable indicators of the type, content, or severity of later stages. However, three discrete factors influence the ease with which an individual successfully integrates a traumatic event into the totality of his experience. These include (1) the extent to which the person grasps and admits the reality of the situation, and acknowledges the emotional, practical, and cognitive consequences of the trauma; (2) the flexibility and effectiveness of the individual's usual techniques for accommodating to stress and crisis; and (3) the availability of external sources of aid and support, and the willingness to make use of them. Evaluation of these factors during the acute phase of a situational crisis is no substitute for assessing the whole person as he responds to the crisis and across other dimensions.

In 1944, after the Cocoanut Grove fire, E. Lindemann described the survivors' emotional responses to the shocking loss of their loved ones. His description of the acute grief reaction has become a paradigm for understanding other situational crises. See Chapter 12 for a summary of his observations.

In the following section, various situational crises that are commonly dealt with by emergency personnel will be discussed: disasters, rape, battered women, and child abuse and neglect. The identification and management of the posttraumatic stress disorder, which represents a deviation from the typical pattern of crisis resolution, is further described in Chapter 13.

Psychological Management of Disaster Victims

Mark R. Proctor, M.D.

1. Introduction

Natural disasters (e.g., floods, earthquakes) as well as disasters attributable to human error (e.g., accidents) or to human design (e.g., war, bombings) are events sufficiently far from ordinary human experience to cause severe psychological stress in the victims. Emergency personnel automatically form part of a disaster rescue team and also see patients in the emergency room presenting with acute or delayed stress symptoms resulting from the disaster. This chapter discusses the specific features of the emergency management of disaster victims.

As advances in communication technology have brought minute-by-minute coverage of catastrophic events into people's homes, there has been a corresponding pressure to study the psychological impact of disasters systematically. Lindemann's study of the victims of the Cocoanut Grove fire in Boston was one of the first such analyses.[1] The massive bombing of cities throughout World War II called attention to the need for information about human behavior in disasters and provided an important stimulus for research during the next two decades. In the early 1970s, efforts were made to standardize the delivery of mental health services for disaster victims. For example, the Disaster Relief Act and Amendment of 1974 formally gave responsibility for providing training and services to the National Institute of Mental Health. The institute sponsors model programs for training professionals and paraprofessionals to deal effectively with the psychological problems of disaster victims. The development of these programs coincides with the continuing growth of literature in this area.[2–6]

2. Psychological Reactions to Disasters

One significant finding emerging from studies of disasters is that few, if any, victims are left untouched by the experience either at the time of the event

Mark. R. Proctor, M.D. • Harvard Medical School, Boston, Massachusetts 02115, and Beth Israel Hospital, Boston, Massachusetts 02215.

or later. The psychological consequences may persist for months, years, or even the duration of a victim's life. Titchener and Kapp, for example, found that more than 90% of the Buffalo Creek victims exhibited measurable sequelae more than two years after the event. It is well known that the effects of a disaster can be minimized for individual victims if the social structure of the community survives intact,[7] but as Erikson has shown, if that structure is itself the victim of disaster, the negative psychological consequences for the individual victim are heightened.[8]

It is clear that one cannot predict from a person's usual level and style of functioning how he will respond to a disaster. In fact, emergency clinicians should be aware of the fact that psychiatric patients do not necessarily have more difficulty than other people coping with disaster.

> An earthquake. Sylmar, California, 1971: One patient, considered the most mentally disturbed patient on his ward, behaved in a more rational and concerned manner during the quake than expected. He dressed another patient who was almost blind, protected him and led him from the building. Observed shortly after leaving the building, he appeared to be in total contact; however, an hour later he returned to his usual psychotic state.[9] (p. 65)

One other crucial finding of disaster research is that although individual responses to disasters vary widely, they nonetheless conform to a consistent pattern over time. This pattern consists of several stages.

2.1. Warning and Threat

If there is prior warning, people try to prepare for disaster. Maladaptive responses to impending disaster include minimizing the potential threat by denying the reality of the premonitory signs, aggrandizing the self's inviolability, and reinterpreting antecedent events as benign and nonthreatening.

2.2. Impact

People respond to the danger at hand; some individuals behave in an adaptive, reality-oriented manner. Maladaptive responses include disorganized behavior and feeling shocked, overwhelmed, immobilized, panic-stricken, confused, or detached.

Fifteen to twenty-five percent of disaster victims remain "cool and collected," evaluating their situation moment by moment and responding appropriately. The victims' awareness is entirely taken up with the present moment, and their behavior is automatic, efficient, and imperturbable.

> An earthquake. Sylmar California, 1971: One hospital aide said: "I felt as if time had come to a standstill. It seemed as if we were the only ones alive in the whole world. No one seemed to be frightened at first. Everyone immediately began to evacuate the patients."[9] (pp. 64–65)

Roughly three-quarters of any population of disaster victims are overtly shocked or stunned at the time of impact.[10] The majority of this group may show signs of confusion and disorientation that can last from minutes to hours, and they may experience an emotional numbness that later gives way to open expression of affect.

> A large fire in an apartment building: One man . . . was unable to describe any feelings, to give any account of what he had seen or done, or how he came to do what he did. Going into a hotel lobby, he at first appeared calm though uncommunicative, unresponsive and preoccupied. He went to use the phone to call some friends and found himself unable to talk, experiencing an acute surge of subjective anxiety. He burst into tears, cried for several minutes, then said he felt better, showing a good deal of trembling and a need to talk of his experience.[10] (pp. 766–767)

The remaining 10 to 25% of disaster victims will have a more dysfunctional reaction to disaster that can include persistent disorientation, confusion, immobilization or feeling overwhelmed by uncontrollable emotions.[10]

2.3. Recoil and Posttrauma

During these phases, the victim manifests the symptoms of a posttraumatic stress syndrome. The disaster is reexperienced in tormenting memories and vivid nightmares. Sometimes, the victim feels that the disaster is actually recurring.

> A tornado. Dallas, Texas, 1957: The appearance of threatening clouds was often . . .
> a precipitating event. One mother described the behavior of her family in cloudy weather by saying, "they just go from window to window watching the clouds." An elderly woman reported: "I just act crazy—just want to dig a hole and get in it," while another made her reaction more overt: "I just go crazy sometimes and run in the house and hide." Another mother reported that her daughter starts vomiting when she sees dark clouds.[11] (p. 137)

Other victims feel numb and develop apathy, withdrawal, memory lapses, and constricted living patterns.

> The Cocoanut Grove fire. Boston, Mass., 1943: A typical report is this: "I go through all the motions of living. I look after my children. I do my errands. I go to social functions, but it is like being in a play; it doesn't really concern me. I can't have any warm feelings. If I were to have any feelings at all I would be angry with everybody"
> . . . The absence of emotional display in this patient's face and actions was quite striking. Her face had a mask-like appearance, her movements were formal, stilted, robot-like, without the fine play of emotional expression.[1] (p. 145)

Fatigue, loss of appetite, multiple somatic complaints, insomnia, and startle reactions are common. Cognitive symptoms include decreased concentration and confusion about the details of one's surroundings and the passage of time. Dysphoria is manifest as depression, irritability, rage, and panic attacks. Survivor guilt and death anxiety may be particularly hard to bear:

> The Buffalo Creek disaster, West Virginia, 1972: "I dreamt about the baby I found with half its face torn off, and the truck full of bodies. Sometimes in those dreams you're running, or trying to get hold of someone to help them out of the mud. Just last week I had that dream. I woke up pulling on my wife. After that you just can't go back to sleep."[12] (p. 4)

3. Assessment

Disaster relief work is typically undertaken in circumstances of extreme disorganization, stress, and hazard. Because of this, disaster victims should be assessed rapidly and treated immediately.

3.1. Identifying Data

The data base should include the disaster victim's name, age, occupation, marital status, and address. In addition, it might also include a list of the disaster victim's family members, close friends, and neighbors. When filed in a central clearinghouse, these data provide the means for reassembling separated families or identifying groups of victims who have special needs.

3.2. History of Disaster Experience

A detailed account of the disaster victim's experience should be obtained. This should include the amount of warning the person had, what the person has seen, heard, and done, and what has happened to him. These data may help the clinician anticipate patients most likely to develop emotional problems.

> The Cocoanut Grove fire. Boston, Mass., 1943: Her recollections of the disaster are that she was walking upstairs from the Melody Lounge and noticed that the fire was sweeping rapidly upstairs. By the time she got up there she already found herself stumbling over many bodies and was afraid that she would not reach the door. . . . She prayed aloud and other people fell in with her prayer. While she was praying she somehow was shoved over piles of dead bodies and finally her hand reached out "into fresh air" . . . The patient has been followed since discharge. She finds it impossible to attend any enclosed public gathering. Visiting a restaurant with her family, she had a vision of fire breaking out, of tables and chairs being tipped over, and left the room in frantic fear without having eaten anything. She had a similar experience of return of memories of the fire when she tried to attend a movie.[13] (p. 817)

3.3. Past History

Sometimes a victim's symptoms and behaviors cannot be adequately explained on the basis of the natural history of psychological responses to a disaster. For example, if a victim is having extraordinary difficulty making use of help, the clinician may want to collect a *developmental history*, which details the patient's experience with important helping persons. Such a history may illuminate the source of the current problem and point the way to a useful strategy for management. Similarly, patients who present symptoms unusual in quality, severity, or persistence should be asked about both their psychiatric and medical histories.

3.4. Mental Status Examination

Because the natural history of emotional reactions to disaster includes the entire range of psychopathological signs and symptoms, the results of any one examination are not likely to help differentiate posttraumatic stress disorders from other psychiatric disorders. The results of repeated mental status examinations over time may be more useful in making this distinction. The clinician should record the time of each examination and note the patient's level of arousal, attentiveness, orientation, and affect. One should also note the presence or absence of hallucinations, abnormalities of thought content and flow, and memory disturbances. Suicidal impulses, although rare in disaster victims, are not impossible and should be discussed, particularly when someone is severely agitated.[13]

3.5. Level of Functioning

The disaster victim's level of functioning should be reviewed. Someone in a denial-numbness phase of a posttraumatic stress syndrome may be so dazed as to be momentarily unable to care for his own needs. Others may be able to interact more productively with relief workers. The availability of support from family and friends should be assessed. Most disaster victims turn to their own social network for help before they turn to relief agencies.

4. Management

Meeting needs for medical care and basic survival (e.g., food, shelter, clothing) takes precedence over the need for psychological support. Once the immediate needs of the victim are met, effective management consists of:

- Alleviating emotional distress and cognitive disorganization resulting from the recent stressful experience.
- Facilitating the victim's realistic appraisal of the event and its consequences.
- Catalyzing effective problem-solving techniques.

Strategies for attaining these goals include the following:

4.1. Encouraging Ventilation

Disaster victims often feel a compelling pressure to be with people and to talk about their feelings and experiences. Providing opportunities for ventilation will help relieve feelings of isolation, helplessness, and vulnerability.

> A school bus crash. Martinez, California, 1976: We listened to families talk of their dead children over and over again. They kept repeating comments such as "I just saw her this morning," "We were saving our money to go skiing together," "She was so good; she went to church every week," "He was going to be a lawyer," "I'll never see her again."[14] (p. 456)

4.2. Providing Information

In a situation that is unfamiliar, chaotic, and terrifying, the disaster victim also experiences equally unfamiliar thoughts and feelings. The conditions of a disaster may prevent him from ascertaining what losses he has in fact suffered—whether, for example, he has lost family members, friends, or property. These circumstances can interfere with a realistic appraisal of the events and lead to agonizing uncertainty:

> The atomic bombing of Hiroshima, 1945: Parents, half crazy with grief, searched for their children. Husbands looked for their wives, and children for their parents. One poor woman, insane with anxiety, walked aimlessly here and there through the hospital, calling her child's name. It was dreadfully upsetting to patients, but no one had the heart to stop her. Another woman stood at the entrance, shouting mournfully for someone she thought was inside.[15] (p. 391)

Accurate information can be a powerful antidote for this kind of distress. When possible, the clinician should give the disaster victim information about what has actually happened. In addition, he can provide information about how people react psychologically, thereby reassuring the victim about his feelings and thoughts.

> The Cocoanut Grove fire. Boston, Mass., 1943: A patient who lost his daughter . . . visualized his girl in the telephone booth calling for him and was much troubled by the loudness with which his name was called by her and was so vividly preoccupied with the scene that he became oblivious of his surroundings. . . . Some patients are much concerned about this aspect of their grief reaction because they feel it indicates approaching insanity.[1] (p. 142)

4.3. Facilitating Problem-Solving

Horowitz has made the observation that "when action is possible, alert perception, planning, and execution top the hierarchy of claims on cognition."[16,17] Victims sometimes react coolly and flawlessly in a critical situation, only to succumb to overwhelming distress later. The converse also appears to be true: Those who are acutely distressed in an emergency often are able to respond when possibilities for action are delineated. Working actively with a disaster victim to identify problems and possible resources and to implement a plan of action can have a powerfully organizing and mobilizing effect. The clinician should also point to successful efforts the victim has made in the past to solve problems.

4.4. Treating Posttraumatic Stress Disorders

Posttraumatic stress disorder—acute or chronic—presents as a cluster of stress-related symptoms that may resemble other psychiatric disorders. If the onset of symptoms is delayed, or if symptoms persist long after the traumatic event, it may be necessary to search for and isolate the pathogenic stressor before the diagnosis of posttraumatic stress disorder can be made. The symptoms of the disorder are specific to the type of precipitating event and to the individual's psychological makeup; they may range from aggressive, violent outbursts to apathetic, self-isolating behavior to anxious, phobic responses. Each stress syndrome should be evaluated, first, for the potential risk it poses to the person and society and, second, for the discomfort and disruption it causes the individual.

If protective measures are deemed necessary, they should be instituted at once. However, for patients with less severe symptoms, management entails helping the person (1) to assimilate the meaning of the precipitating event into his cognitive schemata and (2) to develop short-term adaptive responses to the stress-induced symptomatology. To accomplish these goals the clinician can use techniques that foster inhibition of overwhelmingly intrusive mental events. They include reorganizing the victim's environment to reduce the level of external stress and removing stimuli evocative of the disaster; teaching thought-stopping techniques; and educating the disaster victim about the nature and causes of his stress response. Techniques designed to reduce excessive internal controls and thus promote assimilation of the disaster experience can be used to treat patients who continue to experience numbness and denial. They include encouraging the disaster victim to talk about his experience, providing a group setting for collective reconstruction of the event, and using carefully designed reminders of the disaster to evoke painful memories that may then be explored and interpreted.

It should be noted finally that the treatment of any stress response requires individualization since each psychological reaction is uniquely determined by personality, cognitive style, and past experience. Decisions about continuing psychotherapeutic efforts beyond the first hour of emergency care should be made on the basis of the usual indications for psychotherapy.

4.5. Giving Psychotropic Medication

Parsimony should be the guiding principle in treating disaster victims with psychotherapeutic drugs. Medications should be used only for the treatment of truly disabling anxiety or significant sleep disturbance. Drug treatment always should be closely monitored (see Chapter 4). Maintenance regimens of any drug should not be introduced in the emergency setting unless follow-up plans have been formalized and the patient medically screened.

4.6. Dealing with the Emotional Reactions of Disaster Relief Workers

Finally, the emergency clinician should also be aware of his own reactions to the disaster. In particular, a relief worker's unchecked rescue fantasies may have destructive effects on victims already overwhelmed by feelings of powerlessness, vulnerability, and inadequacy. The emergency worker should not underestimate his own susceptibility to feelings of fear, anger, and grief.

> A school bus crash. Martinez, California, 1976: The staff . . . had to deal with their own reactions as well. These reactions paralleled those of the families, although they were less intense. At times, staff had tears streaming down their faces as they comforted family members. Staff began comforting one another with a hand on the shoulder or an embrace. Most talked of feeling numb and described feeling like a sponge that soaked up the pain and grief of others until a saturation point was reached. . . . No one remained untouched.[14] (p. 456)

Fantasies of omnipotence can also cause emergency workers to misjudge how profoundly draining disaster relief work can be.

5. Conclusion

Because of the rapid pace of events following a disaster and the chaotic, changing circumstances under which disaster victims are seen, emergency clinicians must be prepared to do rapid, highly focused assessments and provide flexible, situation-specific care. They should participate actively with victims to define problems and to implement solutions—not just on a psychological plane, but also around practical issues. Clinicians should bear in mind that crisis work rarely effects major intrapsychic shifts and that relief efforts must instead be focused on the immediate interplay between external reality and psychological forces.

References

1. Lindemann E: Symptomatology and management of acute grief. *Am J Psychiatry* 101:141–148, 1944.
2. Parad HJ, Resnik HLP, Parad LG (eds): *Emergency and Disaster Management: A Mental Health Sourcebook.* Bowie, Md, Charles Press Publishers, 1976.
3. U.S. Department of Health, Education and Welfare: *Training Manual for Human Service Workers in Major Disasters.* Washington, US Government Printing Office, 1978.
4. Cohen REW, Ahearn FL: *Handbook for Mental Health Care of Disaster Victims.* Baltimore, Johns Hopkins Hospital University Press, 1980.
5. Committee for the Compilation of Materials on Damage Caused by the Atomic Bombs: *Hiroshima and Nagasaki.* New York, Basic Books, 1981.
6. Gleser GL, Green BL, Wright C: *Prolonged Psychological Effects of Disaster: A Study of Buffalo Creek.* New York, Academic Press, 1981.
7. Titchener JL, Kapp FT: Family and character change at Buffalo Creek. *Am J Psychiatry* 133:295–299, 1976.
8. Erikson KT: Loss of commonality at Buffalo Creek. *Am J Psychiatry* 133:302–305, 1976.
9. Koegler RR, Hicks SM: The destruction of a medical center by earthquake: Initial effects on patients and staff. *California Med* 116:63–67, 1972.
10. Tyhurst JS: Individual reactions to community disaster: The natural history of psychiatric phenomena. *Am J Psychiatry* 107:764–769, 1951.
11. Moore HE, Friedsam HJ: Reported emotional stress following a disaster. *Soc Forces* 38:135–139, 1959.
12. Lifton RJ, Olson E: The human meaning of total disaster. *Psychiatry* 39:1–18, 1976.
13. Cobb S, Lindemann E: Neuropsychiatric observations. *Am J Surgery* 117:814–824, 1943.
14. Cinca R, Downie CS, Morris M: When a disaster happens: How do you meet emotional demands? *Am J Nursing* 77:454–458, 1977.
15. Hachiya M, quoted by Tyhurst JS: Psychological and social aspects of civilian disaster. *Can Med Assoc J* 76:385–393, 1957.
16. Horowitz MJ: *Stress Response Syndromes.* New York, Jason Aronson, 1976.
17. Horowitz MJ: Phase-oriented treatment of stress response syndromes. *Am J Psychother* 27:506–515, 1973.

Emergency Care of Rape Victims

Maria C. Sauzier, M.D.

1. Introduction

Rape is an act of violence. The rapist uses sex to humiliate, degrade, and inflict pain and injury on a person weaker than himself. The power differential either is inherent (for example, between an adult and a child) or is attained by using threats, physical force, or a weapon. For the victim, it represents an unexpected, brutal invasion of her privacy as well as a life-threatening situation. Rape inevitably produces a psychosocial crisis, with resultant disruption of intrapsychic equilibrium and loss of usual coping mechanisms. Interpersonal relationships are deeply affected; feelings of fear, anxiety, shame, self-recrimination, and guilt are prominent. The emotional crisis may be compounded by actual physical injuries. Skillful emergency management should focus on alleviating the victim's immediate distress, providing medical treatment, psychological support and legal information, and arranging follow-up care.

The crime of rape evokes strong emotion, which may easily override rational considerations. This is compounded by the fact that basic information is not available: Statistics reflect *reported* rather than *actual* rapes or rape attempts. In 1979 approximately 76,000 forcible rapes were reported (statutory rape and other sex offenses are not included in these numbers).[1] The FBI estimates that the numbers of actual rapes are 3 to 10 times the reported numbers. Rape is the fastest-growing violent crime in America, with a 35% increase between 1975 and 1979. The rate of increase is highest in cities, second in suburban areas, and smallest, but significant (4%), in rural regions. There has been a corresponding but far lesser increase in the number of arrests.

2. Definitions

Rape is a criminal act. The legal definition has changed over the past decade and still differs from state to state. In Massachusetts, the statutes were redefined in 1974. Previously, the law described the rapist as "whoever ravishes and carnally knows a female by force and against her will." This description was extended to "whoever has sexual intercourse or unnatural sexual inter-

Maria C. Sauzier, M.D. • Tufts University Medical School, Boston, Massachusetts 02111, and Harvard Medical School, Boston, Massachusetts 02115.

course with a person and compels such a person to submit by threat or bodily injury."[2] The results of this change can be summarized as follows:

- Sexual intercourse (full or partial penovaginal intromission with or without ejaculation) is no longer the only criterion for rape; oral and anal sex, as well as digital or object penetration of the vagina or anus, also constitute the criminal act of rape.
- The actual use of physical force against the rape victim is no longer necessary for the ascription of the legal term *rape*; the threatened use of force is admissible evidence.
- The victim can be male or female.[3]

Statutory rape is a sexual offense against a person who by definition cannot give consent—a minor, for example.

In 1980 Massachusetts created a classification system for sex offenses, often referred to as the "rape staircase," that stipulates graduated penalties. It differentiates aggravated rape (involving serious bodily injury, multiple assailants, and/or other simultaneously occurring crimes such as kidnapping, breaking and entering, or possessing a dangerous weapon), from rape, assault with intent to rape, or indecent assault and battery.[4]

3. Popular Myths versus the Facts

What motivates the rapist and what role the rape victim plays in her own assault are questions that have only recently received attention from professionals.[5–8] In contrast, popular notions about rape have persisted for years, reflecting society's bias. Statements like "Nice girls don't get raped" or Bad girls shouldn't complain" make explicit the condemnatory attitude society has felt toward rape victims. In many cases, this attitude determines not only how the victim is treated by police, hospital personnel, and family members but how she herself regards the trauma. "Did I bring this on myself?" is a common response of rape victims. In a social system in which women are viewed as inferior to men and individuals are rewarded for their ornamental sexual qualities, it is surprising neither that crimes of sexual dominance and abuse are prevalent nor that victims of these crimes are considered complicitous. Because of the sexual nature of rape, it has been taken for granted that the rapist's primary motivation is sexual desire. The rapist is popularly viewed as a hypersexual, frustrated, or sick man who finds himself responsive to a seductive, available woman. He then acts on his sexual impulses and overpowers the woman.

The increasing number of professional papers and books focusing on rape as a violent instead of a sexual act have begun to combat these myths.[9] In 1971 Amir published a study of 646 rape cases and 1292 offenders known to the Philadelphia police over a two-year period from 1958 to 1960. The following highlights some of his findings[10]:

1. 71% of rapes were planned; 90% of group rapes were planned.
2. 93% of rapes were intraracial.
3. 7% of rapes were interracial: 4% white men against black women; 3% black men against white women.
4. 60% of rapists were married and had normal, regular sexual outlets available.
5. 56% of rapes were committed within a residence, although in 48% the rapist had first spotted his victim on the street.
6. 43% of rapes were committed by two or more assailants acting together.
7. The median age of the rapist was 23, with a peak at ages 15 to 19.
8. The age range of victims spanned from 6 months to 93 years.
9. In 85% of rapes, physical force or weapons were used.

Groth and Burgess have challenged the notion that the rapist is motivated primarily by sexual desire.[11-14] They define rape as a sexual deviation and as a pseudosexual act that is more hostile than sexual. Rape may be committed by men who are sexually dysfunctional during the rape (34% of their sample of convicted rapists) or have physiologic symptoms—oligo- or aspermia. Rape is motivated by anger in explosive, unpremeditated rapes or a need for power in premeditated rapes. Rapists often feel helpless. Inadequate and victimized themselves, the use of sexual brutality reassures them about their masculinity. The act affords them an opportunity for fantasied revenge, release of frustration, and a sense of control and power. Some men rape only under extreme stress; others do it habitually as a consequence of a developmental arrest. Rapists do not belong to any one diagnostic category.

4. The Rape Crisis

Sutherland and Scherl[15] were the first to describe a typical pattern of response to the rape trauma. They noted three phases: During the acute reaction phase, the victim manifests shock, disbelief, and severe anxiety. She may be virtually incoherent and very agitated, yet must make critical decisions regarding medical care and reporting to the police. In phase two—outward adjustment—the victim attempts to resume life as usual by denying the rape and suppressing its consequences. This premature pseudoadjustment attempts to protect the self and others from the rape's impact; the victim consequently refuses help that might aggravate her feelings. In phase three, the victim attempts to integrate and resolve rape-related issues. She may become aware of depressed feelings and the need to talk; psychotherapy at this point can lead to understanding, change, and a true working through of the trauma.

Burgess and Holmstrom,[16] in their report on 92 victims of forcible rape, described two phases of adjustment, which they labeled the "Rape Trauma Syndrome." During the acute disorganization phase, the victim manifests both somatic (e.g., muscle tension, gastrointestinal irritability, genitourinary symptoms) and emotional symptoms (e.g., fear, embarrassment, humiliation, anger, and self-blame). During the long-term process of reorganization, the victim may develop nightmares, phobias related to the trauma (e.g., fear of being alone), and sexual dysfunction. She may also change her residence, telephone number, and/or employment.

Rape, as any overwhelmingly stressful event, constitutes a crisis in the victim's life and leads to a decrease in ego functioning, perceptual and cognitive confusion, loss of usual coping skills, use of maladaptive defense mechanisms. This state of crisis is temporary, and can actually lead to the acquisition of new coping skills and psychologic growth.[17-20] Five phases have been described.

4.1. Anticipatory Phase

The first perception of impending danger arouses fear; the person may deny the reality of her perceptions or she may behave inappropriately. "I should have known . . .," "I shouldn't have tried to . . .," "I should have paid more attention . . ." reflect the victim's feeling that she "should" have been prepared.

4.2. Danger-Impact Phase

The traumatic event occurs and the victim reacts to the immediate threat. Events that are sudden, unexpected, arbitrary, and have to be faced alone rather than as part of a group or community are often more devastating to the victim.

4.3. Postimpact Phase

The victim may for the first time experience the full impact of the trauma, and may be overwhelmed by extreme anxiety, fear, helplessness, and confusion. She may also experience somatic symptoms (eating and sleeping disorders), disruption of usual behaviors (difficulty functioning, impaired concentration), preoccupation with the trauma and how she could have prevented it, hostility, and guilt. There often is regression to a more helpless and dependent state at this time. The particular presentation depends on the victim's character style. The victim who seems cool, calm, and collected and feels numb and distant is using denial and reaction formation (the "controlled style"). At the other end of the spectrum is the victim who cries uncontrollably, shakes or laughs inappropriately, occasionally evidencing symptoms such as hysterical paralysis, and feels overwhelmed by her emotions (the "expressed style").[16]

4.4. Rescue and Recovery Phase

This phase gradually leads to the pre-crisis level of functioning. Sometimes a period of "outward adjustment" precedes the true recovery. The victim may attempt to cope by prematurely closing off feelings and memories related to the rape, sometimes electing drastic life changes (e.g., moving away precipitously, abandoning job and friends) in order to "forget."[15]

4.5. Reorganization Phase

This phase, also known as the integration and resolution phase, involves various attempts at problem-solving and working through of the trauma. If resolution of the crisis is unsuccessful, therapeutic intervention may be necessary. Rape victims may develop long-term sequelae, such as repetitive flashbacks, nightmares, mistrust of men, sexual dysfunctions, phobic reactions, and feelings of depression or anxiety. These feelings may be aroused by any event that has a connection (even unconsciously) to the trauma.[21] As in other crises, the long-term reorganization and resolution may lead to psychic gains by stretching the victim's coping mechanisms and enhancing her self-esteem.[19]

The rape victim's actual set of reactions relates to the nature of the crime, extent of physical injury, her personality style and usual coping mechanisms, life-stage, and available supports.[22–25] For example, the young, single woman who is still dealing with separation/individuation may wish to retreat to the safety of childhood, sometimes leading to regressive life choices. Parents can compound this by becoming overly protective. The entire family system may become phobic and self-isolating. Sexual adjustment is another issue: If the young woman had been sexually curious and active, she may question whether she was "bad" or provocative, and whether the rape may have damaged her as a potential lover; this is particularly painful for the raped virgin. Since young women, (ages 17 to 24) are the most common victims (according to FBI statistics of reported rapes), these problems are frequently encountered in rape counseling.

For the older woman, the issues are different: The rape may coincide with the midlife crisis of reassessing goals and plans and struggling with conflicts between dependence and autonomy (e.g., seeing the children leave, starting a career, going back to school). The divorced woman who is raped may feel especially humiliated and guilty because of her already ambiguous social position. How and what to tell her children may present another problem.

Women involved in a long-term relationship may have the added problem of dealing with their partner's reactions. Men who experience anger, shame, or humiliation may unwittingly displace these feelings onto the victim. Unconscious conflicts about homosexuality may become activated by the feeling of having been "had" by the rapist. Counseling can help partners and families express their feelings openly and can be used to inform them about the consequences of rape. It should be emphasized that education before ventilation may lead to superficial intellectual acquiescence while the unexpressed feelings go underground. It is therefore important to first listen to the victim's and her partner's concerns.

Emergency caretakers also experience a wide range of responses, undoubtedly a reflection of their own issues as well as the victim's clinical status. Contact with a rape victim threatens the sense of invulnerability that makes daily living more comfortable. To escape the fear that "it could have been me," one may blame the victim for her lack of judgment. Other concerns add to the stress of dealing with rape victims: Worry about voyeurism or intrusiveness may inhibit detailed history-taking, thus increasing the victim's sense of unspeakable shame. In addition, rape fantasies, which are very common, often get confused with the real event, producing stress in the caretaker and potential blaming of the victim. In fact, rape and rape fantasies are nonoverlapping phenomena, the latter expressing either a wish to enjoy sex without internal conflict (e.g., being ravished by a favorite movie star) or a fear of punishment for forbidden sexual activities (as seen in nightmares).[23] Sadomasochistic countertransference issues may be reflected in wishes to retaliate or brutalize the rapist; these feelings conflict with the caretaker's wish to see himself as an empathic, humane person. Another possible problem is that the counselor may identify with the victim to such an extent that discussing the rape creates a corresponding feeling of victimization. All such responses can undermine genuine empathy, leaving the victim emotionally isolated or pushed out of treatment prematurely.

Professional stress is an acknowledged problem for rape counselors. Admitting the difficult nature of the work and sharing the feelings and conflicts either with a supportive individual or in a team setting may diminish the stress. Some conflict and emotional discomfort are inevitable, but not to the extent that objectivity and professionalism are sacrificed.

5. Management

Managing rape victims involves coordinating psychological, medical, and legal efforts. While the patient's major emotional need is to regain control over her life and to restore her sense of dignity, medical procedures must be performed and legal options considered. A particularly important and difficult decision for the victim is whether or not to report the rape to the police. The emergency staff should know the legal options available in their state so that the victim can be given information and supported in her decision.

Emergency personnel should foster the patient's active participation in the treatment process, explain what will happen next, and respect the patient's need for privacy. The emergency ward nurse usually becomes the primary contact person or advocate for the rape victim[26,27]; she performs the initial assessment and acts as coordinator of all medical, psychological, and medicolegal interventions. She orients the victim to the emergency setting, explains the procedures, and should remain with the victim during all phases of the examination. Relatives and friends should be encouraged to support the victim but should be asked to leave during history-taking and medical examinations, unless the victim requests otherwise.

Rape victims are traditionally women who have been raped by one or more men. This makes their first encounters with other men particularly difficult, especially if the situation suggests any power differential or loss of control.[28,29] This situation requires particular sensitivity by the gynecologist performing the pelvic examination or the police officer collecting information. The presence of the coordinating nurse is always helpful in this regard.

Because of the complicated medical–legal interface, many emergency settings have formalized treatment procedures as "Rape Protocols."[30,31] Along with standard rape examination kits, the protocol should be accessible to personnel at all times. What follows is an outline for a typical rape protocol; it may be modified to fit local needs, resources, and legal requirements.[30,31]

5.1. Initial Assessment

Gather identifying data, including names of persons who should be contacted. A detailed explanation of the emergency room protocol should be offered at this time so that the patient may give her informed consent to all necessary examinations.

Determine the chief complaint: i.e., whether immediate medical treatment is required or whether psychological symptoms predominate. A brief history should be obtained and initial observations of the victim's emotional and physical status should be recorded.

5.2. Medical Examination

Although many victims come to the ER for a medical examination and gynecologic treatment, this nevertheless can be a very difficult experience for them.[32]

5.2.1. Medical History

A standard medical history should be taken. Special attention should be given to problems that might affect treatment: allergies, use of medication (present and past), penicillin or psychotropic medication sensitivities, major illnesses and operations, migraines, hypertension, strokes, seizure disorders, venous disease, coagulation disorders, and so on. A gynecologic history should include onset of menstruation (and menopause if applicable), last menstrual period, use of contraception, last intercourse near the time of rape, history of venereal disease.

5.2.2. History of the Assault

History-taking has medical as well as legal implications, especially if the victim has decided to report the rape. If not, the victim may decide to report it later or the record may be subpoenaed. Because the medical record is admissible as evidence during court proceedings, it is necessary to make the record legible, complete, precise, and nonprejudicial; it should contain an account of the incidents as described by the victim in her own words and an accurate description of all collected and observed data, particularly her emotional state and signs of force, penetration, and/or ejaculation. A diagnosis of "reported sexual assault" or "reported rape" is a nonprejudicial designation with no prior judgment about the assailant's guilt.[3] Areas to be covered include:

1. Date, time, and location of the reported rape.
2. Threats of violence or retaliation.
3. Use of force, restraints, or weapons.
4. Signs of trauma or struggle.
5. Description of the victim's clothing and signs of violence (tears, rips).
6. Evidence of blood, semen, mud, or other foreign matter.
7. Description of all sexual acts completed or attempted. The victim may be too confused and/or ashamed to volunteer this information and may need to be asked about specific acts, types of penetration, or insertion of foreign bodies.
8. Ejaculation and site of ejaculation.
9. Description of all activity since the rape, especially pertaining to the collection of evidence (douching, showering, bathing, contraceptive jelly, urination, defecation, change of clothing, etc.).
10. An account of preattack injuries.
11. Use of drugs or alcohol (this pertains to the issue of consent: to what degree was the victim conscious or unconscious at the time of the assault).

In addition to the above, the examining physician should note his observations and impressions of the victim, including signs of emotional trauma.

5.2.3. Physical Examination

The physician should examine the victim's entire body, with special attention to those areas that she complains about. The clinician should note all signs of physical trauma, including abrasions, lacerations, bruises, swollen areas, fractures, teeth marks, broken nails, etc. Findings should be described in words as well as by marks on a body chart. If necessary, X rays should be ordered.

5.2.4. Collection of Medicolegal Evidence

This part of the examination should be completed by the nurse and the physician (usually a gynecologist). If the victim is unsure about reporting the rape, she should be encouraged to allow the collection of evidence in case she eventually decides to report the crime. The following guidelines should be followed:

1. Clothing should be examined for evidence of semen, blood, and foreign matter, and saved in a labeled *paper* bag. Plastic bags promote moisture retention, which in turn leads to the formation of mold and mildew, thus distorting evidence. The bag should be given to the police if the rape is reported. The contents of the bag and the receipt for its transfer to police should become part of the medical record.
2. Foreign matter from clothing or body (soil, sand, clothing fibers) should be collected in labeled and sealed envelopes and should indicate where the material was found.

3. If the victim struggled with her assailant, fingernail scrapings should be similarly collected and placed in a labeled and sealed envelope.
4. Any loose hair adhering to the patient's body or clothing should be collected. If indicated, the patient's pubic hair should be combed with a plastic comb to gather loose foreign hairs which are sealed in an envelope labeled "foreign pubic hair"; a second sealed and labeled envelope should contain a sample of the victim's pubic hair (at least three hairs with follicles gathered by vigorous combing or plucking).
5. Dried specimens of semen on clothing or skin can be tested by placing a saline-moistened swab on the area for 15 seconds and then testing the swab for the presence of acid phosphatase. This evidence can be gathered up to six months after the alleged rape occurred.
6. The acid phosphatase test should be performed on any body cavity reported to have been penetrated (vagina, rectum, mouth).

5.2.5. Pelvic Examination and Collection of Laboratory Specimens

Special care should be taken to ensure that the victim does not perceive the examination as a revictimization. This may be the first pelvic examination for a surprisingly large number of patients. The entire examination should be performed in the presence of the nurse. First, the outside genital and anal area should be checked for trauma or erythema; if necessary, pubic combing can be performed at this time.

An unlubricated speculum should be used for the pelvic examination and all slides and specimens labeled with a diamond-tip pen, recording the patient's name, hospital number, and date (two to three slides per orifice). Specimens should be sufficient for both routine gynecologic laboratory tests and special studies, as follows:

Wet mount for motile sperm should be employed. Immediately after the examination, the physician should examine specimens from the vulva, vagina, and cervix (wherever penetration occurred). One or two intact spermatazoa are generally considered evidence of penetration. Their quantity (per high-powered field) and their motility should be noted. Absence of sperm does not rule out the possibility of ejaculation or penetration since the alleged rapist may be oligospermic or aspermic.

Pap smears taken from the endocervix, exocervix, and posterior fornix may help to detect sperm; they are sometimes seen in the stained material.

Gonorrhea specimens should be collected from the cervix, rectum, or pharynx (if appropriate) and placed on Thayer-Martin plates for immediate incubation. Gonorrhea can be identified in cultures within two hours.

Blood group antigens are secreted in semen, saliva, and sweat by most people; care should be taken not to contaminate the sample with the examiner's secretions (use gloved hands). A cotton-tipped swab is placed on any area that may contain the assailant's secretions, then smeared on a piece of filter paper, air-dried, and placed in a labeled envelope. Dried stains can also be used with a saline-moistened swab. These specimens are given to the police for special testing.

Once the lab specimens are collected, a bimanual pelvic examination should be performed. When necessary, blood samples should be taken for drug and alcohol screening, blood type, VDRL, and a beta-subunit test if there is a question of early pregnancy. In addition, the examiner should record his assessment of the victim, including external appearance, emotional state, etc.

5.2.6. Chain of Evidence and Integrity of Findings

To secure the legal validity of the evidence and the test samples, the clinician should establish a written chain of evidence. Each change of hands should be recorded—proving that the evidence was at all times in someone's possession (e.g., locked in a cabinet in the ER, transferred to a specific person in pathology, or given to a police officer). Each item should be labeled in permanent ink with the victim's name, hospital number, date and time of collection, collector's name, and site of collection. Samples sent to the lab have to be hand-carried and registered. The alleged victim's consent to this procedure must be recorded and signed in the medical record.

5.2.7. Medical Treatment

Rape can have medical consequences: physical injury, venereal disease, and pregnancy. Treatment should begin in the emergency room, with physical injuries treated first and tetanus immunization reviewed.

Venereal disease, which occurs in about one out of 30 victims, can be treated prophylactically as follows:

- Procaine Penicillin: 4.8 million units IM (effective for most strains of N. gonorrhea and incubating syphilis).
- Tetracycline: 5 mg PO every six hours for five days. Given to penicillin-sensitive patients (effective for most strains of N. gonorrhea; for incubating syphilis a 12-day course is recommended). It is contraindicated for pregnant women because of possible teratogenic effects.
- Minocycline: 50 mg PO four times daily for five days. Given to penicillin-sensitive patients who wish to avoid the gastrointestinal side effects of tetracyclines. It is also contraindicated in pregnant women.

Pregnancy is a risk that should be calculated carefully, on the basis of menstrual history, previous conceptions, and use of contraception. Since the risk of pregnancy after one unprotected intercourse is only 1% to 5%, the patient should be reassured. If the risk is relatively high, however—that is, if the patient was within five days of ovulation and was using neither birth control pills nor an intrauterine device—she should be told about the following options:

Estrogen therapy: The so-called "morning after pill" has not been approved by the FDA and may cause various adverse effects such as nausea, vomiting, breast tenderness, and delayed menses. It is not entirely effective;

pregnancy occurs in approximately 3 per 1000. In these pregnancies the risk of ectopic implantation or fetal malformation is increased. It can be given in various forms but must be started within 72 hours of intercourse.[27,33,34]

- Ethinylestradiol 5 mg PO once daily for five days.
- Premarin 25 mg PO daily for five days.
- DES is not recommended.

In the rare instances requiring intravenous medication:

- Premarin 25 mg IV daily for three days.
- Premarin 50 mg IV daily for two days.
- Trimethobenzamide hydrochloride (Tigan) 250 mg three to four times daily as necessary can be used to alleviate nausea and vomiting. Since these side effects are quite distressing, some patients interrupt estrogen therapy.

Therapeutic abortion: If pregnancy is indicated by the beta-subunit test (maximal accuracy reached within nine days after conception), the victim should be informed that she has the option of a therapeutic abortion. She can either wait to have a vacuum or surgical curettage at approximately six weeks of pregnancy or can elect to have a menstrual extraction, which may be performed within two weeks after a missed period.

Intrauterine device insertion: This should be completed within 48 hours of the rape; its effectiveness, however, has not been well documented.

Whatever form of treatment the patient chooses, she should be apprised fully of the risks and benefits and she should sign consent forms for the chosen treatment plan.

5.2.8. Other Medical/Legal Points

If the victim remains undecided about reporting the rape to the police, all evidence, including the medical record, should be kept in a hospital safe. If the victim does not wish to report the rape, it is nonetheless possible to file a third-party report in some states. The victim remains anonymous, but the report gives the police information about the specific details of yet one more rape. Such information can serve to "harden" the picture of the particular rapist who uses an identifiable *modus operandi*.[30]

5.2.9. Counseling

A rape victim has just survived a potentially life-threatening trauma and is in a state of crisis. Her response to this trauma depends on her character structure and on the particular events she has just experienced. Counseling involves helping the rape victim to recover her precrisis equilibrium and evaluating the likelihood for psychological or interpersonal difficulties. In some settings, specially trained rape counselors are available, either as part of the emergency team or at a local rape crisis center.

In the emergency room, the counselor may meet the victim either before or after the medical and gynecological examination. When and where no counselor is available, the nurse takes a more active role in providing support and information. If no rape crisis team is locally available and the patient needs further psychological help, referral to a local mental health center or therapist should be discussed with the patient.

The rape victim is likely to be overwhelmed by feelings of helplessness, fear, anxiety, guilt, or shame, and should be encouraged to express these feelings. The counselor should help her acknowledge the fact of the rape and to explore her most prominent concerns. These may be fears about future safety or the attitudes of spouse, family, friends, and society in general; she may worry about possible retaliation by the rapist if she reports the assault to the police, and question her own role in the attack—whether it was something specific to her or her behavior. The counselor should be prepared to offer support and reassurance, and to provide realistic information about rape and its aftermath, the psychological reactions to be expected, and legal options. Above all, the counselor should support the rape victim through the crisis period so that she can leave the ER with an increased sense of self-control, self-respect, and assurance.

5.2.10. Arrange Follow-Up

Follow-up options should be clarified before the patient leaves the emergency room. She should be given names and telephone numbers of her counselor or of outside therapists. She should be informed of the importance of scheduling a gynecologic exam within two to six weeks with the ER physician or her private physician, and given fact sheets about rape and safety. She should be left with the feeling that she can return for help at any time. Transportation home or to a supportive environment should be arranged, using the police if necessary.

6. Conclusion

Rape is by definition a crime of violence perpetrated usually against a single, helpless individual. In effect, however, it is a crime against society, for it violates the most basic human values that society has collectively espoused: the right to personal dignity, self-determination, and privacy.[35] Through no fault of her own, the rape victim has temporarily lost these rights. In the few hours following the rape, she must take the first in a long series of steps toward reestablishing her sense of dignity and freedom, and restoring her faith in the fundamental decency of other people; emergency room personnel are critical participants in that first step.

References

1. Federal Bureau of Investigation: *Uniform Crime Reports: Crime in the US, 1979.* Washington, US Government Printing Office, 1980.

2. *Massachusetts General Law Annotated*, 1980, Chapter 265.
3. Richmond AE: Rape law and the judicial process, in McCombie S (ed): *The Rape Crisis Intervention Handbook*. New York, Plenum Press, 1980, pp 79–97.
4. *Massachusetts General Law Annotated*, 1980, Chapter 459.
5. McCombie S (ed): *The Rape Crisis Intervention Handbook*. New York, Plenum Press, 1980.
6. Brownmiller S: *Against Our Will: Men, Women and Rape*. New York, Bantam Books, 1976.
7. Burgess AW, Holmstram LL (eds): *Rape: Victims of Crisis*. Bowie, Md, Robert J. Brodie, 1974.
8. Nadelson C, Notman M: Psychoanalytic considerations of the response to rape. *Int Rev Psychoanal* 6:97–103, 1979.
9. Groth AN, Birnbaum HJ: The rapist: Motivations for sexual violence, in McCombie S (ed): *The Rape Crisis Intervention Handbook*. New York, Plenum Press, 1980, pp 17–21.
10. Amir M: *Patterns of Forcible Rape*. Chicago, University of Chicago Press, 1971.
11. Groth N: *Men Who Rape: The Psychology of the Offender*. New York, Plenum Press, 1979.
12. Groth N, Burgess AW: Rape: A sexual deviation. *Am J Orthopsychiatry* 47:400–406, 1977.
13. Groth N, Burgess AW, Holmstrom LL: Rape: Power, anger and sexuality. *Am J Psychiatry* 134:1239–1243, 1977.
14. Groth AN, Burgess AW: Rape: A sexual deviation. *Am J Orthopsychiatr* 47(3):400–406, 1977.
15. Sutherland S, Scherl DJ: Patterns of response among victims of rape. *Am J Orthospychiatry* 40:503–511, 1970.
16. Burgess AW, Holmstrom LL: Rape trauma syndrome. *Am J Psychiatry* 131:981–985, 1974.
17. Parad HJ (ed): *Crisis Intervention*. New York, Family Service Association, 1965.
18. Lindemann E: Symptoms of acute grief. *Am J Psychiatry* 101:141–148, 1944.
19. Caplan G: *Principles of Preventive Psychiatry*, New York, Basic Books, 1964.
20. Bassuk E: A crisis theory perspective on rape, in McCombie S (ed): *The Rape Crisis Intervention Handbook*. New York, Plenum Press, 1980, pp 121–131.
21. Katan A: Children who were raped. *Psychoanal Study Child* 28:208–224, 1973.
22. Nadelson CC, Notman MT: Psychological responses to rape. *Psychiatr Opinion* 14:13–18, 1977.
23. Notman MT, Nadelson CC: The rape victim: Psychodynamic considerations. *Am J Psychiatry* 133:408–413, 1976.
24. McCombie SL: Characteristics of rape victims seen in crisis intervention. *Smith Coll Stud Soc Work* 46:137–158, 1976.
25. Burgess AW, Holmstrom LL: Coping behavior of the rape victim. *Am J Psychiatry* 133:413–417, 1976.
26. Burgess AW, Holmstrom LL: The rape victim in the emergency ward. *Am J Nursing* 73:1740–1745, 1973.
27. Gilmore BS, Evans JW: The nursing care of rape victims, in McCombie S (ed): *The Rape Crisis Intervention Handbook*. New York, Plenum Press, 1980, pp 43–59.
28. Silverman D: First do no more harm: Female rape victims and the male counselor. *Am J Orthopsychiatry* 47:91–96, 1977.
29. Hallek SL: The physician's role in the management of victims of sex offenders. *JAMA* 180:273–278, 1962.
30. Appendices, in McCombie S (ed): *The Rape Crisis Intervention Handbook*. New York, Plenum Press, 1980.
31. McCombie SL, Bassuk E, Savitz R, Pell S: Development of a medical center rape crisis intervention program. *Am J Psychiatry* 133:418–421, 1972.
32. Klapholz H: The medical examination: Treatment and evidence collection, in McCombie S (ed.): *The Rape Crisis Intervention Handbook*. New York, Plenum Press, 1980, pp 59–60.
33. Wertheimer A: Examination of the rape victim. *Postgrad Med* 71:173–180, 1982.
34. Braen GR: *The Rape Examination*. North Chicago, Ill, Abbott Laboratories.
35. Hilberman E: The impact of rape in the woman patient, in Notman M, Nadelson C (eds): New York, Plenum Press, 1978.

16

Emergency Care of Battered Women

Ronnie F. Ryback, M.S.W., A.C.S.W.

1. Introduction

The numbers of battering victims presenting to emergency settings have increased in the past decade. Currently, there are an estimated 2.8 million battered women in the United States, constituting more than half the married women in this country.[1] These figures do not include women who are beaten by boyfriends and lovers, or a staggering number of unreported or unidentified cases. Women who fear the stigma of public humiliation and the very real danger of retaliation by husband or lover are reluctant to identify the actual cause of their injuries or distress and most often present to the emergency room as unwitting victims of accidents, not abuse. This chapter deals with both those women who identify themselves as battering victims and those who deny the assault; in both situations, the general principles of emergency care are described.

2. Definitions

Domestic violence, or, more specifically, the battered woman syndrome, has many definitions. Medically, a battered woman is someone "who has suffered serious or repeated physical injury from the man with whom she lives."[2] The severity of the injuries falling within the definition's purview range from those requiring no medical attention to those necessitating hospitalization. Legally, each state has its own criteria: In Massachustts, for example, domestic violence is defined as the "occurrence of one or more of the following acts between family or household members:

1. Attempting to cause or causing physical harm.
2. Placing another in fear of imminent physical harm.
3. Causing another to engage in sexual relations by force, threat of force or duress."[3]

3. Background

Historically, the use of physical force by a man to control a woman's behavior has been commonplace. The Old and New Testaments, the Talmud,

Ronnie F. Ryback, M.S.W., A.C.S.W. • Beth Israel Hospital, Boston, Massachusetts, 02215.

and the Koran contain passages that dictate the total subjugation of a wife to her husband.[1] In the United States, laws permitted wife-beating for correctional purposes until the late 18th century, when the Married Women's Act was passed. Laws prohibiting wife-beating were not implemented in Italy, Scotland, or Iran until the 1970s.[4,5] Most states now permit women to initiate criminal proceedings against abusive husbands or lovers, but the laws are often both ambiguous and cumbersome. In a social structure that denies women full and equal status, domestic violence is just one of many forms of routine oppression.

4. The Victims, Their Families, and the Abusers

The problems of battered women concern not just the women themselves but their husbands or lovers, the relationship between the two, the children who are bound to the family system either as witnesses or victims, and the larger social system, which includes extended families, friends, schools, police, courts, hospitals, and social and psychiatric agencies. Battering and domestic violence occur across all socioeconomic, racial, ethnic, and educational lines. A higher incidence associated with a particular demographic profile may reflect only a weighting in the reporting statistics, not the actual frequency of occurrence.[6–8]

According to a study by Star, Clark, Goetz, et al.,[9] a typical battering victim has a devastatingly low self-concept, tends to withdraw from society, and experiences a high degree of isolation and passive dependence on others. She usually reports a history of poor relationships in her early life, frequently describing her father as alternately violent and seductive. As a child, she may have witnessed, or been the victim of abuse and has consequently learned to accept physical aggression as a problem-solving method. She may have viewed early marriage as a way out of her unhappy childhood home. As a result, she frequently has had little or no work experience and limited social opportunities. She may therefore be withdrawn and anxious in new situations, reluctant to make changes, and literally immobilized by her financial and emotional dependence on her husband.[10–12]

Study of the abuser reveals a man who is generally not psychotic, but immature and lacking in self-control, confidence, and realistic marital expectations. He tends to blame his wife for the marital strife, claiming that she is the cause of his violent behavior. The abuser's low self-esteem renders him incapable of viewing himself positively, and it is therefore up to the spouse to make him "feel like a man." His frustrated expectations, wishes, and demands can trigger an explosive outburst; violence becomes the normal route for achieving his way and for resolving conflict. Like the victim, the abuser was often exposed to violence in childhood. As a consequence, signs of characterologic depression may appear in adulthood.[10,13,14] In spite of these typically problematic personal and interpersonal characteristics, abusive men tend to elicit protective, sympathetic feelings from their spouses during periods of relative nonviolence. These women can still point to their husband's attractive features. Rather than holding them responsible for their violent behavior, they describe them as childlike, dependent, and remorseful, men whose histories of neglect and abuse have caused their current problems. Threats to commit suicide or homicide are commonly made by these men when the woman tries to break out of the relationship, thus entrapping both spouses further in the cycle of frustration, violence, remorse, and pity.

The battering cycle follows a relatively typical course in which the tension over some precipitating event begins to mount. Women may resort to self-degrading, inappropriate forms of pacification to avoid or postpone the violence. If these efforts prove futile, violence erupts, sometimes at the provocation of the woman, who can no longer tolerate the anxiety of waiting for the inevitable. In the postviolence phase, the abusive man may express profound remorse and behave affectionately and solicitously toward his wife. This phase may be dramatized by the appearance in the emergency setting of a distraught husband hovering over his recently abused wife. The husband's seductiveness during this period seems to bind the woman more tightly to the relationship, allowing her to seem unconcerned about the potential for future violence.[12,15]

The beatings usually start early in the relationship, during the first months of marriage or during the first pregnancy. The precipitating factors include arguments over money, extreme jealousy and possessiveness, sexual problems, alcohol and drug abuse, disputes over children, unemployment, the woman's desire to expand her role (e.g., to work outside the home), and pregnancy.[16] Although these are commonly considered as precipitants, they cannot be regarded as the causes of violence. Disagreement exists about the etiology of domestic violence. Popular mythology, for example, depicts the victim as causing, engaging in, and needing violence: "She asked for it—she wanted it, otherwise she'd leave." "If she were a better wife, he wouldn't abuse her." Violence is, according to these theories, sought by the woman as punishment for her fantasized badness.[17] In contrast, other theories portray the man as resorting to violent forms of oppression to compensate for his felt inadequacies; relative to the humiliated, abused victim, the abuser is powerful and dominant. From the standpoint of social systems theory, domestic violence erupts when roles or positions in the family are threatened. Men, for example, who have failed to achieve or maintain their status as head of the household are more likely than their female counterparts to respond to stress with physical violence. And women who are isolated from outside social networks, who are overwhelmed by helplessness and dependence, are likely to remain locked within a violent dyad.[5,6,16]

5. The Emergency Presentation

Regardless of the etiology of domestic violence, it must be emphasized that whenever a beating occurs, it constitutes a crisis for the victim. She may be seriously injured. She has experienced a brutal, humiliating assault that threatens not only her self-respect but also her respect for and trust in her husband. If she has been chronically abused, she may be perpetually apprehensive, guilty, ashamed, hopeless, and desperate, but still paralyzed by fear and indecisiveness. Like other victims, she may feel absolutely numb; and worst of all, she may be unable or unwilling to identify herself as a victim of abuse.

> Alison was a 24-year-old mother of two children. During her five-year marriage, she had been beaten regularly, requiring emergency treatment for bruises and cuts on her arms, legs, and back. She denied that the injuries were the result of beatings—until a particularly brutal assault to her face. At that point, she reported the truth. "I just looked in the mirror and saw my swollen face and said to myslef, "This is it, I'm not taking this anymore.' I started to scream and couldn't stop. . . ."

Other victims, however, have been living in a nightmare for a long time and have adopted a coping stance that effectively numbs them to their circumstances.

> Sophie came to the emergency ward for multiple slash wounds from a razor used by her husband "to keep her in line." She recounted the events leading up to the argument with great calmness, requesting only that her wounds be sutured so that she could return home to her five children. All attempts to offer help were rejected. "I've gotten used to this. If I tried to leave, he'd kill me and the kids. . . ."

Other victims may present to the ER with physical injuries, somatic complaints, or psychological symptoms, but deny a violent origin. If the physical injuries are not specifically reported as abuse-related, the opportunity for effective intervention may be lost. The emergency clinician should, therefore, pay special attention to available cues: the nature of the injuries, the emotional responses of the injured person, the interaction of the suspected victim and her spouse or lover. Black eyes, strangulation marks, cigarette burns, bites, upper body bruising, signs of forced sexual intercourse, lacerations, or abdominal bruises in a pregnant woman should be regarded with a high degree of suspicion. Similarly, if the patient's emotional response does not seem to fit the proffered explanation for the injuries, it can be assumed that she is hiding some part of the truth. She may seem overly anxious or fearful, evasive, depressed, or guilty, while simultaneously insisting on a benign or accidental cause for her injuries. A highly charged emotional atmosphere surrounding the victim and her suspected abuser would not make sense if the injuries were truly accidental.

If there is a high index of suspicion, but the injured person seems reluctant to admit the truth, she should be interviewed privately, assured that her responses will be kept confidential and encouraged to vent her feelings. A direct question such as "Did someone hit (cut, burn) you?" may relieve the victim of the responsibility for volunteering difficult information. If the question elicits a negative response, the answer should not be challenged. Instead, other opportunities for acknowledging the abuse should be provided.

The emergency clinician's task is far easier if the victim identifies herself. The intervention can then be directed beyond immediate treatment to longer-range preventive management. Without admission of abuse, however, the ER can only provide relief for the current injuries and distress.

6. Assessment and Management of Identified Victims

Assessment and management should be an overlapping, ongoing process of evaluating and treating the patient for physical injuries and psychological trauma. The emergency intervention usually involves five phases: orienting the victim to the emergency setting and informing her of treatment procedures; obtaining a medical and psychiatric history; examining the victim; treating the physical injuries; and counseling the patient. These steps may be carried out sequentially or concurrently, or they may overlap.

During the orientation phase, the victim should be informed about legal, medical, psychological, and social resources available in her community. She should not be pressed for a decision about her participation but merely informed of all the choices regarding alternative housing, protective measures, legal recourse, and psychosocial intervention. Emergency procedures should be explained to the victim so that she knows what to expect. Consent or refusal forms should be provided.

A standard medical and psychiatric history should be obtained, but with emphasis on the evaluation of the patient's current and previous coping mechanisms, the available support network, her level of functioning, and her perspective on the cycle of abuse. Battered women have a high incidence of depression and make frequent suicide attempts (e.g., self-poisoning and/or self-mutilation, overmedicating with antidepressants or tranquilizers). Homicidal potential and alcohol and drug use also should be assessed. If children are involved, their safety must be evaluated. If there is evidence that the victim and/or the children are at risk, are unable to function appropriately, and need protection, custodial arrangements should be considered. If necessary, a care and protection document should be filed for children of battering victims who may themselves be neglected or abused (see Chapter 17). The physical examination should focus on acknowledged and unacknowledged areas of injury, checking for the following: lacerations with sharp instruments; external or internal injuries from punches, kicks, or falls; strangulation marks around the neck; burns or scald marks; bite marks and infected areas; fractures (nose, mouth, vertebrae, pelvis, skull, or ribs); dislocations; retinal damage associated with blackened eyes; head injuries (skull fractures, subdural hematomas); acute anxiety that presents as palpitations, hyperventilation, gastrointestinal complaints, migraine headaches; obstetrical complications (bleeding, cramping, premature labor).

As part of the physical examination, pulse, temperature, and blood pressure should be routinely obtained, and necessary X rays or laboratory tests should be ordered. When the nature and severity of the physical injuries have been assessed, treatment should be explained to the patient and promptly undertaken.

Counseling is perhaps the most difficult and delicate aspect of the treatment process. The victim may be suffering physically as well as emotionally. She will undoubtedly be distressed by the intensity and range of her feelings, which include:

- Loss of control and helplessness arising from feeling at the mercy of another's violent outbursts. Women report that some attacks are unwarranted, even unexpected. The victim may appear passive and submissive and may feel "acted upon"—unable to gain control over her situation. She may be immobilized by fears about her own violent fantasies and aggressive impulses toward the abuser.

    Cheryl was a 29-year-old college professor and mother of three children. She had been married to Bill for five years. As his drinking increased, so did his violent threats. For the past year he had been beating her. She finally sought help after she purchased a gun. "I'm really afraid that I'm going to kill him" was a feeling that prompted her to come to the ER.

- Fear, not just for her future safety but for that of her children, is a very real part of the victim's experience. Because admitting the violence may lead to retaliation, the victim should be reassured that her responses are confidential. To assess the immediate danger, direct questions about guns or other weapons, drugs, alcohol, or medications of any kind should be asked.
- Anger is experienced by all victims at least on some level. If it is not directed at the abuser, it may manifest itself as depression, with concomitant guilt and self-blame. Some women may identify with the aggressor's projections, feeling that they are beaten because they are bad.
- Shame may be evinced in an elaborate effort to cover up the beating, to fabricate explanations for the injuries, or to ensure hospital complicity in keeping the beatings secret.
- Doubts about sanity may result as victims of chronic abuse become increasingly isolated and identify with the abuser's projected characterization. Reality testing is compromised, and victims begin to believe that the abuser's taunts are true and that their own excessive anxiety, fear, and/or depression are signs of mental instability.
- Ambivalence about the abuser is standard. The victim may hate the abuser, have violent fantasies against him, and yet retain positive feelings about "the other side of him"—his little-boy quality and charming, affectionate nature. She may express protective or sympathetic feelings about the abuses suffered by him during childhood or at the hands of the world during adulthood.

The battering victim should be encouraged to talk about her feelings. She should be helped to acknowledge the reality of her situation and her reaction to it. She may be so enmeshed in her problems, fears, and dependency needs that there seems no way out; through the technique of labeling, the clinician can help to compartmentalize and focus on small parts out of the larger, bewildering whole. Focusing reduces the victim's anxiety in the face of seemingly overwhelming chaos. As part of this process, the clinician should anticipate and acknowledge the ambivalent feelings the victim may have toward her spouse. Her willingness to change or leave the relationship should be assessed: Is there evidence that realistic plans are being made or are capable of being made? Is revenge an issue? Does the victim recognize that there is a pattern of violence, not just isolated events, and that violence is not an appropriate solution to domestic arguments? Social networks and support systems are vital to the abused family. Supportive family members, friends, clergy, employment affiliations are valuable resources to the victim. They may help the victim extricate herself from the abusive cycle. Factors such as ongoing risk to her and the children, availability of alternative living arrangements, willingness to leave, and capacity to operate outside the abusive dyad play a part in determining not only how the victim reacts during each crisis but if she will be able to follow through beyond the emergency intervention. It is, therefore essential that the victim's frame of reference and position be acknowledged. She should not be pressured into making a decision for which she is emotionally unsuited. Instead, she should be helped to see reality, especially her strengths, rights, and value as a human being.

It is unlikely that the abusive cycle can be broken during a single emergency visit, but it is possible that the first step toward righting a troubled and dangerous relationship can be taken. This may occur if, by the end of the intervention, the victim and the abuser can accept the difficulties in their interactive pattern and make a commitment to subsequent longer-range treatment. Referral to private therapy, mental health agency, or other community service should be made from the emergency room. If this is not possible for the couple, the victim should be encouraged to seek help alone in extricating herself emotionally and physically from the abusive cycle.

7. Conclusion

Unlike other medical and psychiatric emergencies, domestic violence challenges the clinician in a unique way. The clinician has in his power the capacity to make rapid, accurate assessments, effect prompt, successful treatment, and help the patient get through the immediate crisis. But what is not directly within his power is the single factor that determines the patient's long-range welfare— the willingness of the victim to acknowledge the cycle of abuse and accept help. By the end of the emergency intervention, the clinician must either have helped the victim to see the destructiveness of the violent episodes and their inherent risks or he must stand back and allow the victim to return to the violent relationship. In effect, emergency personnel are forced to accept real limits to their interventions even when human responsibility might dictate otherwise.

References

1. Langley R, and Levy RC: *Wife Beating: The Silent Crisis.* New York, EP Dutton, 1977.
2. Pahl J: The general practitioner and the problems of battered women. *J Med Ethics* 5:117–123, 1979.
3. Abuse Prevention Act (1978) *Massachusetts General Laws,* Chapter 209A.
4. Martin D: *Battered Wives.* San Francisco, Glide Publications, 1976.
5. Dobash RE, Dobash R: *Violence Against Wives.* New York, The Free Press, 1979.
6. Gilles R: *The Violent Home.* Beverly Hills, Sage Publications, 1974.
7. Grambs M: Wife-beating as an American pastime. *Behavior Today,* February 1977, pp 5–6.
8. Davidson T: *Conjugal Crime: Understanding and Changing the Wife-Beating Pattern.* New York, Hawthorn Books, 1978.
9. Star B, Clark C, Goetz K, et al: Psychosocial aspects of wife battering. *Soc Casework* 60:479–487, 1979.
10. Gaylord JJ: Wife battering: A preliminary survey of 100 cases. *Br Med J* 1:194–197, 1975.
11. Walker LE: Battered women and learned helplessness. *Victimology* 2:525–533, 1978.
12. Hilberman E, Munson K: Sixty battered women. *Victimology* 2:460–471, 1978.
13. Elbow M: Theoretical considerations of violent marriages. *Soc Casework* 58:515–526, 1977.
14. Scott PD: Battered wives. *Br J Psychiatry* 125:433–441, 1974.
15. Walker LE: Treatment alternatives for battered women, in Chapman J, Gates M (eds): *The Victimization of Women,* vol 3. Sage Policy Series on Women. Beverly Hills, Sage Publications, 1978.
16. Carlson B: Battered women and their assailants. *Soc Work* 22:455–460, 1977.
17. Liebernecht K: Helping the battered wife. *Am J Nursing* 78:654–656, 1978.

Child Abuse and Neglect

Florence Sullivan, M.S.W., and Rosemary Evans, M.S.W.

1. Introduction

According to estimates recently published by the National Center on Child Abuse and Neglect, more than three million children in the United States were subjected to abuse or neglect during a one-year period. Although only one-third of those children were actually reported to child protective services, one-third of these were seriously neglected and one-third were severely injured. Two thousand children died, averaging six victims a day. Many children who survive are irreparably hurt; they are left with permanent physical damage or emotional impairment. All 50 states have enacted protective legislation requiring that suspected cases of abuse be reported to a designated agency. In addition, each state had provided extensive services for abused or neglected children. There are telephone hotlines, crisis centers, outpatient facilities, family service networks, and specially designed treatment modalities such as family therapy and parent aid and training programs. The key to interrupting the pattern of abuse and neglect in our society, however, is not merely to add more services but to find and identify the victims and connect them with services that can help.

2. Dynamics of Child Abuse and Neglect

There are four types of abuse and neglect: physical abuse, sexual abuse, emotional or psychological abuse, and neglect. In general, because abuse and neglect are not typically found in the same family, they must be seen as different phenomena. In abuse, an active, albeit violent, response is made to a child. In neglect, there is usually no response; the child's needs remain essentially unmet. Abuse takes place episodically in the context of ongoing care. Neglect, however, is a chronic pattern in which the needs of the children are routinely ignored. Situations of neglect have typically carried a poorer prognosis than their abusive counterparts. The following profiles may explain these findings.

Abuse is typically focused on one child, the so-called scapegoat, who is either different or perceived to be different by the abusing parent. The parent

---

Florence Sullivan, M.S.W., and Rosemary Evans, M.S.W. • Judge Baker Guidance Center, Boston, Massachusetts 02115.

usually has had a history of childhood abuse, has learned to respond to stress with violence, and suffers from low self-esteem. He tries to counter these feelings with excessively high performance standards for himself and his child. When the "abusive potential" is high in a particular parent and there is an identified scapegoat, it may take no more than a minor stress—a small act of disobedience on the part of the child, a disappointment, a conflict or frustration for the parent—to produce a violent episode. Violence may be followed by a period of remorse, with increased attention and affection for the child; it may also be followed by a quiescent period during which the tension in the family again begins to build. In either case, abused children develop chronic anxiety. They are often wary of adult contacts and may be very withdrawn or aggressive. They may present with emotions or behaviors unusual for normal home conditions, but quite explicable in view of an early life of abuse.

> Mr. Adams, age 35, is the married father of five boys; Charles, the youngest (age 2) is mildly retarded. Mr. A. is a successful CPA. He came into treatment six months ago because he was losing his temper and had begun to beat his wife. The Adams family moved to this community one year ago and had few friends. Both parents seemed overwhelmed by the needs of their children. Mr. A. complains that his wife seems to let them get away with everything. He feels his wife does not appreciate his efforts to support and care for the family. This week, Mr. A. came into his therapy session markedly upset, saying that he had hurt Charles the night before.

This case illustrates many of the early danger signs of potential abuse, including a highly motivated, perfectionistic man; a passive wife incapable of protecting herself; a "different" child, e.g., mildly retarded; no relatives and few friends; a nonsupportive, nonharmonious marital relationship; and ignorance of appropriate discipline methods.

In contrast, neglect is a chronic pattern. The parent or caretaker does not respond to the needs of the child. The household may be chaotic, the lives of the parents disorganized, the parents themselves apathetic, depressed, and hopeless. A child is not singled out for neglect; rather, the personal, social, educational, and medical needs of all the children are largely ignored. Negligent parents perceive themselves as unsuccessful, failures at living. They tend to be isolated, without social resources, and unwilling to use available supports.

> Mary is age 6, the oldest of three children, and a first-grader at the local public school. Her teacher, Miss Brown, has been concerned about Mary and asked for a consultation with the school psychologist. Miss Brown reports that Mary is a frail, often unhappy-looking child. She is small for her age. She seems unable to concentrate on her work, though she has tested at low normal intelligence. She is having difficulty learning to read. Miss Brown is most concerned about Mary's isolation in the classroom. She appears uninterested in the overtures other children make, and she takes no initiative. Mary attends school regularly and brings lunch with her, but is often late without explanation. Her parents have not responded to an invitation for a conference.

The teacher and psychologist agree that neglect could explain Mary's affect and behavior. The data supporting such a view include undersized, unhappy-looking child; frequent, unexplained tardiness; inability to concentrate on schoolwork; withdrawal and failure to socialize with children or seek comfort from adults; mother is young and has three small children; and no parental response to school outreach.

3. Legal Issues

The laws about child abuse and neglect vary from state to state; their purposes are to document the extent of the problem and to ensure that appropriate resources are mobilized. Each state has a *mandatory reporting law* that defines abuse and neglect, those required to report suspected cases (i.e., mandated reporters), the agency designated to receive and investigate such reports, and the penalty for failure to report. Legal requirements supersede the professional ethic of confidentiality. The issue for a mandated reporter is not *if* a report should be made but rather how to handle it with the family. Generally, protective service work is more effective when the family knows who made the report and has been told by the reporter in advance.

In Massachusetts, the law states who must report cases of suspected abuse or neglect, but the designated agency (Department of Social Service) defines abuse and neglect as follows:

Abuse—A physical injury or emotional injury by other than accidental means that causes or creates a substantial risk of death or protracted impairment or physical or emotional loss or impairment of the function of a bodily organ; and the commission of a sex offense against a child as defined in the criminal laws of Massachusetts.

Neglect—A condition in which a caretaker responsible for the child either deliberately or by extraordinary inattentiveness permits the child to experience avoidable present suffering or fails to provide one or more of the ingredients generally deemed essential for developing a person's physical, intellectual, and emotional capacities, such as:

- Adequate food, clothing, shelter, education, or medical care, though financially able to do so or offered financial or other reasonable means to do so; and proper supervision or guardianship.
- Steps to avoid physical dependence of a child upon an addictive drug at birth.

In Vermont the following definitions appear in that state's reporting law:

Abuse—Physical injury or injuries inflicted upon a child by a parent or other person responsible for his care by other than accidental means, or any other treatment, including sexual abuse, which places that child's life, health, development or welfare in jeopardy or which is likely to result in impairment of the child's health.

Neglect—The abandonment of a child by his parents, guardian, or other custodian.

Massachusetts law differentiates between mandated and nonmandated reporters. Mandated reporters are those who must report cases of suspected abuse/neglect, under penalty of a fine of not more than $1000 for failure to do so. Nonmandated reporters are all other persons not designated as mandated who may also report cases of suspected abuse and neglect. Mandated reporters are not liable in any civil or criminal action by reason of such report. Nonmandated reporters are also not liable in any such proceeding if the report was made in good faith. Mandated reporters include any physician, medical intern, medical examiner, dentist, nurse, public or private schoolteacher, educational administrator, guidance or family counselor, probation office, social worker, foster parent, or policeman.

The law requires that when any mandated reporter in his professional capacity has reasonable cause to believe that a child under the age of 18 is suffering serious physical or emotional injury resulting from abuse, including sexual abuse, or from neglect, including malnutrition, or who is determined to be physically dependent upon an addictive drug at birth, he shall report such condition to the department immediately by oral communication and written report within 48 hours.

The Department of Social Service has the responsibility to (1) investigate all reports of child abuse and neglect, (2) determine whether or not abuse or neglect has occurred, and (3) develop a treatment plan with the child in or out of his own home, temporarily or permanently.

In addition to the mandatory reporting laws, all states have established means for bringing such matters before the court. The latter are referred to as "Care and Protection" (C & P) laws. While most reported cases are resolved without court intervention, the department can file a C & P if a family has not cooperated with the department's efforts to provide a safer home for the child and/or if the department is seeking removal of the child from the home. The court may then order the parents to cooperate with the department in specific ways or sanction the removal of the child from the home, either temporarily or permanently.

Sometimes a C & P is brought before the court by a petitioner other than the department (e.g., a private citizen, agency, or group). The complaint must describe why the petitioner believes that the child is in need of care and protection. In response, the department must investigate the case immediately and report back to the court. If the judge feels the child may be in immediate danger, the child may be placed in temporary custody of the department, the petitioner, a relative, or a private agency or group deemed suitable while awaiting the report from the department. The case then proceeds as if a report of suspected abuse or neglect had been originally filed with the department; however, the court may decide to supervise the process more closely.

4. Evaluation and Intervention

In addition to evaluating and treating life-threatening injuries or the chronic ravages of neglect, the clinician should try to identify the abusive/neglecting pattern; this is critical to the success of the emergency intervention. Sometimes parents acknowledge the abuse or neglect openly. In other situations, the child reports violence or neglect. And in still others, both parents and children conceal the reality underlying a pattern of injury or neglect. The task of the emergency clinician is considerably lessened if the fact of abuse or neglect is acknowledged. However, the parents should not be unduly pressured to explain the cause of injury. Instead, the emergency clinician may need to rely on some common clinical indicators associated with abuse and neglect (see Table 1).

The children of neglect are often harder to identify than the children of abuse. In severe abuse, there may be signs of physical injury: burns, bruises, welts, bites, or fractures. In chronic cases, it may be the repetitiveness or frequency of poorly explained injuries that indicates abuse. In neglect, however, there may be no overt signs; the child may appear listless, fatigued, and apathetic. Although not necessarily dramatically underweight, the child may nonetheless appear undernourished and pale, with dull eyes, skin, and hair. The clothing may be ill-fitting or inappropriate. It may be the total picture of the child, including affect and behavior, that signals neglect, not any one indicator.

Building a short-term therapeutic alliance with the child and his parents is the essence of effective emergency work with families who display destructive patterns. If no alliance can be made, not only is immediate crisis management threatened but the opportunity for longer-term resolution is reduced. Supportive, nonjudgmental interviewing techniques are essential. During the emergency visit, the child should be encouraged to talk in private, as should each of the parents. The interviewer should work on several levels at once by addressing practical issues, assessing the psychological status of both parent and child, identifying available supports and psychosocial stressors, discharging the charged emotional atmosphere through talk, and preparing the parent and family for future departmental action.

The ambivalent feelings of both parent and child should also be explored. Although the child may long for relief and the parent may long to be rid of his burden, both fear even a transient separation. Often both experience feelings of love and attachment along with anxiety, anger, and—in situations of neglect—apathy and helplessness. The clinician should convey that these feelings are valid and acceptable.

Emergency workers should assess the amount of stress on a family and their capacity to deal with that stress. To protect the child, the emergency worker must sometimes act quickly and decisively; he may, for example, need to do the following immediately:

1. File a report of suspected abuse or neglect and request an immediate response (in Massachusetts, within four hours). On nights and weekends this report should be filed through the hotline.
2. File a C & P. The court will bring the department in within 24 hours and may provide temporary custody in the interim.
3. Arrange for a child to be taken to the local emergency shelter.

Table 1. Physical and Behavioral Indicators of Child Abuse and Neglect[a]

Type of CA/N	Physical indicators	Behavioral indicators

Physical abuse	Unexplained bruises and welts
	  on face, lips, mouth
	  on torso, back, buttocks, thighs
	  in various stages of healing
	  clustered, forming regular
	    patterns like
	  articles used to inflict (e.g.,
	    electric cord, belt buckle)
	  on several different surface
	    areas
	  regularly appear after absence,
	    weekend or vacation
	
	Unexplained burns
	  cigar, cigarette burns, especially
	    on soles, palms, back, or
	    buttocks
	  immersion burns (socklike,
	    glovelike, doughnut-shaped on
	    buttocks or genitalia)
	  patterned like electric burner,
	    iron, etc.
	  rope burns on arms, legs, neck,
	    or torso
	  infected burns, indicating delay
	    in seeking treatment
	Unexplained fractures/dislocations
	  to skull, nose, facial structure
	  in various stages of healing
	  multiple or spiral fractures
	
	Unexplained lacerations or
	  to mouth, lips, gums, eyes
	  to external genitalia
	  in various stages of healing
	
	Bald patches on the scalp
		Feels deserving of punishment
		Wary of adult contacts
		Apprehensive when other children
		  cry
		Behavioral extremes:
		  aggressiveness or withdrawal
		Frightened of parents
		Afraid to go home
		Reports injury by parents
		Vacant or frozen stare
		Lies very still while surveying
		  surroundings
		Will not cry when approached by
		  examiner
		Responds to questions in
		  monosyllables
		Inappropriate or precocious
		  maturity
		Manipulative behavior to get
		  attention
		Capable of only superficial
		  relationships
		Indiscriminately seeks affection
		Poor self-concept

Physical neglect	Underweight, poor growth
	  pattern, failure to thrive
	Consistent hunger, poor hygiene,
	  inappropriate dress
	Consistent lack of supervision,
	  especially in dangerous
	  activities or long periods
	Wasting of subcutaneous tissue
	Unattended physical problems or
	  medical needs
	Abandonment
	Abdominal distention
	Bald patches on the scalp
		Begging, stealing food
		Extended stays at school (early
		  arrival and late departure)
		Rare attendance at school
		Constant fatigue, listlessness, or
		  falling asleep in class
		Inappropriate seeking of affection
		Assuming adult responsibilities
		  and concerns
		Alcohol or drug abuse
		Delinquency (e.g., thefts)
		States there is no caretaker

(Continued)

Table 1. (*Continued*)

Type of CA/N	Physical indicators	Behavioral indicators
Sexual abuse	Difficulty in walking or sitting Torn, stained, or bloody underclothing Pain, swelling, or itching in genital area Pain on urination Bruises, bleeding or lacerations in external genitalia, vaginal or anal areas Vaginal/penile discharge Venereal disease, especially in preteens Poor sphincter tone Pregnancy	Unwilling to change for gym or participate in physical education class Withdrawal, fantasy, or infantile behavior or knowledge Poor peer relationships Delinquent or runaway Reports sexual assault by caretaker Change in performance in school
Emotional maltreatment	Speech disorders Lag in physical development Failure to thrive Hyperactive/disruptive behavior	Habit disorders (sucking, biting, rocking, etc.) Conduct/learning disorders (antisocial, destructive, etc.) Neurotic traits (sleep disorders, inhibition of play, unusual fearfulness) Psychoneurotic reactions (hysteria, obsession, compulsion, phobias, hypochondria) Behavior extremes (compliant, passive; aggressive, demanding) Overly adaptive behavior (inappropriately adult, inappropriately infantile) Developmental lags (mental, emotional) Attempted suicide

[a] From Lauer et al.[10] (p. 10).

5. Follow-Up

After filing a report, the clinician should follow up on the treatment plan. He should see that the department has in fact made contact with the family. If he feels the department is making the wrong decisions, the clinician may choose to act as an advocate of the family. Alternatively, he can offer additional services to the family if they are consistent with the department's plan.

6. Summary

The role of emergency personnel is to identify possible abuse and neglect, report it to the proper agency, and provide immediate treatment for the child.

These tasks should be handled in a nonthreatening, supportive, empathic manner and should involve not only the child but the broader family unit. The clinician should help the parent (and the child) to see the report as a helpful act that can mobilize needed resources. The family should emerge from this contact with a sense of hope for the future and a concrete plan for the creation of a safer home for the child.

Bibliography

1. Bassett LB: How to help abused children and their parents. *RN Magazine* 37:2–8, 1974.
2. Brandt, RST: *Manual on Sexual Abuse and Misuse of Children.* Boston, New England Resource Center, Judge Baker Guidance Center, 1975.
3. *Child Abuse and Neglect: A Handbook.* Boston, Children's Advocates, 1979.
4. *Child Abuse and Neglect: The Problem and Its Management,* vols 1, 2, 3. Washington, US Department of Health, Education and Welfare, 1975.
5. Gil DG: *Violence Against Children: Physical Child Abuse in the United States.* Cambridge, Harvard University Press, 1973.
6. Helfer RE, Kempe CH (eds.): *Child Abuse and Neglect: The Family and the Community.* Cambridge, Ballinger, 1976.
7. Justice B, Justice R: *The Abusing Family.* New York, Human Sciences Press, 1976.
8. Kempe RS, and Kempe CH: *Child Abuse: The Developing Child.* Cambridge, Harvard University Press, 1978.
9. Kinard EM: Mental health needs of abused children. *Child Welfare* 59:451–462, 1980.
10. Lauer JW, Laurie IS, Salus MK, et al: *The Role of the Mental Health Professional in the Prevention and Treatment of Child Abuse and Neglect.* Washington, US Department of Health, Education and Welfare. National Center on Child Abuse and Neglect, 1979.
11. Martin HP (ed.): *The Abused Child: A Multidisciplinary Approach to Development Issues and Treatment.* Cambridge, Ballinger, 1976.
12. Newberger EH, Daniel JH: Knowledge and epidemiology of child abuse: A critical review of concepts. *Pediatr Ann* 5:140–144, 1976.
13. Schmitt SC (ed.): *The Child Protection Team Handbook: A Multidisciplinary Approach to Managing Child Abuse and Neglect.* New York, Garland Press, 1978.
14. Schmitt BD, et al: *Guidelines for the Hospital and Clinic Management of Child Abuse and Neglect.* Washington, US Department of Health, Education and Welfare. National Center on Child Abuse and Neglect, 1979.
15. Steitz SK, Straus MA: *Violence in the Family.* New York, Harper & Row, 1974.

VII

Patients and Clinical Syndromes 5
Special Populations

18

Psychiatric Emergencies in Children and Adolescents

Daniel W. Rosenn, M.D.

1. Introduction

According to recent estimates, at least 30% of the visits currently being made to hospital emergency rooms involve patients under the age of 18 years.[1] One such survey has shown that emergency room visits for minors increased by 127% from 1958 to 1968 compared to a less than 50% increase in overall services for the same period.[2] In the last decade, teenagers accounted for approximately 15% of all general hospital psychiatric emergencies. Although there is a corresponding trend toward increased drug dependence and abuse, adolescent emergencies comprise all diagnostic categories.[3,4]

Despite the increasing numbers of children and adolescents requiring emergency care, the development of these services has not kept pace with demand. In 1977, for example, only 43 of the 501 hospitals in the United States providing psychiatric services offered emergency services for adults, and of those, very few extended emergency psychiatric care to children and adolescents.[5] In a similar survey of outpatient treatment facilities for families, it was found that only 17% of the 314 clinics belonging to the Family Service Association of America provided child emergency services; of the remaining 143 clinics belonging to the American Association of Psychiatric Services for Children, over two-thirds did not offer child emergency services at all.[6] Although the Community Mental Health Centers Act of 1963 stipulated that emergency services were to be provided, as late as 1970 half of the federally assisted community mental health centers responding to survey questions reported that they were serving *no* children in crisis treatment.[7]

The problem of limited resources for the psychiatric emergency care of minors is considerable in its own right, but it is worsened in part by a deficient conceptual framework. Adults who regularly interface with children, such as physicians, nurses, teachers, clergy, police, and parents, have no standard approach for evaluating psychiatric emergencies involving children and preadults. Mental health professionals have agreed that life-threatening behaviors (suicidal and homicidal states) and psychotic decompensations represent true

Daniel W. Rosenn, M.D. • Harvard Medical School, Boston, Massachusetts 02215, and McLean Hospital, Belmont, Massachusetts 02178.

emergencies, but the list has now been expanded to include school phobias, firesetting, running away, and other crisis states.

In general, a childhood psychiatric emergency involves far more than a child's symptoms. The foundation for an emergency situation is laid when a child abruptly loses the ability to use adaptive skills, inner restraints, or appropriate behavior, and is further compounded when, as Morrison and Smith have stated, "the significant adults around the child can no longer help him master his anxiety and can no longer provide temporary ego support and controls."[8] (p. 17). In addition, the community has traditionally reserved the right to define and manage situations that it regards as harmful or dangerous to children, even when it means overriding the judgment and/or perceptions of the children and parents involved.

For practical purposes, any urgent request for help from child, parent, teacher, welfare worker, pediatric ward nurse, fire department personnel, or court officer should be considered an emergency. A high level of fearfulness, disorganization, or helplessness in a child, or the abrupt onset of bizarre, inappropriate, or unusual symptoms should also warrant immediate attention. And any change in the child's environment that might threaten his safey or well-being should be considered a potential crisis.

2. Description of Childhood Psychiatric Emergencies

Currently, there are very few broad clinical surveys that describe childhood psychiatric emergencies. Most studies have tended to collate the experience of a single facility, thus introducing a demographic bias. For example, urban general hospitals report a disproportionately high number of adolescents with drug intoxications or dyscontrol reactions. Child clinics affiliated with social service departments may see a large number of abuse or neglect cases on an emergency basis preparatory to foster-home placement. In spite of the inherent bias in these clinical surveys, however, it is generally agreed that the two most common categories of child and adolescent emergencies are suicidal or marked depressive behavior and assaultive or other antisocial behaviors. Other types of emergencies reported include mood disturbances with and without somatic correlates, psychotic symptoms, school refusal, and running away.[9–12] In addition, these studies tend to confirm that girls generally are seen more frequently for emergency consultation than boys by a ratio of 3 to 2. This ratio reflects the marked surge in suicidal behavior among girls at around age 14. Otherwise, there is a relative preponderance of suicidal behavior among latency-age males over their female counterparts, which accounts for preadolescent boys appearing for emergency consultation three times more frequently than preadolescent girls.

3. General Considerations

Evaluating and managing preadult psychiatric emergencies have certain inherent difficulties. The majority of childhood psychiatric emergencies are generally managed either by pediatricians or by pediatric emergency facilities,[13] but a small proportion are seen first in the traditional emergency unit. In the latter case, the front-line emergency staff must often rely on consultation with child specialists.

Dispositions in childhood emergencies are time-consuming and cumbersome, since they may involve the entire social network of the patient. Diagnoses and formulations are problematic; presenting symptoms overlap many diagnostic categories, and traditional classification may have no treatment value. "Hyperaggressive behavior" in a 10-year-old may indicate depression, anxiety, impulse-control disorder, or incipient psychosis. The chief complaint may not come directly from the child at all but may involve complicated interactional patterns within the child's social system. If there are definite psychiatric symptoms, they may represent a primary disorder or they may be entirely situation-specific, or they may be secondary to a medical condition; severity and type of symptoms manifested by a child are not necessarily reliable indicators of etiology or outcome. In short, the urgency of the typical childhood crisis makes rapid, accurate assessment and effective management a very difficult clinical task.

Assessment within the rushed, pressured emergency setting requires a structured approach to problem-formulation. The task is to figure out *what* the problem is, *who* has it, *whether* it is treatable, and *how* it is best treated. Since almost all children have episodic symptoms, the emergency evaluator must assess the overall dimensions of the symptoms, and the role they play within the child's personal life and his interpersonal connections:

> *Abnormality*—How different is this behavior or symptom from the child's usual baseline of behavior and from typical patterns among children of the same age, race, gender, culture, and class?
>
> *Impairment*—How much suffering, social constraint, or handicap does the symptom present to the child and his family?
>
> *Threat*—How dangerous is the behavior or symptom for the child and for his family or environment, and for his ongoing emotional well-being?

To answer these questions, the clinician needs to employ a developmental approach to child assessment, that is, to measure the emergency patient's particular symptoms or behaviors against the phase-specific concerns and patterns of other children at the same developmental stage. Pruett, for example, describes the emergency referral of two young siblings who had witnessed the shotgun murder of their mother by their father.[14] To understand, and thereafter to resolve, the traumatic experience from the children's perspective, it was necessary to determine the phase-related preoccupations that colored the children's perception and understanding of their mother's death. This kind of developmental perspective is the cornerstone of child evaluation.

Although the mechanics of managing an adolescent psychiatric emergency may resemble those used with adults, adolescent emergencies must be regarded as a class in their own right, dependent on, and related to, the specific features of the adolescent's developmental stage. Techniques for engaging the adolescent patient, evaluting the symptoms, and formulating treatment strategies are particular to this population, although they may be borrowed from the clinician's work with children to some extent and may overlap with techniques employed for adult emergencies as well.

4. The Emergency Intervention

The hospital emergency room is not an easy setting for an upset child or his family. During the waiting time, the family should be encouraged to prepare the child for the interview, and may be made more comfortable by being placed in an empty treatment room or visiting area.

The order and grouping of persons to be interviewed is generally controversial, but it can be resolved by using three criteria: the severity or dangerousness of the patient's symptoms, the age of the patient, and the information potential of persons accompanying him. It is vitally important that no youngster who is confused, suicidal, violent, or likely to run away be left unattended. Similarly, the age of the child may preclude separation from his parents. A preschooler, for example, should not be separated from both parents during the early phases of the emergency evaluation except in cases of failure to thrive, suspected child abuse, or where the patient could be traumatized by significant information from the parents or accompanying adults. Finally, if the child is brought to the emergency room by a welfare worker, policeman, neighbor, or teenage peers, it may be practical to talk with these persons before interviewing the patient. These cautionary notes notwithstanding, it is a general rule of thumb to obtain information and initial impressions from the triage nurse, intake aide, or clinic receptionist first. Next, the child and the parents should be interviewed together. Family members and/or the preschool patient can be interviewed separately as the evaluation proceeds, depending on the clinician's sense of unacknowledged trouble in the parent–child relationship. It is appropriate to begin the interview with latency-age children and parents together, and then to see the child and parents separately. It may be necessary to see the adolescent without his parents initially in order to diminish his phase-related suspiciousness and to establish an alliance with him independent of his parents. The patient's parents can be seen separately or can be asked to join the patient during his interview. Diagnostic sessions that put the patient and some or all of his family members together are extremely revealing and may provide explanatory clues to the patient's symptomatic behavior.

4.1. Interviewing Techniques

Because there are so many excellent books and papers that describe evaluation and history-taking in child psychiatry,[15–19] only a few general guidelines will be presented: It is best to structure the expectations of patient and parents positively, but realistically. The child should be addressed on his own level. He should be told what kind of doctor he is seeing, and the interview should be structured to encourage the child's expression of feelings, preoccupations, and concerns rather than facts and historical details. Parents or other accompanying adults can ordinarily supply information about history and presenting symptoms.

4.2. Using Play

If a child is communicating well verbally, it may be superfluous to play with him. For younger children and uncommunicative school-age youngsters, however, it is often useful to introduce toys during the evaluation. The clinician's collection of toys can be highly personal and individualistic, and need not include elaborate, expensive, or numerous items. For children 8 years and younger, an adequate set of diagnostic playthings would include a small doll house with some furniture (beds and a toilet are key items) and a set of little family dolls; a bit of plasticene; crayons; a doctor kit; a large rubber doll; and a scary rubber animal whose mouth opens, like an alligator or a shark. For children a little older, a few army men or space invaders, some "matchbox" cars, and a small, three-dimensional puzzle will be enough. Preadolescents and teenagers are usually offended by being offered toys. Sharing a soda or a candy bar may diminish anxiety more effectively than play.

Play is of undeniable diagnostic value, but it can have powerful therapeutic efficacy as well. The following vignette provides a graphic illustration:

> A 3-year-old girl was brought to the ER at 6:00 p.m. She had just been bitten on the right leg and left hand by a neighbor's dog. Her wounds were washed and dressed. The child received a tetanus shot and a lollipop. She whimpered throughout the procedures and seemed somewhat dazed. She was sent home with aspirin and diphenhydramine (benadryl) for sleep. The mother called the ER at 1:15 a.m. The child had fallen into a deep sleep for a few hours but had awakened screaming. She seemed terror-stricken and kept shouting "no, no!" A sympathetic ER nurse advised the mother to take the child into her bed, reassure her that she was safe, and "get her to talk about what had happened." The mother called back 1½ hours later. Her efforts to get the child to talk seemed to increase her terror. At 7:00 a.m. the mother and child once more appeared in the ER, equally frantic. They were seen together immediately. The clinician then invited the child to play with some toys. The child was uninterested in the toy doctor's bag and the Band-Aid box, but soon took the rubber alligator and the family dolls. She played out the same drama over and over. Each time, she had the alligator attack the family dolls. She would then hit the alligator, kick it, throw it against the wall, and finally put it outside the door. After a few seconds, she would retrieve the alligator from the hall and repeat the whole sequence again. The clinician watched quietly and occasionally uttered a phrase or two such as, "She's so mad at the alligator," "She would like to throw him away," "She's really hurting him back," and "That will teach that animal." The child would nod excitedly after each comment. The mother just watched. After about 25 minutes, the child's activity level

dropped off, she smiled at the resident, yawned a few times, put her head in her mother's lap, and promptly fell asleep.

4.3. Administering the Mental Status Examination (MSE)

The formal organization of the mental status examination for children is similar to that for adult patients: general appearance (clothing, hygiene), speech, affect and mood, thought content and flow, judgment, insight into problems (capacity to accept responsibility for some part of the difficulty, or propensity to project and externalize blame), cognitive and physical development, relationship with parents, peers, school, and examiner, and ability to play and fantasize. Techniques for children are different than for adults, however; subtracting serial threes, for example, is an abstract operation appropriate for assessing adult functioning but is not necessarily appropriate for children. To evaluate attention span and other functions, the clinician should adapt to the twists and turns of the session:

EXAMINER: You were just telling me about your brothers and sister; how old are they all?
CHILD: Mary is 18 and John is 13 . . . uh, I think Peter's gonna be 11.
E: Hmmm. Mary is pretty old. How many years older than John do you think she is?
C: I guess she's 6 years older.
E: Yup. She's really a lot older than Peter, since he's only 11. Let's see, 11 from 18 works out to be . . .
C: Seven.

Similarly, orientation to time and place can be evaluated by discussing the scheduling of favorite TV shows. Short-term memory tests can be built into games that are part of the normal flow of the interview. Hallucinations and delusions are difficult to assess in children because of the fuzzy boundaries between reality and fantasy, but direct questions can help.

CHILD: My Raggedy Ann told me not to go to sleep.
EXAMINER: Do you *really* believe a doll can talk?
CHILD: Well, maybe it didn't *actually* say it, but still, I'm not going to go to sleep tonight.

Communicating effectively with a child does not require adopting childish characteristics like exaggerating facial expressions or using particularly infantile phrasing. It does mean adapting the adult presence to the specific developmental age and personality of the child. The structured protocol of the MSE should give way to a spontaneous, free-flowing process of data collection whose product can be formally reorganized later.

4.4. Clarifying the Problem for the Family

As the clinician develops a working hypothesis of the case, he should begin to convey a selected portion of his findings to the family. It may be helpful to start with a brief review of the family's account, with affects labeled and pertinent information placed in causal sequence. The clinician might then offer his view of the crisis in plain, nontechnical language. The following is an example of such a review based on an initial 50-minute interview:

EVALUATOR: I'm glad you finally decided to come in for help today. I know it hasn't been easy talking about these things, but you've really been quite good at giving me a picture of what things have been like. It sounds like Jimmy had been doing well until a few months ago when you and your husband split up. He was mixed up and scared. He began to wet the bed and act like a younger child than 8 years old. And then he began to steal things from your house and the drugstore. Spanking him didn't help. You've been pretty upset and lonely yourself and you told me you haven't had a lot left over emotionally to give to the kids. Yesterday, when the principal called and said Jimmy took his teacher's wallet almost in front of her nose, it was the last straw. It sounds like you have got to your wits' end with him and you wonder if he's going to grow up to be a criminal.

In cases where the emergency interview lasts for more than an hour, it is customary to let the family take a brief break. Later, the family should be asked to discuss their reactions. The response contains vital information about the family's ability to understand and accept the previous explanations, and their readiness to follow recommendations for further treatment.

4.5. Planning a Disposition

The goal of the emergency intervention is not to do an exhaustive diagnostic assessment, to develop a complete formulation of the case, or to effect change within the family system. It is instead to gather enough information about the status of patient and family to ameliorate the immediate distress effectively and to plan for further definitive treatment. The following are possible disposition alternatives:

- Commit to a locked psychiatric facility.
- Arrange voluntary commitment to psychiatric hospital or pediatric ward.
- Refer for immediate medical treatment (e.g., in cases of rape, child abuse, delirium).
- Extend the evaluation in the emergency setting.
- Refer to outpatient department, private psychiatrist or facility, or crisis clinic.
- Treat and discharge at the end of the emergency session.

The need for hospitalization and/or medical referral is discussed later in this chapter. For those children who are referred to a clinic, the clinician should remember that the compliance rate for referrals from an emergency setting is less than 50% and is even lower for adolescents. The method of referral is therefore critical; parents should be given the name of the outside clinic and therapist and a definite appointment time. Later, the emergency room interviewer should call to see if the appointment has been kept.

4.6. Summary

In short, an effective intervention for children must include at least[11] (1) prompt diagnostic evaluation of the child and his family; (2) clarification of the factors that provoked the crisis; (3) active involvement of the parents in a treatment plan to alleviate the child's distress and to give him adequate protection, ego support, and external control; (4) referral to an appropriate inpatient setting for the children who require admission; referral to other clinicial facilities for children who need continued study and short-term therapy; (5) collaboration with community agencies, clinics, and/or schools that have responsibility for the child.

5. Classification of Psychiatric Emergencies in Childhood and Adolescence

Table 1 is not an exhaustive list of all childhood and adolescent disorders that might present as a psychiatric emergency. Indeed, given the right combination of precipitating conditions, almost any set of psychological symptoms can erupt with crisis proportions. The scheme in Table 1 groups the most prominent childhood symptoms according to the need for immediate, urgent, or prompt diagnostic action, respectively.

Class I emergencies require immediate assessment. If there are organic signs with the psychiatric symptoms, e.g., disorientation, fever, stiff neck, or extreme lassitude, immediate pediatric consultation is essential. The psychiatric clinician should communicate directly with the pediatrician, particularly when the presenting symptoms include confusional states, rage reactions, or suspected child abuse. In the absence of clear organic signs, the clinician must arrange for the child's protection as soon as possible. Those situations that involve the potential for serious injury to the child as the indirect result of his own actions should be considered Class I emergencies. For example, in some cases of run-away behavior, where the likelihood of prostitution or deliquency is clear-cut, the clinician may need to utilize police or hospital security force and arrange for appropriate temporary legal guardianship to contain an otherwise unmanageable and unsafe adolescent (see Chapter 3).

Class II situations, although not requiring immediate attention, do cause considerable distress and may therefore necessitate prompt action. Families with Class II crises should be seen within 24 to 36 hours of application, or sooner if the distress becomes too severe.

Class III crises can usually be scheduled for evaluation within a few days of the referral, depending on the amount of disturbance or anxiety within the family.

The classification scheme in Table 1 includes symptoms and conditions of childhood and adolescence that are considered genuine psychiatric emergencies, on the one hand, and pseudoemergencies, on the other. There are, in addition, other situations that arise within the child's domestic framework that

Table 1. Classification of Psychiatric Emergencies in Childhood and Adolescence

Class I. Potentially life-threatening emergencies
  A. With immediate risk to the child
    1. Suicidal behavior
    2. Self-destructive acts: refusal to take insulin in the juvenile diabetic, severe starvation in anorexia nervosa, repeated removal of IV line in the hospitalized child, etc.
    3. Physically abusive behavior by parents or caretakers
    4. Extreme neglect by parents or caretakers
    5. Acute confusional states, e.g., acute psychotic reactions, toxic (or other organic) confusional states leading to loss of ability to behave safely
    6. Certain runaway reactions (see text)
  B. With immediate risk to others
    1. Acutely violent states, e.g., rage reactions, episodic dyscontrol conditions, psychotic agitation, panic states (including homosexual panic)
    2. Hyperaggressive behavior, e.g., intentional homicidal behavior accompanying severe character and impulse control disorders, particularly when a helpless victim such as a younger sibling or aged grandparent is involved
    3. Firesetting
Class II. States of heightened disturbance requiring urgent intervention
    1. Rape or traumatic sexual abuse
    2. Being victim of, or witness to, a horrifying event, e.g., assault/murder, kidnapping, car crash, natural disaster
    3. Death of parent or sibling
    4. Severe anxiety attacks of whatever cause
    5. Recently disclosed incest
    6. Witnessing a potentially overstimulating event, e.g., sexual deviation
    7. Debilitating conversion reactions and group hysteria
    8. Interference by parents in the medical treatment of a seriously ill child, e.g., threatening to sign out a hospitalized child, hindering ward management of a hospitalized child
Class III. Serious conditions requiring prompt but not necessarily immediate intervention
    1. School refusal
    2. Crises in the lives of parents that
      a. remove them emotionally from the child, e.g., acute parental depression following the birth of a defective child, or
      b. bring into question their ability to care for the child, e.g., acute medical or psychiatric illness
    3. Impending hospitalization for which the child has not been prepared, especially if it involves surgery and invasive procedures
    4. Impending divorce or marital separation for which the child has not been prepared
Class IV. Pseudoemergencies (situations in which intervention is demanded but not medically warranted)
    1. Ignorance of proper mental health channels
    2. Parents attempting to punish or frighten child for misbehavior
    3. Interagency struggle, e.g., between school and welfare department over case disposition
    4. Effort by parents or lawyer to relabel criminal activity as a "psychiatric disorder" to avoid or alter legal consequences
    5. Long-standing, chronic antisocial behavior that caretaker or school decides finally to address, e.g., breaking "one too many windows"
    6. Frustration of mental health consumers (parents, school, community agency) with an inefficient, overburdened child guidance clinic, e.g., 6-week waiting period in a community clinic where there are no alternative resources
    7. Wish for a (favorable) second opinion by angry parents who have just received an unwelcome psychiatric diagnosis from a private physician or clinic
    8. Request for an "emergency" psychiatric consultation from a pediatric ward officer after the medical evaluation is completed and the patient is ready for discharge
    9. Wish to transform a psychosocial crisis into a medical emergency by using a general hospital emergency room instead of a mental health facility, because suspicion, shame, or fear militate against acknowledging that a crisis is psychiatric, and not strictly medical.

catapult the child directly into the Class I emergency. For example, an acutely intoxicated or psychotically confused parent who appears at a medical clinic with dependent children jeopardizes the safety of the children. Unless voluntary arrangements can be made for the children through other family members, the hospital lawyer may need to obtain a temporary restraining order from the court preventing the impaired parent from taking the children.

Similar situations arise when the caretaking abilities of parents are compromised by specific crises: terminal medical illness, major depression, or marital disturbance. If the parents' physician or therapist considers the implications of the parental crisis for the children, an early referral can be made to a family guidance clinic, in-hospital, or community-based social service department before the child becomes symptomatic.

There is no rigid stratification within the classes of Table 1. Just as suicidal behavior is susceptible to gradations in severity, so are childhood reactions to stress or hospitalization. In general, Table 1 serves as a guide for assessing urgency, but it should be used in combination with the following two criteria: the inherent pathogenicity of the precipitant, and the degree of reactive distress experienced by the child and/or parent.

The inherent pathogenicity of the traumatic precipitant may not be directly measured by the appearance of symptoms in the child. Even in the absence of symptoms, any particularly violent, unanticipated, grotesque, or overstimulating event involving the child as participant or witness should be taken very seriously. Childhood defenses of denial, repression, and reaction formation consolidate quickly, so that emergency evaluation should take place as soon as possible to forestall premature encapsulation of traumatic experiences. The emergency intervention may require only one or two sessions. For planned, but unavoidable, traumas such as hospitalization involving surgical or dental procedures in young children, preparation is absolutely essential. Many hospitals anticipate the emotional turmoil and offer preadmission programs designed to help children and their parents master the hospital experience.

The degree of reactive upset experienced by the child and/or parent is a second guide to the urgency of a childhood crisis. Patients with anxiety states involving panic or extreme agitation should be seen without delay.

> A 10-year-old girl saw a movie in which one of the characters dies in agony of botulism. Within hours, the child developed a full-blown food phobia and would take only liquid nourishment. The following day she became panic-stricken that her parents might eat contaminated food. She was seen that afternoon and on each of the next three days by the same member of the crisis team of a university hospital's child psychiatric unit. Her anxiety gradually abated and she successfully completed an eight-session course of short-term psychotherapy.

Not all severe reactive upsets manifest as conspicuous or dramatic psychological states. For example, in quiet, withdrawn children, strong emotions such as guilt or shame may present with few overt signs. Detection may be more difficult, but the symptoms are no less serious for the child.

Thomas, a 9-year-old studious, conscientious altar boy, was discovered by his mother in homosexual play with a neighbor's young child. Thomas cried only briefly when confronted by his parents, and stayed in his bedroom the rest of the day working on his stamp collection. He was polite but distant with his father and refused dinner, saying he wasn't hungry. His parents discovered him the next morning in the bathroom in the process of swallowing aspirins.

Intake workers, mental health professionals, and other clinical figures in the child's social network must be sensitive to covert emergencies in the first three classes. Not only can relatively ordinary childhood symptoms become critical in a short period of time, but genuinely urgent situations can be missed, deliberately minimized, or unconsciously denied by parents, caretakers, or other adults in child-custodial roles.

Class IV situations are neither overt nor covert emergencies. At times, a parent who utilizes the emergency room for other routine medical services may bring in a child with a nonurgent emotional problem. In other cases, families who have received excellent emergency care for true psychiatric emergencies may resort to the same service for less urgent matters. Occasionally, families use the emergency room to prove a point, or to dramatize a "crisis."

A middle-aged accountant and his wife came to the ER Sunday morning at 9:00 a.m. with their 15-year-old daughter meekly following behind. They had discovered her smoking marijuana in her bedroom. The father angrily demanded that "some doctor impress her with how this stuff can rot her brain and that she ought to know better." The clinician spoke to the three for 30 minutes, allowing the parents to ventilate their anger and anxiety. He acknowledged that the three of them had a problem with communication, and that they could be helped in outpatient family therapy. The family agreed, although the daughter did so reluctantly. Follow-up contact indicated that they had kept the appointment.

Whatever the motivation underlying the use of emergency room services for nonurgent situations, it is important to bear in mind that there is stress or pressure in at least some segment of the child's life. The "emergency" cannot be dismissed by the interviewer, but should be evaluated and clarified for the family. If necessary, a more appropriate placement can be recommended. Although the rate of compliance in these cases is low, it can be increased by careful family management during the emergency intervention, and by attentive follow-up efforts.

6. The Specific Syndromes

What follows is a discussion of some specific clinical syndromes classified in Table 1. In Table 1 these syndromes were organized hierarchically: that is, according to their potential to threaten the life, safety, or well-being of the child and/or others. To fit this classificatory scheme, each syndrome was lifted from its etiological base, its demographic roots, and its diagnostic labels and was evaluated solely from the standpoint of risk potential. In truth, however, each syndrome has its own intrinsic symptom spectrum from mild to severe, and each covers a multiplicity of pathogenic and etiologic factors. The discussions that follow amplify the points condensed in the framework of Table 1.

7. Suicidal Behaviors in Children and Adolescents*

7.1. Introduction

Suicidal behavior accounts for approximately 30 to 40% of all acute emergency referrals among children and adolescents today.[20] Approximately one million or more American children develop suicidal crises, behaviors, and preoccupations every year, according to the Institute for Destructive Behavior. Clearly, therefore, suicidal behavior among children and adolescents must be reckoned as a serious psychiatric condition, not only from the standpoint of its potential risk but as a reflection of profound emotional turbulence in the preadult population generally.[21-29]

7.2. Suicidal Behavior in Preschool Children

The incidence of suicidal activity in the 6-and-under age group is quite low; that is not to say, however, that suicidal behavior is nonexistent.[30-35] At the Beth Israel Hospital clinic, for example, several preschoolers were treated over the past few years for clear suicidal symptoms. Two children (ages 4 and 5) tried to jump from windows, and one (age 6) intentionally darted into traffic and later tried to strangle himself. A fourth, a 5-year-old boy, attempted to use his life-threatening allergic reaction to chocolate as a suicidal bargaining point. The boy had hidden a Hershey bar with the intention of locking himself in the bathroom and eating it unless his divorcing parents stopped fighting. To demonstrate his resolve, he had on one occasion deliberately licked the chocolate bar, developing a mild periorbital and buccal edema.

Life-threatening behaviors are not uncommon among very young children. Many youngsters are "accident-prone"; as very small children, they crawl on ledges or dart into traffic; they are fascinated by flames, sharp-pointed objects, and household chemicals, exploring many of these with their hands and mouths despite otherwise disagreeable taste, texture, or toxic consequences. Many of these youngsters gradually develop responsibility for their own body management, but for a small subgroup, the early propensity for self-destructive acts evolves and escalates as the child matures.

* This section is condensed from material by Daniel Rosenn: *Lifelines: Clinical Perspectives on Suicide.* Suicide in children and adolescents, in Bassuk EL, Schoonover SC, Gill A (eds.): New York, Plenum Press, 1982.

It is not always easy to distinguish between the influence of intrinsic genetic or constitutional factors and environmental factors in the evolution of self-destructive behavior. It is safe to say, however, that in almost every case of childhood suicidal activity the home environment is troubled. That is not to say that environment is a necessary cause of childhood suicidal behavior, only that it is a strong, perhaps universal correlate. The distressed, chaotic homes of some suicidal children are often characterized by unpredictability and inconsistency; they are often the scene of violent hatred, and not infrequently of actual child abuse. Self-destructive behavior such as hair-picking, skin excoriation, and self-burning are not unusual, and appear to occur in response to excessive corporal punishment. Green has suggested that these children may come to regard themselves with the same hostility as their parents, thus forming the nucleus of a "bad" self-image.[36]

Despite rejecting, ambivalent caretaking, many of these suicidal children are intensely attached to their mothers and experience severe anxiety at times of separation. Some clinicians have suggested that there is a splitting of the internalized maternal object: The actual mother is regarded as good, while the child sees himself as bad, worthy of punishment.[31,37–41] As Margolin succinctly puts it, "the young child would rather feel bad and be taken care of by the 'good' mother than feel good and be taken care of by a 'bad' mother.[40] (p. 312). The world external to the child remains benign and safe in the child's belief system if the mother's essential goodness can be maintained.

Because some youngsters identify with unconscious or conscious punitive wishes of parent(s), they may feel driven to carry out these subtly communicated urges. A depressed and delinquent 9-year-old, for example, tried to strangle himself at the beginning of the school year and was hospitalized. For Christmas, only a few months later, his family gave him the board game "Hangman." In a similar case, a premed college student who had taken several overdoses of low lethality was given the Physicians Desk Reference (PDR) by his father as a birthday gift, "so he could learn the ins and outs of medications before getting to medical school."

7.3. Suicidal Behavior in Latency

In general, childhood and adolescent suicidal behavior has been treated as a single topic, indeed a single phenomenon, and since the completed suicide rates for preadolescents are low (153 reported deaths in 1978 between ages 5 and 14), it has been the custom to dismiss the preadolescent group and focus on adolescents. In fact, however, clinical experience and several recent surveys[42–44] suggest that suicidal preoccupation/ideation in preadolescence is higher than one would expect from the numbers of completed suicides alone. At the Beth Israel Child Psychiatry Clinic between 1979 and 1981, for example, 9% of all latency-age children at the time of intake presented with an actual attempt or clear suicidal ideation. Add to these data the number of patients who disclosed suicidal thoughts during the course of treatment, and the figures begin to approach those published in several recent studies which indicate that as many as 33% of latency-age children in an outpatient psychiatry clinic had suicidal symptoms.[45] Given the low suicide completion rate in latency, it is obvious that intent and lethality of attempts or gestures are low also. They do not remain low, however; long-standing suicidal preoccupation and depression in latency-age children may continue into adolescence or adulthood, when repeated attempts are made.[46–48] In a report of 31 completed suicides in children between the ages of 13 and 14 in England and Wales, 46% had previously displayed suicidal behaviors.[49] Children with untreated depression and suicidal preoccupations may form the subgroup of suicidal adolescents and adults who are at highest risk.

7.4. Depression in Childhood and Adolescence

Not all childhood or adolescent suicidal behavior is correlated with depression, nor is childhood or adolescent depression defined by clearly recognizable signs and symptoms. DSM III and other recent studies have attempted to elucidate diagnostic criteria from a phenomenological standpoint.[50–54] At the basis of this approach is the recognition that childhood depression is not a monolithic entity, but undergoes its own characteristic development from one stage of childhood to the next. Depressive symptoms are parallel to, and interwoven with, corresponding developmental phases, and are thus influenced by age-related advances in symbolic representation, language, and cognitive operations.[55] The conceptualization of childhood depression, therefore, has shifted from focus on broadly applicable symptom sets to distinctive epigenetic states. Mood, the central locus and determinant of childhood depression, is profoundly influenced by cognitive and affective characteristics at various developmental stages.[58] The evolution of depressive symptomatology can be structured theoretically as follows: the physiologically generated states of dysphoria in newborns; despondency secondary to unmet anaclitic needs in infancy; withdrawal and misery in reaction to deprivation or object loss in early childhood; a sense of chronic, but realistic, sadness in children whose environments are narcissistically unsatisfying; and finally, feelings of internally generated self-deprecation not directly related to external events. The latter stage appears to be an early or rudimentary version of pathological depression and despair in adults.

Not all suicidal children exhibit recognizable depressive symptoms whose core is an expressed or experienced mood disturbance. Some children display what have been called "childhood depressive equivalents."[57,58] These "equivalent" symptoms include hyperaggressive and antisocial activity, school refusal, truancy, and lack of academic motivation. Although they are referred to as "depressive" equivalents when they are linked with suicidal preoccupation and/or behavior, they are not strictly and exclusively indicative of childhood depression. When suicidal latency-age children were compared with a carefully matched control group of nonsuicidal, psychiatrically disturbed children, no significant difference could be found between the groups with respect to the incidence of stealing, firesetting, running away, sleep disturbances, or other hyperaggressive reactions.[59] The emergency clinician should, nonetheless, be alert to the possibility that the symptom constellation described above does represent a depressive disorder with suicidal potential.

Diagnostic distinctions are not easy to make in the assessment of symptomatic children and adolescents; awareness of the distinctions among childhood psychiatric disturbances is critical to emergency assessment, however. One such distinction is between acute, reactive depression and chronic characterological depression. When a child presents with severe withdrawal, it is important to differentiate between depressive withdrawal as an acute or episodic reaction and schizoid withdrawal as a chronic and characterological stance. In the latter case, there is usually a retreat not only from social situations but from reality itself; the fantasies of these children are commonly bizarre and idiosyncratic.[60] In depressed, suicidal children the most common fantasies and feelings are being unloved, unwanted, and discarded. These go well beyond ordinary latency-age fantasies about adoption and substitute families. The following example is illustrative:

> A sad and lonely 7-year-old was asked during an acute psychiatric evaluation to draw a picture of his family. He spent 20 minutes laboring over his house and detailing his father, mother, and sister. He failed to draw himself. When asked if anyone was missing from this family, he thought for a few moments, then all at once brightened and drew his cat. When it was finally suggested that he had left himself out, he desultorily began drawing a figure of a boy, but soon lapsed into apathy. Finally, he put his crayon down, leaving an unfinished, nondescript figure.

This case highlights a by-product of the depressed child's perception of himself as neglected and unwanted: namely, a deep involvement with pets or other potential sources of affection. When asked to whom they feel closest, many of these suicidally depressed children give the name of a pet, a television or movie idol, God, a particular saint, or even a deceased relative.

7.5. The Child's View of Death

The argument that "suicidal behavior" is not a correct label for the self-destructive activity of children is based on the idea that they do not comprehend the finality of death sufficiently to choose it as a primary consequence of their actions. While it is true that death is incompletely understood by children, there is no practical relevance or benefit in calling "suicidal behavior" an incorrect label for a child's self-destructive acts. Children can and do die as a result of their own deliberate actions; whether or not they intend to die is not the primary or exclusive determinant of lethality.

The child's conception of death changes and evolves as he ages. Before age 5 or 6, the child tends to see death as reversible and temporary, translatable into understandable states like sleeping or playing possum. Between ages 5 and 7, a cognitive shift occurs with respect to causal relations, and the idea of death is correspondingly refined. Disappearance from life, removal to a final place, and being seen no more are attributes of death that seem to arise quite spontaneously in latency-age children regardless of religious training or conviction. In a classic study of 378 normal preadolescents, Nagy found that most latency age children personified death in some way.[61] While to some it was Evil, to many—perhaps for age-appropriate defensive reasons—death was perceived as Good, congruent with a peaceful and pleasant Heaven. Many investigators see the typical childhood tendency to romanticize or idealize death as potentiating suicidal ideation.[58,62–64] The disturbed child may view death as a return to a conflict-free state, a reunion with a lost parent or relative, a way of recovering a fulfilling, satisfying existence, or a method for inducing sorrow, grief, and remorse in the "surviving" family members. Ackerly has termed the propensity for latency-age suicidal children to regard death as a route to a glorious rebirth the "phoenix myth."[31]

Not infrequently, ambivalent suicidal behavior in both adults and preadults has at its affective and cognitive core a realistic or age-appropriate comprehension of death interwoven with, and offset by, a magical belief in the person's immortality.

> A 19-year-old college sophomore was seen in our hospital emergency room after overdosing on a tricyclic antidepressant. Despite the fact that she said she took an antiemetic immediately prior to the overdose to increase the lethality of the attempt, she later admitted after emerging from coma that "I knew I would not really die. My body is stronger than the medications."

In the face of the elaborate intrapsychic defenses commonly erected against the fear of death by children and adults alike, the intellectual capacity to understand its finality seems of relatively small moment in the suicidal process. What is clear and highly relevant, however, is that suicidal children are more preoccupied with thoughts of death and dying than are either healthy children or psychiatrically disturbed nonsuicidal children. Suicidal children spend considerably more time contemplating death and fantasizing about doom and destruction than their counterparts.[59] Moreover, both mothers and fathers of hospitalized suicidal preteenagers have been shown to have significantly more self-destructive ideation than parents of psychiatrically hospitalized nonsuicidal controls. It is also common to find the presence of suicidal behavior or preoccupation with death in siblings and extended family of self-destructive children.[29,32,65]

Suicidal male preadolescents appear to have more serious psychopathology, their attempts tend to be more lethal, and their completion rates are higher than those for preadolescent females. Jumping from heights seems to be the most common latency-age suicidal behavior, followed by running into traffic, ingestion of toxic substances, and hanging.

The immediate precipitants of suicidal behavior in preadolescents can be a catastrophic event, such as the death or loss of a parent, events that form part of an intolerable, but chronic pattern, or seemingly inconsequential events that are profoundly significant to the child such as parental rebuke, mild disciplinary action, or poor grades. The identification of precipitants has led to the overgeneralization that suicide in children and adolescents is either impulsive or the result of an overwhelming recent event. In fact, however, most latency and adolescent suicidal activity occurs in the context of long-standing family and intrapsychic conflicts; without those predisposing conditions, even overwhelming events are unlikely to trigger a suicidal episode.

7.6. Suicidal Behavior in Adolescents

The incidence of suicidal activity shows a sharp increase for young adults between ages 12 and 14, and a logarithmic increase throughout the remaining teenage years. There is undoubtedly a significant correlation between these data and the fact that psychological issues shift abruptly with the onset of puberty, making the early adolescent years turbulent and confusing. Nevertheless, there has been no satisfactory explanation for the correlation. A few of the many simplistic theories in current usage are as follows:

1. *Adolescents are supervised less than children.* The fact is that supervision *per se* does not seem related to diminished suicidal behavior. Many adolescents and children make their attempts in close physical proximity to parents or caretakers. In early latency, a typical suicidal attempt is for the child to drop his mother's hand and dart into a busy street. Jacobziner found that the mother was present physically in approximately 30% of 294 teenage suicidal ingestions.[25] Lack of supervision is important primarily when it reflects the emotional absence or lack of investment on the part of the parent.

2. *A corollary idea is that suicidal behaviors increase during adolescence as young people leave the safety of the home.* The majority of adolescent (and childhood) attempts in fact occur in or very near the home.[23] Although the parent may not be present at the time of the attempt, the return of the family member is often anticipated for rescue or remorseful discovery.

3. *Adolescents have more means available to kill themselves than children.* Thirty percent of adolescent attempts are by ingestion of pills: Aspirin and tranquilizers are preferred and are usually obtained from the home medicine cabinet. During the past decade, adolescents have increasingly used firearms and street drugs, notably narcotics and barbiturates, for self-destructive purposes. Again, these are generally accessible means, as almost half of all American households have a firearm. Conversely, while suicide by intentional car crash is impossible for latency-age children, running in front of a car is not. Therefore, accessibility of suicidal means can only be a partial explanation for the increasing adolescent suicide rate.

4. *Adolescents are extremely impulsive.* Although some investigators describe teenage suicide as spontaneous and impulsive, the majority of authors agree that most adolescent suicides are the culmination of many years of maladaptive behavior coupled with self-destructive preoccupations.

5. *Adolescents are more capable of making a plan and carrying it out than*

children. This explanation is probably accurate as far as it goes because it acknowledges the teenager's growth in intellectual and problem-solving capabilities. The external reality of the adolescent's world (e.g., accessibility of cars, guns, drugs; increased strength) is not the primary cause for the increase in suicidal behavior at puberty. The 8- to 12-year-old child also has similar opportunities, limited impulse control, and the physical ability to make an attempt, but does not do so with the same frequency as the adolescent.

It must be concluded, therefore, that it is the internal changes during adolescence that impel some adolescents toward suicidal behavior as a solution to conflict. The opportunities for self-destructive activity provided by the adolescent's external world are secondary contributors to this type of behavior.

The internal changes occurring during adolescence are extremely complex. Rapid physical development, shifting biological forces, and endocrinological changes exact corresponding revisions in the psychological structures of childhood. As personality features, coping mechanism, identifications, and psychic defenses undergo change, the adolescent experiences confusion, emptiness, and occasional despair. For the particularly troubled adolescent, there is a lowered threshold for self-destructiveness when exacerbated by destructive environmental factors. This may lead to the development of active suicidal behavior.

The adolescent's developmental process has been likened to a normative crisis; the process is inherently painful, but if it is successfully mastered, it produces a more stable personality configuration. Indeed, one of the fundamental challenges to the adolescent is the emergence of adultlike aggressive and sexual drives, requiring the abrupt transfer of libidinal ties from parent to peers and other nonincestuous persons. This process of detachment from parents can produce anxiety and feelings of unendurable loss in seriously troubled adolescents. When the previous parental relationship is already deeply ambivalent, the separation process may cause the adolescent to feel trapped between intensely hostile feelings, on the one hand, and deep symbiotic needs, on the other. Avoiding the mother in order to spare her from the adolescent's rage may also be experienced as abandonment just at the time she needs protection—thus the tug of war between both sides of the adolescent's magical, unconscious, dualistic wishes.

Larry W., a 17-year-old high school junior, was brought to the emergency room after his mother and two brothers discovered him in a semicomatose condition. He had overdosed on medication belonging to his 54-year-old mother, who had been treated for breast cancer over the preceding several years. The father had deserted the family when Larry was 4. For the next 10 years, the mother worked at two jobs to hold the family together. The caretaking was shared by an aunt and an inconsistent, relatively uninterested grandmother. Larry's mother was aloof, rigid, and a stern disciplinarian; she openly disapproved of his school performance, and of his behavior in general. She had unrealistic expectations for herself and was frequently depressed, although never overtly suicidal. She often engaged

Larry in discussions about the point of living. Over the past few months she had become increasingly despondent and had been taking her medication erratically. Larry, in turn, had begun refusing to go to school or would leave early, expressing the fear that he would come home and find her dead. In the months before his suicide attempt, he ran away from home several times, fought repeatedly with his brothers and classmates, and failed several subjects.

The history of Larry and other adolescents who have attempted suicide share common themes. Chronic, repeated separations or losses are prominent features of the clinical picture: For example, in an intensive investigation of 50 suicidal teenagers, it was found that 72% had grown up with either one or both of the natural parents absent from home because of divorce, desertion, or death.[29] Twice as many of these teenagers had been raised by nonparent caretakers than had teenagers of a representative control group. Teicher found that 20% of suicidal teenagers had a parent who attempted suicide, and 40% a parent, relative, or close friend.[29] Thus, while many adolescents experience object loss in childhood without becoming suicidal, self-destructive teenagers have generally experienced object loss *and* exposure to suicidal thought, talk, or behavior within their immediate environment.

Another component of the teenager's generally increased vulnerability for suicidal behavior is the pervasive change in his relationship to his own body. Sexual feelings begin to be experienced with adult urgency; physical development is rapid and dramatic. Some adolescents find their sexual urges and developing bodies abhorrent, and feel they cannot successfully control their feelings:

> Sara, a 13½-year-old girl, was admitted to a psychiatric ward after over-dosing and slashing her arms. She had been involved in sexual activities with her stepfather for several years but had consistently refused him since the onset of puberty six months before. One week before her suicide attempt the stepfather was arrested for having intercourse with the patient's sister. During the arraignment, Sara's previous sexual activity was revealed, pre-cipitating the suicide crisis. Sara experienced her pubescent body as be-coming like that of her passive, unloving mother, with whom she was in-tensely, hatefully identified.

Suicide can be seen in this and similar cases as just punishment for the alien, bad body, while the true self remains intact—"dying means killing the body but not necessarily the mind."[66]

In summary, it can be said that suicidal behavior intensifies during adolescence for various interrelated reasons. Profound biological and physical changes create a developmental crisis unlike any other. At the same time, the individual is struggling with issues of identity and separation compounded by the emergence of adult sexual feelings. This struggle is mirrored cognitively by the adolescent's confusion of concrete and abstract logic, on the one hand, and is reflected in the facile switch between childhood and adult emotional patterns, on the other.[67] During this phase, ideas, including suicidal fantasies, can seem real and hypothetical at the same time. While the adolescent is struggling with these powerful internal drives, he is also being buffeted by societal pressures that make violence, disaffection, and alienation a way of life among some adolescent subcultures.

7.7. Prediction

It is virtually impossible to predict suicidal attempts prospectively; there are no reliable predictive indicators. With the exception of cases where threats have been made in advance of the attempt, the first suicidal act often comes as a surprise to parents, school personnel, and pediatricians. Since "keeping things secret" is an age-related phenomenon, late latency and adolescent patients may deliberately suppress talk or behavior that would otherwise provide clues to the danger.

Retrospectively, it is usually possible to identify prodromal signs for youthful suicide attempters. "Active" signs such as running away, truancy, drug abuse, cultism, defiance, and delinquency are often cries for help, as are "passive" complaints such as chronic stomachaches, muscle pulls, headaches, visual problems, and nausea. Medical complaints represent an implicit request for emotional relief and are often a prominent feature of the clinical picture for other members of the suicidal adolescent's family. In Teicher's previously mentioned study, it was found that in 48% of adolescent suicide attempts, a sibling or parent was treated for a serious medical or emotional problem within the five-year period before the attempt.[29] While seriously stressful in itself, the sibling's or parent's illness forces an indirect shift in the family's regular roles and responsibilities.

Many suicide attempts occur outside the adolescent's usual or familiar environmental structure, especially when the adolescent has brought about his own isolation through family embarrassment at a pregnancy, expulsion from school, or chronic truancy. Other breaches in the adolescent's social network are common to the history of teenage suicide attempts, such as chronically impaired peer relationships or extreme peer dependency. When such tenuous or overvalued relationships flounder, a suicide attempt is not unusual.[29,61]

7.8. Acute Treatment and Management Approaches

The principles and techniques of emergency intervention for adult patients are highly relevant to suicidal preadults, but they do not represent the totality of management principles for this patient population. The clinician working with acutely disturbed children and adolescents must consider the child as an individual within his developmental phase and within his social system.

7.8.1. Developmental Approach

Various factors are common to the assessment of suicidal children and adults, namely, impulsiveness and aggressive drive of the patient, concreteness, lethality and intent of the plan, seriousness of the precipitating crisis, and security of the support network. In addition, however, the clinician must address issues, circumstances, and developmental phases specific to the preadult patient. For example, separation and loss have been found to be among the most prominent psychogenetic factors in preadult suicidal activity. The treatment plan should consider:

- the nature, object, and permanence of the loss.
- the developmental level of the child, the age-dependent tasks being mastered at the time of the loss, and the impact the loss has had on the child.
- the quality of the child's object relations, in fact and fantasy.
- ego strengths of the child, i.e., intelligence, capacity to regulate affects, to reality-test, and to accommodate experience.
- the security, strength, and supportiveness of the child's social environment, i.e., the family's tolerance of, and sensitivity to, the child's symptoms; the interactive pattern among family members.

7.8.2. Need to See beyond the Symptom

One of the most common errors in management by clinican and parents alike, especially with the preadolescent population, is failing to give credence to the help-seeking motives of the attempt. Suicidal verbalizations and behaviors are often so transparently manipulative that adults may not even see the child's desperation until it escalates. The threat to life may be small at first, but if the attempt is unacknowledged, the long-term threat to life and well-being may be very great.

Likewise, physicians, particularly pediatricians, must constantly probe for masked self-destructive motivation underlying the "accidents" of their latency and adolescent patients. For example, in any "accidental" ingestion of medication or toxic substances in a child more than 5 years old, suicidal intent must be assumed.

No matter how minor the suicidal attempt, the clinician must additionally remember the child "as the bearer of the family's symptoms." In our clinical experience, we have noticed repeatedly that covert child abuse is frequently associated with suicidal activity in preschoolers and young school-age children, as is the presence of parental or sibling suicidal behavior with suicidal behavior in young children.

7.8.3. Hospitalization for Children and Adolescents

The safety of the suicidal child or adolescent is the primary clinical concern. Hospitalization may be the only treatment option for patients who are actively suicidal or at high risk. When a child is hospitalized, especially if it is on a nonpsychiatric ward, the room should be made suicide-proof: The clinician must carefully assess window accessibility and must remove potentially dangerous objects such as discarded tubing, pull-strings on toys, and, of course, sharp or pointed objects.

Although hospitalization provides a temporary respite from situational pressures and may produce a sense of security, it is undoubtedly stressful to some children. When separation from the parent is especially traumatic, marked depressive symptoms can occur. If the suicidal youngsters have developed intensely dependent transference attachments to ward personnel, or if the home situation is turbulent, suicidal feelings can reemerge at discharge. It is essential that the family be actively involved in the therapeutic process during the child's hospitalization. If a destructive familial pattern persists, alternative placement of the child must be considered.[62]

Suicidal ideation in psychotic children or adolescents is extremely serious and is almost always an indication for hospitalization, even in the absence of suicidal behavior. Medication may be required, at least initially, although childhood psychoses are generally more refractory than adolescent- or adult-onset psychoses. Latency-age children who are both psychotic and suicidal carry a grave prognosis.

7.8.4. Outpatient Management

Many preadult suicide attempts are clearly manipulative. The child is hoping the attempt will alter the environment in which he lives; it is essential that outpatient treatment specifically address those environmental stresses. Systems work, especially family therapy, is the preferred modality, but it may be necessary to extend the therapeutic process indirectly to cover the child's extended social network, including teachers, guidance counselors, principals, probation officers, or outreach workers who are actively involved with the child.[22,30] If the ancillary members of the social network can come to understand the child's motives and wishes, they can deal with him and his family more adaptively.

7.8.5. Psychotherapeutic Considerations

Individual psychotherapy is essential to treating the suicidal preadult, but it is unlikely to be successful unless combined with systems work. A difficult, but absolutely critical, aspect of the work with adolescents is forming a therapeutic alliance. Under the best of circumstances, healthy adolescents have trouble talking to adults, and adults have trouble talking to teenagers. Under the worst of circumstances, when the teenager is suicidal, angry, clinging, withdrawn, impulsive, or suspicious, the alliance is particularly difficult to negotiate. Therapeutic techniques employing sarcasm, ridicule, criticism, or pious judgment are absolutely contraindicated. A natural, flexible stance is preferable to a passive, effaced, inactive approach or a falsely supportive, empathic style. Timing is essential; it is better to develop a positive working relationship before interpreting transference phenomena or using confrontational techniques.

Whenever the effectiveness of the therapy is seriously threatened and suicidal risk is exacerbated, the suicidal teenager may need to be hospitalized. The constancy and intensity of inpatient psychotherapy can strengthen the working alliance and turn around the chances for successful long-term outpatient work.

8. Homicidal Behaviors in Children and Adolescents

8.1. Introduction

Juvenile violence appears to be increasing at nearly twice the rate for adult violence. In 1975, for example, although males between 5 and 20 years of age represented only 8.5% of the population, they committed 35% of violent crimes. During the past decade, the rates for antisocial or aggressive acts among young women have increased markedly. Now more than 20% of all violent crimes are attributable to young females. Of the 6,100,000 arrests made in the United States in 1974 for violent crimes such as homicide, rape, and aggravated assault, over 27% were committed by males and females under the age of 18.[68] These figures account for only the crimes that are reported and the offenders that are caught. The actual statistics are undoubtedly much higher. The mortality rate among preadults is increasing dramatically. The frequency of violent deaths by accident, homicide, and suicide is declining among all age groups except for adolescents.[69,70] Suicide and homicide account for the greatest number of deaths in adolescence, and in parallel fashion, suicidal and homicidal behavior account for the majority of emergency psychiatric visits among children and adolescents—as many as 60–70% in some studies.

8.2. Development of Aggression

Theories about the development of aggression vary. Behaviorists focus on aspects of aggressive behavior that are learned or conditioned by the operation of environmental stimuli. Psychoanalytic theories have emphasized the instinctual origins of aggression, and sociobiologists have looked at it as a survival mechanism. Psychophysiologists have studied control and dyscontrol mechanisms activated by changes in brain chemistry or chemical intoxication. Others have investigated transgenerational patterns of aggression. In the absence of a unified conceptual framework, the following guideline is useful: Violence in children and adolescents, except in the service of self-defense, should be considered pathological.

8.3. Literature Review on Youthful Homicide

The literature on youthful homicide generally focuses on specific cases exclusive of control-group comparisons. Nevertheless, it may be useful to summarize the most important conclusions.

In Bender's classic report of 33 children and adolescents who had killed, there were 11 boys and 2 girls in the 10-and-younger group.[71] Four of these had caused death by firesetting, four had been involved in drownings, two children had stabbed their victims, and two had repeatedly beaten their victims with a heavy instrument. Three of the youngsters were mentally retarded males.

Bender concluded that these 11 children did not fully intend to kill their victims and, with the exception of the mentally retarded youths, had apparently reacted with extreme shock to the deaths. The fatal incidents followed a clear history of psychiatric disturbance (or retardation) in all 11. Subsequent to the deaths, all of these children evinced more severe disturbance, even threatening to kill again. One child was implicated in the death of other children only months after the first incident.

In Bender's series, prior psychiatric evaluations had been carried out in 50% of the cases. The recommendations were almost universally disregarded, even when the official findings indicated that the child was seriously dangerous. In her conclusion, Bender isolated the following four factors: (1) poor impulse control in an otherwise disturbed youngster, (2) immediacy of a victim, (3) easy accessibility of a weapon (or hazardous situation), (4) lack of supervision. Homicidal risk would be considerably potentiated by the presence of organic brain damage, abnormal EEG, childhood schizophrenia, compulsive firesetting, and other violent symptom matrices.

8.4. Sibling Murder by a Young Child

Sibling rivalries and resentments are almost universal aspects of childhood. It is rare, however, for these hostile impulses to result by accident or design in the death of a sibling. For the most part, fratricide and other youthful homicides correlated with exposure to brutality by the young assailant.[72-74] Sibling deaths generally occur under two different sets of conditions. Under one set, based on a study of five infant homicides, Adelson[75] found that the deaths occurred because of the particular vulnerability of the immature infant, and that the majority of the assailants were "apparently normal boys who displayed the commonly encountered combination of childhood hostility, jealousy and 'playfulness.'" In these cases, the victim was envied by the older child for his special position and hated for displacing the older child.

Tooley[76] proposed a second set of conditions for sibling murder; the older child, not the infant, is felt to be the favored child, acting out the mother's murderous wishes against the younger children. Two cases in point follow.

> One young child had deliberately set fire to her younger brother, had tried to put Clorox down the throat of her infant sister, and had set fire to the baby's bedclothes. The other child, a 6-year-old boy, had also set fire to his younger sister's dress on two occasions and had deliberately held her head under water until stopped by an adult who was swimming nearby. Neither mother was disturbed by the attacks, dismissing them as childish mischief.

These two children were not hyperaggressive and impulse-ridden. On the contrary, they were described by Tooley as "cool, canny beyond their years, quite well-controlled and self-sufficient." They did well in school, were liked by peers, were self-possessed and attractive. Unlike the typical homicidal child, these children were articulate and playful. Their attacks, on the other hand, were clearly intentional; although they did not regard death as entirely irreversible, they did understand the idea of absence. They wished to get rid of the younger siblings who were overburdening their mothers and the household. Psychological testing and long-term psychotherapy revealed that the primary motivation for the acts was to protect the mothers from the demands of the smaller children. The youngsters felt no pleasure in the homicidal act or strong animosity toward the victims. The mothers, for their part, seemed to condone and even encourage these acts.

8.5. Homicidal Tendencies in Adolescents

The most common psychiatric conditions coexisting with latency-age murder or homicidal impulses are conduct disorders, organic brain damage, schizophrenia, marked mental retardation, and psychosocial abuse or deprivation. These same disorders appear to underlie adolescent homicide as well, but the prodromal period is more clearly defined in the latter group.

Malmquist studied 20 adolescent murderers ranging in age from 13 to 18 in order to establish common features with possible predictive value for juvenile homicide.[77] Among his key findings were the following:

- Prior to the murder, a clear-cut shift in mood occurred involving deep pessimism, brooding, self-hatred, and requests for help such as asking to be admitted to a psychiatric hospital, or begging for help from a friend or family member. These requests were often ignored, misunderstood, or minimized.
- There was an unexpectedly high incidence of somatic preoccupations that intensified during the prodromal period. Headaches were especially common; several youths had overt somatic delusions.
- The victim was usually an acquaintance or family member on whom the murderer was particularly dependent. The precipitant was often threatened loss or modification of the relationship.
- In several cases, the teenage male was directly incited by girlfriend or mother to commit the murder. In others, covert or explicit homosexual advances by the victim were sufficient to trigger the assault.

Malmquist concluded, however, that he could not use these findings to predict adolescent murder. He observed, as have other investigators,[78–81] that there is a close association between homicidal and depressive symptomatology—that is, feelings of worthlessness, self-depreciation, and guilt. The murder, as Malmquist indicated, was often immediately preceded by a failure of affective controls, evidenced by periods of crying, sobbing, marked brooding, or inappropriate and unrestrained laughter.

King studied nine teenagers (8 boys and 1 girl) who had committed homicide.[2] Although only one was diagnosed psychotic, all shared a history of violence at home, with unpredictable and inconsistent parenting. He observed that an inability to communicate effectively in these youngsters correlated with an exaggerated need for compensatory action:

> Among our youths, a most disabling defect in their development was . . . their inability or disinclination to master prevailing language. They had not learned to read well or to deal effectively with symbols. . . . To sustain omnipotence, they strove to reduce the symbols of communication . . . to the primitive experience of terse speech, and, ultimately, action. Terseness and action warded off talk and the cognitive challenge of reason. They attempted to make action the language of communication.[82] (p. 138)

Although action was an acceptable substitute for talk and reasoning at home, it was not tolerated at school. Many of these homicidal teenagers were unable to master basic verbal and cognitive skills; their verbal productions were immature and constricted, their capacities to use fantasy, symbolism, and allegorical play virtually nonexistent, and their ability to displace and sublimate undeveloped. Ordinary substitutes for competitive and aggressive action such as team sports or games were of no value to these youngsters, so that they continued to discharge aggression in explosive, assaultive violence.

8.6. Predictive Symptoms

Investigators have tried to delineate previolent signs with reliable predictive value. Perhaps the most familiar of these symptom constellations is the so-called violent triad: cruelty to animals, firesetting, and enuresis. In their study of violent and nonviolent criminals, Hellman and Blackman found that the symptom triad appeared in 75% of the violent group, while one symptom or more of the triad appeared in only 28% of the nonviolent group. The authors concluded that a history of the three symptoms in childhood might be well predictive of adult violence.[83]

Other authors challenge the triad's predictive value. One study produced a new "quintet" of childhood signs common to adolescent and adult violence: (1) fighting, (2) temper tantrums, (3) inability to get along with others, (4) school problems, and (5) truancy. On the basis of literature analysis, extensive clinical interviewing, and case studies, these five symptoms were found to occur in the histories of violent criminals two to three times more frequently than the triad of enuresis, cruelty to animals, and firesetting. The authors pointed out, however, that some of these behaviors occur in every child at some point, and are not therefore absolute predictors of later violence. They did suggest that the quintet was a more reliable predictor than the triad and that the two together indicated serious emotional disturbance very likely to result in violent behavior.[84]

In another study,[85] Sendi and Blomgren compared the frequency of symptom-predictors in the histories of 10 teenagers who had committed homicide, 10 who had attempted or threatened homicide, and 10 adolescent controls chosen randomly from the population at a psychiatric hospital. Firesetting, cruelty to animals, and enuresis were equally distributed among the three groups, and the triad itself was not present in any subject at all. The study concluded that the triad and each of the individual symptoms were not significant predictors within the investigated population. Instead, the 10 who had committed murder were found to have a high incidence of diagnosed schizophrenia (60%), with a long history of schizoid adjustment, intense maternal symbiosis, and sexual immaturity. This group was higher in measured intelligence and school achievement than the group that had attempted or threatened homicide. The latter, in contrast, showed a high degree of organic brain pathology, tended toward greater impulsiveness than either the murderers or the controls, and suffered from episodic discharge of primitive and explosive aggression.

The authors concluded that while there were marked differences in the previolent psychopathology between the two violent groups (schizoid, symbiotic, regressive patterns in the adolescent murderers vs. impulsive, minimally brain-damaged, episodically aggressive patterns in the adolescents who had attempted or threatened murder), pathogenetic environment factors were common to both violent groups. They generally shared chaotic home lives, brutal rejection by the fathers, and family endorsement of violence.

8.7. Parents and Families of Violent Youth

Many violent young people spend their formative years in a destructive interpersonal system marked by unstable marriages, periodic desertions, violent parental fights, unwanted pregnancies (including the index patient), problem drinking, discipline that is either too harsh or nonexistent, and unusually cruel treatment of the youngster in particular. It is not uncommon for violence and hostility to be the prevailing interpersonal mode within the households of homicidal youngsters, not only between sibling and sibling but between husband and wife, and parent and child. It is the common language, a mirror of the familial mood and a reflection of the deficiency of alternative communication styles.

8.8. Neurological Dysfunction and Violence

It is commonly agreed that perinatal trauma, head injury, infantile convulsions, and postencephalitic states are often associated with explosive rage in later life. Although temporal and limbic lobe seizures have been implicated in episodes of violent behavior, the exact relationship between epilepsy and juvenile violence is unclear. Psychomotor epilepsy occurs far more frequently among juvenile delinquents than in the general population: Over 18% of incarcerated teenagers had probable psychomotor seizures compared to an estimated 0.5% incidence among the general population. Moreover, the severity of the epileptic symptoms correlates directly with the seriousness of the violent behavior.

Habitually hyperaggressive people without clinical epilepsy have a very high incidence of nonspecific organic brain dysfunction with EEG abnormalities. In about 40% of these patients, the propensity to violent behavior emerges in early childhood and declines in about the fourth decade.[87] Violent behavior beginning during the preschool and latency periods is usually indicative of psychosis and/or organic brain disease.[88] Fewer than 20% of these violent children become well-adjusted adults. By the time they are 18 years old, 20% have become (or continue to be) psychotic, and 40% display aggressively antisocial behavior throughout their lives.[89] In either case, the prognosis for this group is poor. Although it is extremely difficult to determine whether neurological dysfunction or environment contributes more to periodic violence in habitually aggressive youngsters, the clinician should assess and treat environmental stressors in neurologically impaired children as carefully as in other groups of disturbed youth.

8.9. Emergency Management of the Violent Child and Adolescent

The emergency clinician uses many of the same principles for managing the violent or acutely agitated youngster as he does for the adult patient. (see Chapters 2 and 6). It may be unnecessary to resort to mechanical or chemical restraints for a child, but if he cannot be brought under control, it is best to enfold the child from behind, using the floor and a wall as supports. If the child is flailing, kicking, or biting, all four extremities must be held down and the child's head steadied until he is quiet. The clinician should reassure the child during the process:

> I will not hurt you, and I won't let anyone else hurt you. You are safe with me, and I won't let you hurt yourself or anyone else. I know how scary this is, but we will work on it together. When you can stop kicking, I'll take my legs off yours. When you feel ready, tell me and I will take my hands off your wrists. I'm not mad at you; I'm glad you are calmer and I hope we can begin to figure out how to help you.

Once the violence has been contained, and the child reassured, the evaluation can proceed to the question of organicity, either chemical/toxic or medical. For example:

> An 11-year-old girl was brought to the ER after attacking an unknown adult on the street with her fists. On admission to the ER, she seemed dazed, and one pupil was markedly larger than the other. While vital signs were taken and a neurological examination begun, the child had another episode of uncontrollable rage, attempting to bite and scratch staff and parents. The patient was restrained physically and transferred to the pediatric neurology ward for extensive testing.

Since violence can erupt at any moment, the clinician should pay special attention to the following:

1. Episodes of prior violence, the precipitant, setting, weapon, victim, seriousness of the injury, intent, remorse, threatened repetitions, etc.
2. Factors reducing controls or diminishing impulse inhibition: use of alcohol or street drugs (especially PCP, substances containing bella-

donna, alkaloids, amphetamines, gasoline, and glue, and some sedative-hypnotics). Mental retardation at times promotes hyperaggressive behavior; psychosis seriously exacerbates violent tendencies, especially if there are auditory hallucinations instructing the child to kill or destroy.

3. Intent and impulsiveness; the vast majority of acutely violent and out-of-control preadults do not intend to kill anyone, they are more concerned with the feeling of being out of control and the fear of "doing something awful." Premeditated homicidal activity is rarely seen on an emergency basis, and would be disguised if it were. The evaluator should determine the frequency and nature of violent fantasies and impulses, the availability of weapons, the patient's own sense of his impulse control, and the existence of a concrete victim and plan.

4. Intrafamilial struggles; family members themselves often contribute to aggressive behavior by directly or subtly provoking violence. If the violent patient has reason to believe that he will be attacked, punished, or displaced by the potential or intended victim, the likelihood of violence is very high. Young children and elderly family members are particularly vulnerable.

5. The risk of suicide or suicidal behavior in conjunction with, or immediately following, homicidal activity is very high for adults[78–81] and is similarly elevated for adolescents who have been hospitalized because of aggressive behavior.[90]

All details of the assessment should be checked against information supplied by other family members or friends. While an adolescent will usually understand the interviewer's questions but may be unwilling to answer them directly, a younger child may be willing to answer questions but is unable to grasp their content easily. It may be necessary to elicit information indirectly by inquiring about favorite TV shows or movies, as in the following fragment of an interview with a 10-year-old child. The child was being evaluated for putting a cat in a clothes dryer. When asked to describe his favorite TV show, the boy began to tell about Saturday afternoon wrestling.

B: That Man Mountain, he's wicked huge. I once saw him twist a guy's head right off.
MD: Right Off! Really?
B: Yeah, really . . . well maybe not completely all off, but there was blood everywhere, and guts and stuff, really neat . . . and this old woman was yelling and screaming and. . . .
MD: What old woman?
B: . . . .and they got about 200 cops with clubs and Man Mountain just mowed them down. It was incredible. And then the Claw came out and slammed him in the back with the claw. You should have seen it go in. I'm saving up for tickets for August 15.
MD: Pretty wild. Sounds like the kind of thing that could give anyone bad dreams.
B: Yeah, well . . . sure.
MD: How about you?

B: I had one where I was in the ring in front of everyone and my mother and sisters
were right in the front row. This is the weird part, this giant dude comes up, he looks
really strange, with a hatchet, but I ram the rope post right into his chest, except he
keeps coming anyway, and. . . .

A child or adolescent who manifests high homicidal potential generally
requires hospitalization. When in doubt, the emergency room clinician should
admit the patient for a thorough evaluation, even on an involuntary basis.
Homicidal and suicidal children under the age of 17 can be admitted against
parental wishes under the same statutes as those governing adult commitment.

9. Firesetting

9.1. Introduction

Firesetting must be considered a true psychiatric emergency simply because of its potentially lethal consequences. Paradoxically, however, firesetting
emergencies constitute fewer than 5% of the acute intakes in an emergency
facility, and do not begin to reflect the very heavy incidence of youthful firesetting in the general population. In 1980, for example, in Boston alone,
children were responsible for setting 308 building fires, 48 vehicle fires, and
2133 fires in rubbish piles, vacant lots, fields, etc.[91] Popular opinion and the
professional community alike often fail to respond to firesetting in itself as
sufficient reason for psychiatric evaluation, unless it is combined with other
aggressive symptoms like fighting, stealing, or truancy. It should be considered
a serious symptom, however, and a genuine psychiatric emergency.

In spite of attention variously focused on the libidinal versus the aggressive
features of firesetting, the symptom fits no single diagnostic category. Youthful
firesetters conform to no uniform profile, seem to exhibit ranging personality
types with multiple psychodynamic histories. There are a few general features,
however: Firesetters tend to be male rather than female, come from unstable,
deprived home situations usually with absent fathers, and typically show poor
impulse control and impaired ego integration.[92-95]

9.2. Relationship of Firesetting to Developmental Level

Children of all ages seem to be fascinated by fire, and may at times even
play with fire. Firesetting is a deliberate activity motivated by different impulses, from merely curious play to consciously destructive intent. Most preschoolers who play with fire do so in the context of normal exploratory behavior
and inability to grasp the potentially serious consequences of their actions. The
critical part in the acute evaluation of preschool firesetters is to assess the level
of parental supervision and generaly safety in the home environment.

A 4-year-old boy was brought to the ER with a large second-degree burn
on one leg, the accidental result of playing with a cigarette lighter left on

the coffee table at home. Three months previously he had been seen for a puncture wound in one foot, the accidental result again of playing barefoot in the alley next to his house. During the interview, it was discovered that much of the caretaking was done by two older sisters, ages 11 and 8. The mother was divorced, worked at two jobs, and was away from the house most of the day. Arrangements for a homemaker were made, with day care for the child and an after-school program for the older siblings. No further treatment was necessary.

As the case demonstrates, simple curiosity and unsupervised access to matches can turn child's play into a serious situation, or a repetitively dangerous pattern. Most young children can be discouraged from firesetting either by arranging for adequate child care, as in the first case, or by training parents to manage the child more effectively, as the following case illustrates.

A distraught mother came to the pediatric walk-in clinic with her 5-year-old daughter. Despite the mother's prohibitions and a warning spanking, the child persisted in lighting matches in the cellar. This anxious and confused mother asked the clinician whether she ought to burn the child slightly with a match "to show her what could happen." The mother had a friend who handled a similar problem by taking her small son to see a burn unit at a local hospital, but the child then developed nightmares and became terrified of hospitals. The mother was advised to set a special time aside to show her daughter how to light matches safely. The child was allowed to light matches herself every day, but only at a special time when the mother could supervise. After a few days, the child's curiosity was satisfied and the problem vanished.

9.2.1. Latency

Repeated firesetting in school-age children is a serious symptom. For this age group, pathological incendiarism seems to be directly related to a hostile, rejecting home situation. Yarnell, for example, found that latency-age children (6–8) tended to set fires in or near their homes, often in a deliberate effort to punish a parent or a sibling.[94] The destructiveness of the fire seemed of paramount concern to these children, and of far more importance than the libidinal gratification obtained from igniting or viewing the flames. These children showed little or no interest in playing with matches, even when they were given the opportunity to do so.

Vanersall and Weiner found that their sample of 20 youngsters could be grouped according to differences in personality structure.[93] The first cluster (45% of the total) was composed of extremely deviant personality types ranging from developmentally retarded, infantile, or borderline children to frankly psychotic youngsters. These children were hyperactive and highly impulsive. The second group (40% of the total) functioned at a significantly higher level than the first. They appeared neat, compliant, and eager to please, although their behavior had an obsessive, slightly phobic quality, and the children themselves seemed depressed. Firesetting was frequently compounded by stealing. The third cluster (15% of the total) functioned at the most adaptive level of all, were primarily passive-aggressive personality types, and were "resourcefully manipulative." None of the 20 children had satisfactory relationships with peers, and all evidenced loneliness, poor self-esteem, and extreme jealousy. *Not one of the 20 came from a home with a consistently available father*, and in most cases, the mother–child relationship was pathological. Parenthetically, it should be added that only 3 of the children were originally referred for firesetting.

9.2.2. Late Latency and Adolescence

In Yarnell's study of 60 firesetters, he posited that firesetting among adolescents symbolically represented, or became a displacement for, sexual activity,[94,96] in contrast to latency-age firesetters who had experienced sexually precocious or deviant activities. Many adolescents who were otherwise immature socially and sexually set fires in pairs, the partnership having either unconscious or sometimes explicit homosexual overtones. The firesetting episodes were well planned and evoked intensely excited feelings, which were enhanced by watching the arrival of the fire trucks and the fire-fighting efforts.

Lewis and Yarnell went on to speculate about the specific psychodynamics involved in adolescent firesetting.[96] They concluded that the firesetting incident is an effort to discharge extreme inner tension, brought on by external stress burdening an already severe character disorder. The fact that these youngsters choose firesetting to discharge tension rather than some other method, such as wrist-slashing or excessive masturbation, is highly idiosyncratic and determined by multiple factors.

For some adolescent firesetters, the fire itself appears to have magical retributive/restorative qualities. These youngsters report primitive fantasies filled with rage, destruction, dismemberment, and conflagration; thought processes and reality testing may approximate psychotic agitation or profound dissociation, with the adolescent appearing regressed and disorganized. The fire is ignited often in an almost dreamlike state.

Macht and Mack[95] felt that firesetting was not simply the breaking through of an impulse in an impulse-ridden teenager: The meaning of the act itself was bound to particular aspects of some key relationship. To substantiate their thesis, they studied four adolescent firesetters, showing that the syndrome included the following key activities: firesetting, signaling for help, waiting for the firemen, watching and sometimes assisting with extinguishing the fire. Not least of the intense motivations underlying the act was the potential friendship with the firemen. In each of the families of the four patients, the father was absent. The firesetting might, therefore, have been a symbolic "call from the overburdened adolescent to the absent father." Additionally striking was the fact that all four fathers (or surrogate fathers) had occupations associated with fires; one father, for example, worked as a furnace stoker in a boiler room. When he had abruptly deserted the family, it was to go to sea to work as a fireman in the ship's engine room. The father in the second case had been a

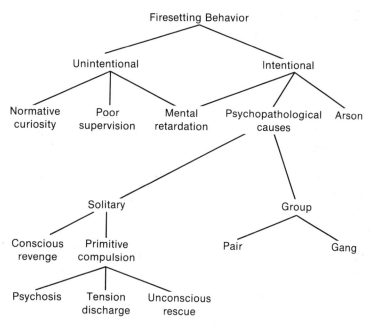

Figure 1. A decision tree for diagnosing firesetting.

gas burner repairman, and his duties involved lighting the burners. The third boy had helped his father dispose of junked cars by pouring gas over them and setting them ablaze. Two of these three boys had developed close relationships with firemen, while the fourth patient studied had actually been adopted by a fireman. The adoptive father died suddenly, and the firesetting escalated. When he was questioned about the firesetting and his thoughts while doing it, this boy replied,[95] "I want it to burn, but I don't want it to burn. . . . I wouldn't want anybody to get hurt. . . . I used to worry about my father falling off one of the fire engines and getting killed. . . . I do things to people I like, I don't know why. . . . I used to think of him [father] when I set fires. I could picture him right in front of me staring at me . . . telling me not to light the fire. . . ." (p. 284).

While there are striking similarities among the histories of young firesetters, each set of dynamics is highly individualized and can be understood only by understanding the specific roots.

9.3. Emergency Assessment and Management

The psychiatric management of the firesetting youngster can be effective only if the clinician addresses the psychological mechanisms underlying the symptomatic behavior. To structure the interview, the following decision-tree format should be used (see Figure 1).

The first approach is to establish the intent behind the act. If the fire was not set intentionally or to achieve a specific end, the clinician should consider the possibility that poor parental supervision, access to matches, and curiosity contributed to the incident, and could do so again. The therapeutic intervention in this case should address the lack of supervision and inadequate parental management.

If the firesetting proves to be intentional, the clinician should determine if it was done for profit, or for some other reason. Firesetting for profit—arson—is a criminal offense to be treated within the criminal justice system. While it is true that some youthful arsonists may have psychiatric symptoms, arson is not considered a psychiatric disorder.

If the firesetting is intentional, and motivated by psychopathology rather than profit, it is important to determine the general context of the behavior: whether the act was performed alone, with one other youngster, or as part of a gang; the emotional tones of the experience; and the fantasies behind the action.

As a general rule, there is a distinction between solitary and group firesetting. Gang fires are a sociopathic or sociosyntonic phenomenon. The teenagers involved generally do not do well in outpatient psychotherapy or in a psychiatric hospital. Firesetting may be only one of many deliquent acts, leading eventually to criminal apprehension and conviction. Another version of gang firesetting is radical or political terrorism employing fire-bombing or explosive devices. These adolescents may end up in the emergency room involuntarily because of injuries and burns sustained accidentally.

Youngsters who set fires deliberately, as a result of emotional problems, need to be evaluated and treated psychiatrically. There is often little correlation between the seriousness of the fire and the seriousness of the child's psychopathology; firesetters who are capable of planning and staging a serious fire are likely to be less impaired than youngsters who are poorly organized and regressed. The clinician should specifically evaluate the degree of planning involved and the consequent degree of remorse, the level of impulse control (as manifest in the presence or absence of other symptomatic behaviors such as stealing, cruelty to animals, sexual deviations, suicidal activity), level of ego organization, thought content and reality testing, and parental involvement in the symptomatology—whether as exacerbating or moderating influences.

The clinician should base his dispositional decisions on specific findings, bearing the following guidelines in mind: Organized firesetting accompanied by little remorse indicates a conduct disorder or antisocial personality. This is especially true for teenagers who set fires with one other friend, or for latency-age children motivated by revenge or persecution. Children and adolescents of this type do not necessarily require hospitalization so long as they and their families adhere to outpatient treatment plans.

Solitary firesetters whose ego organization and reality testing are generally poor may require hospitalization. When these children are borderline or overtly psychotic, firesetting may be only one of many symptoms signaling a deeply rooted emotional disorder. Hospitalization may be the only safe modality in which to begin treatment.

To summarize, it should be emphasized that the better ego organization of the youngster, the clearer the precipitant and/or motive, and the more effectively motivated the parents, the better the prognosis for outpatient psychotherapy.

10. Runaway Children and Adolescents

10.1. Introduction

Current estimates put the number of child and adolescent runaways in the United States at close to one million each year. Runaways tend to be young adolescents, the majority of whom are under 16.[97] Most flock to large cities; a much smaller percentage choose rural communes. Police estimate that at any one time there may be as many as 20,000 runaway youths in New York City alone. In the Times Square area, about 1000 identified pimps have control of close to 7000 teenage girls in a prostitution and pornography industry involving $1.5 billion a year.[98]

The first community shelter for runaways was opened under the direction of James Gordon. His profile of the adolescent runaway depicted a broken home and a generally abusive atmosphere from which the youngster was trying to escape.[99] Most observers agree that today's runaway children leave home to escape a destructive home life, not to embrace a religious or counterculture life-style.

The majority of runaway teenagers are never seen for psychiatric evaluation; those who are seen, however, represent a large proportion of the preadult psychiatric emergency evaluations, perhaps as many as 13%, according to some surveys.[100] In latency, there are twice as many male runaways as female runaways, but the pattern is reversed in the larger teenage population where female runaways are two to three times more frequent than male runaways.

10.2. Psychodynamics at Various Developmental Stages

Running away is not necessarily evidence of psycopathology. Preschoolers occasionally wander away from home because of curiosity, limit-testing, and normal separation/individuation processes. These youngsters are otherwise active and outgoing. Others in this age group run away to escape maternal overprotectiveness, or to break out of extremely chaotic living conditions. Repetitive or extreme runaway reactions warrant investigation of the home situation. For example, Steven, a 4-year-old, was found wandering naked at night in the street. It was his third runaway attempt. A court-ordered investigation revealed an alcoholic step-father and an overwhelmed, Valium-dependent mother. When Steven was placed in a foster home, his running away stopped.

10.2.1. Latency

Running away is a common school-age behavior and an even more common threat, prompted by anger at parental limit-setting or jealousy of a sibling. Children of this age fantasize about finding a "better home," where adults and children live together in an ideal atmosphere of warmth and support. Following an argument where the child feels particularly helpless, he may communicate his intention to leave, pack some belongings, and go to a friend's or grand-parent's house. Most of these episodes do not reach emergency proportions since the child returns home on his own or is persuaded to do so by his family. If the parents are sufficiently threatened by their child's drive for autonomy, however, so that they either mollify the child and soften the limits or punish and restrict him harshly, then the foundation is laid for more pathological re-actions later.

Another common runaway situation among this age group is the adopted child's quest for the idealized biological parents. The emergency intervention can be structured to help the adoptive parents respond to the child's quest with sympathy rather than regarding the search as a repudiation of their own love.

10.2.2. Late Latency and Adolescence

In this age group, the causes of runaway reactions tend to be complex, variable, and, in some cases, pathological. Repetitive or serious running away can best be understood within the context of the interpersonal system.

Stierlin[100,101] has distinguished three types of pathological family styles: binding, expelling, and delegating. He has linked these styles with at least four characteristic runaway reactions. The key determinant in these links is the adolescent's relationship with the dominant parent.

1. *Binding families* try to keep the adolescent at home in a physical and emotional sense by reinforcing or exploiting dependency needs, by interfering with the developing sense of autonomy, and by promoting regressive separation guilt. Two characteristic runaway patterns emerge from these families:

- Abortive runaways, who attempt to break loose but are thwarted by their own pathological ties to the family. They frequently engineer their return by loitering near police stations, neighbors, or parents' friends. One 15-year-old presented herself to a local ER complaining of abdom-inal pains, and promptly gave the staff her father's office phone number.
- Schizoidal runaways, who ordinarily have no place to go, no peers, and no friends at home. These runaways may be subject to acute psychotic decompensations during which thinking is idiosyncratic, often bizarre. Their parents are described as cool and aloof, but very possessive. One 15-year-old boy was found in the men's room of an urban bus station where he had been "hiding out" for two days. Overcome by panic, he slashed his arms with a broken bottle and was rushed to a nearby hospital by police.

2. *Expelling families* typically neglect or reject their children. They can appear to be normally concerned about, and giving to, their children, but in fact simply do not care. Others actively drive the children away by harshly or even sadistically punishing them. These families produce:

- Casual runaways, who, in contrast to the abortive or schizoidal runaways, separate with remarkable ease from the parents. These tough teenagers appear to be precocious socially and sexually. They are survivors in the runaway culture, although their object relations are shallow, exploitative, and transient.

3. *Delegating families*, according to Stierlin, are both expelling and binding at the same time. While ostensibly wishing to have the teenager remain part of the family, they "delegate" missions to fulfill certain unconscious impulses of their own. These families generate:

- Crisis runaways, who remain intensely and ambivalently preoccupied with their families, even though they may remain away for weeks. Their "missions" may satisfy the parent's wish for forbidden sexual or aggressive gratification, compensatory achievement, or punishment via risk-taking or criminal activity.

10.3. Acute Management of the Runaway

A runaway emergency may present in one of three ways: The runaway teenager comes to the ER or crisis clinic during a runaway episode, the parents of a missing runaway seek counseling and advice, and the parents bring in a returned or threatening runaway for family work.

Teenage runaway alone. The first step is to provide immediate help, and to promote a working alliance toward longer-term resolution of the problem. Immediate help might include treatment for veneral disease, malnutrition, skin or dental diseases, parasites, and/or pregnancies. If the patient is in no immediate danger, the clinician can move to arrange temporary placement at a runaway center, religious organization, group home, foster family, or social welfare facility. If the intervention is too radical (e.g., urging the child to return home), the runaway typically bolts from the ER.

After an alliance has been established, the clinician must determine whether or not to return the runaway to his home or to contact his parents. The safest course is undoubtedly the one that helps the teenager to weigh the decision from his own perspective. Getting as much detail about the home situation, the teenager, and the runaway episode can make the difference between a successful intervention and another failure. For example, it is essential to know how long the patient has been away from home, how well planned the "trip" was, whether it was undertaken alone or with friends, whether there was a triggering incident or a chronic pattern of abuse and neglect at home, how he has survived, and whether he has been exploited or involved in criminal behavior.

Abortive and crisis runaways are very likely to cooperate with the clinician's suggestion, even to permit contact with parents. Casual runaways rarely come to the ER, unless for purely manipulative reasons. They have usually broken primary ties years before, and are extremely difficult to treat in any psychiatric setting, especially as outpatients.

Schizoidal runaways are very hard to reach, even harder to assess. They seem disorganized and may be very depressed. A mental status examination is indicated for all runaways, but particularly for this group because of the high incidence of psychosis and suicidal ideation. If the runaway is disturbed enough to neglect or abuse his own welfare, hospitalization may be required.

Parents alone. In the days immediately following the runaway child's disappearance, parents are often overwhelmed with guilt and anger. This is a time for direct guidance and concrete advice: Attempts to find the child should be instituted promptly, police should be notified, and friends of the teenager called. Since friends often know exactly where the child has gone, parents should be advised to use patience and not resort to angry threats or bribes. Inquiries should also be made at various runaway shelters and clearing houses. Parents need support and an opportunity to begin reviewing anger, ambivalence, marital conflict, and family dynamics that may have contributed to the runaway. Family sessions can begin if there are other children at home, and can serve as a foundation for reintegrating the returned child. It is useful to discuss strategies for managing the child without pushing him farther away, or setting up a repetitive pattern for the future. Anger, threats of reprisal, and guilt-provoking barbs increase the likelihood that the child will leave again, but a submissive, guilty, or martyred stance sets the stage for future runaway episodes as well.

Parents and returned runaway together. It is essential that the family be seen together shortly after the runaway's return in order to forestall the return of old family patterns. The therapeutic goal is to alter the basic interactional style underlying the runaway episodes. It may be useful to begin with the concrete demands and counterdemands surrounding the running away and return, since these inevitably highlight the family's dynamics. Some families benefit from short-term, highly structured crisis intervention; others require some combination of longer-term family work, with individual treatment for the adolescent. When teenagers run away to escape internal turmoil and stress, they may need residential treatment in order to contain the symptomatic activity.

11. School Refusal

11.1. Introduction

Excessive school absenteeism can be caused by a number of different factors: illness, truancy, negligent parents, transportation problems, and some emotional disorders. School refusal, which is one aspect of childhood anxiety disorder (DSM III), is rarely the presenting complaint in a hospital emergency room. There are usually other more conspicuous problems, such as chronic somatic complaints with no discernible medical cause, suicidal threats, or acute psychotic decompensation. School refusal as a symptom in itself accounts on the average for approximately 10% of the typical child guidance clinic's crisis referrals.

Absenteeism is routine to almost every child's school experience. In middle-class school districts, for example, latency-age children and adolescents average about six to nine missed school days per year.[102,103] In large urban schools serving lower socioeconomic strata, the average number of missed days is considerably higher—a figure that parallels the increasing truancy rate in these areas. In general, a student who misses three weeks of school per year should be evaluated for a school avoidance disorder unless the child is suffering from a demonstrated medical condition or there are other extenuating circumstances preventing regular attendance.

School refusal or school phobia as a psychiatric symptom can be the product of complicated family psychopathology, as the following case demonstrates.

> A 42-year-old married mother of three was brought to the ER at 10:30 a.m. by her own 61-year-old mother. The younger woman was suffering from an attack of chest pain, light-headedness, and difficult breathing. Her 11-year-old son accompanied them. The child seemed unconcerned about missing school that day, and in fact had already missed several weeks while helping his mother during her "attacks." The medical examination proved unremarkable, as it had for other similar episodes. A psychiatric consultation was requested. School absenteeism proved to be one symptom within a serious multigenerational family conflict.

The first step in the emergency assessment of school avoidance is to rule out true medical illness, and thereafter to determine the psychosocial etiology. Associated with school avoidance are truancy, difficult home conditions, realistically distressing school situations, and genuinely phobic reactions. The most common cause of excessive absenteeism for children over 10 is truancy. Truant children are distinct from phobic children in the ease with which they leave home, presumably setting out for school. This type of behavior is often associated with other antisocial or deliquent behaviors. Unlike the true school phobics, these children generally have a history of misbehavior.

Other causes of excessive absenteeism are realistically distressing school situations and difficult home conditions. Children who are continually teased, beaten up, or otherwise victimized at school develop avoidance behaviors, even going to extreme lengths to escape from conditions they fear. When the threat of victimization is removed, however, these children return easily to school. Other children may be absent excessively because of an unusually dependent parent who treats her loneliness, physical illness, or crippling anxiety as an excuse to keep the child home. What clearly differentiates these cases of school absenteeism from genuine school phobias is the typical ease with which the former children can separate from their primary attachment figure(s).

The clinical history of school phobia begins with the child's marked reluctance to leave for school; exposure only escalates the child's anxiety and reluctance, often to the point of panic. Despite emphatic pressure from school authorities, punishment from parents, peer pressures, and the child's sincere wish to attend school, he is consistently overwhelmed by massive, intractable anxiety as he gets ready to leave home. Often the anxiety manifests as headache, stomachache, vomiting, diarrhea, dizziness, weakness, or achiness, none of which has a demonstrable organic etiology.

> John, a 7½-year-old child, was brought to the pediatric ER of a large urban hospital by his exasperated grandmother. That morning the child had been complaining that he felt "sick to his stomach," had a sore neck, and was shaking. The day before he had complained of diarrhea and pains in his side. The child appeared cheerful and unconcerned. Physical examination, CBC, sedimentation rate, throat and stool culture, and an infectious mononucleosis screening proved negative. During the clinical interview it was discovered that the boy's mother had run off 10 days before. The night before his symptoms began, she had phoned from California promising to come home "any day now."

The somatic symptoms typically begin when it is time to leave for school, on Sunday night, or at the end of a holiday. They disappear once the child is allowed to stay at home, during the summer months and long vacations.

A third variation of the clinical picture is scattered absenteeism, the result of chronic school phobia to which the child has made only a marginally effective adaptation. The child in this case is only periodically managing to control his separation anxiety, so that school absence is scattered but cumulative.

There is no clear-cut profile of the school-phobic child and no higher incidence among boys than girls. There are discernible trends, however: School phobia seems to occur with greater frequency among the youngest and oldest children, among the higher socioeconomic strata, and among upwardly striving middle-class families. The disorder seems to conform to family groupings and crosses generational lines.[104–106]

The dynamics of the school phobic child usually involve a mutually dependent, hostile relationship between mother and child. The mothers may be deeply committed to their children but have lifelong, unresolved dependency needs themselves. Most have a typically hostile, ambivalent interaction with their own mothers. The fathers, according to most studies, appear unable to assume effective and responsible paternal roles, behaving instead like anxious, hovering maternal figures.[105,107,108] Parents of the phobic child deliver duplicitous messages: "You must go to school, but maybe you had better stay home." Within this bind, the child is virtually paralyzed, highly vulnerable to the fear of abandonment, on the one hand, but unconsciously furious at the parent, on the other.

11.2. Relationship to Developmental Level

School phobias occur at any age and developmental stage. Fleeting episodes are probably a regular part of any childhood and may even extend through boarding school or college years. Pathological school phobia has identifiable features, however, and these are specific to the three developmental levels of childhood.

11.2.1. Prelatency

During the first few years of life, separation anxiety is expected, and adaptive. By the age of 3 years, most children have completed the process of separation/individuation and can master structured separations with minimal distress. For some children, however, vulnerability in this area becomes particularly evident at the time of nursery school or kindergarten. These children may appear happy, outgoing, and active at home, but careful investigation reveals weaknesses in the development of autonomy: history of sleep disturbances, inability to tolerate baby-sitters, sleeping in the parental bedroom (or bed) for several years. The parents may report having had no vacation together (without the children) since the birth of the child. It is not uncommon for the mother to be especially attached to the school-phobic child, either because of her own unresolved dependency needs or because the child is perceived as unusually vulnerable. Difficulties in conceiving, carrying, or delivering the child, life-threatening neonatal illness, recent divorce, or death of the mother's parent are sufficient to set up an overprotective mother–child relationship.[109,110]

The presenting style of school phobia in the prelatency child may not involve symptoms until separation from the parent has occurred. Anxiety or terror may not be evident before or during separation, but the affected child may be withdrawn, whiney, or alternately clingy and aloof at the day care center or nursery school.

> Sharon, a 3-year-old Japanese-American girl would enter her nursery school each morning without overt distress, but within a few minutes would gravitate to the edge of the group. She could often be seen sitting forlornly at the periphery of a room looking out the window. Although she was able to interact well with the adult aides or teacher, her mother reported Sharon would regularly burst into tears in the car on the way home, and would follow the mother around the house for several hours, crying inconsolably.

11.2.2. Latency

While a young child with school phobia can be withdrawn from the phobic setting—nursery school or day care—until he "outgrows" his fears, elementary school offers no such escape. The phobic symptoms intensify accordingly: Trepidation, terror, humiliation, self-reproach, and defensive somatization become part of the clinical picture. School phobia at this point is compounded by the developmental stage, as the pressure mounts to disengage from parents and move toward peer relationships. The wish to relinquish the nuclear bonding of early childhood conflicts with the fear of doing so. The precipitants of the "first" episode are typically minor events; the birth of a sibling, for example, the vacation of parents, minor illnesses in the mother, or a German police dog en route to school are the conspicuous corollaries for a complicated, unconscious displacement pattern.

The longer the child is permitted to avoid school, the more deeply entrenched the avoidance behavior becomes. The child begins to show impairment in crucial areas of development, and pathology spreads to most areas of ego function.

11.2.3. Late Latency and Adolescence

In early and mid-latency, school phobia is most likely to present as an acute, intensely symptomatic syndrome. The adolescent presentation is less abrupt, following a period of gradual withdrawal, increasing sullenness, and defiance. The cynical, critical posture with respect to school yields to panic and immobility as the syndrome develops. If the youngster is pressured to return to school, reluctance turns to refusal. Children of this type have commonly had earlier periods of school refusal and a long-standing history of subclinical emotional troubles. Because adolescence involves a second individuation process, the push toward separation frequently impels a precariously balanced youngster and family into a pathological position.

11.3. Prognosis

The acute onset of school phobia in the younger child has a generally favorable outcome. In one study, 90% of treated children under the age of 11 made a successful school adjustment in contrast with only 35% of older children.[111] Other clinicians, however, have established a success rate in the neighborhood of 90–95% even for older patients.[105,112] However, Coolidge et al. have found that school-phobic children who were treatment successes continued to lead constricted, phobic, passive lives 10 years later.[112] This was particularly evident among the males, who were culturally unable to hide their dependent, fearful traits, unlike their female counterparts, who could conceal extreme dependency within their marriages, which usually allowed displacement of the binding attachment from parents to husband.

11.4. Emergency Management of School Refusal

Although there are reportedly several techniques for the treatment of school phobia, the following steps, which have been modified from the work of Lassers et al.,[113] are extremely useful:

1. The child who presents with school refusal in combination with a physical complaint should have a pediatric evaluation. Medical illness should be ruled out as a matter of course. When there is no medical justification for keeping the child at home, neither parent nor child can continue to use the physical symptom in the service of ambivalence about school-imposed separation.

2. The clinician should assess parental involvement in the symptom. If the mother is inordinately distressed or panicky, and seems overidentified with the child's phobic reaction, the diagnosis of school phobia secondary to pathological family dynamics is almost certainly confirmed.

3. The interviewer should do a mental status examination, particularly with adolescent patients, to rule out the presence of psychosis, impending psychosis, or depression. Managing these and other psychiatric symptoms takes precedence over treating school avoidance behavior.

4. The clinician should gather as much detail as possible about the phobic syndrome, what it means to the patient and family, who sympathizes with it, and who opposes it.

5. The family dynamics and structure should be examined independent of the symptom: i.e., who is allied with whom, and who is dominant. If necessary, the clinician may have to enlist the aid of a strong or influential member of the family's social system (e.g., relative, neighbor, clergyman, or pediatrician) who can exert therapeutic leverage. This person will work closely with the therapist during the intervention phase.

6. Once the details about the patient, syndrome, and family are known, the clinician should negotiate the acute treatment plan with the family. Reassuring the family, altering environmental factors, and cajoling the child are likely to be ineffective unless the family sees the symptom as a result of mutual separation anxiety. As the reasons for the symptom are clarified, the major treatment objective is introduced—the child *must* return to school. If the family refuses all reasonable efforts to enlist their cooperation, the clinician may need to communicate his intention to involve the local courts via a truancy petition, or a "child-in-need-of-services" petition. Residential school placement or hospitalization are other options to ensure interruption of the school-phobic cycle, and may be required if the child and parents cannot effect a return to school on their own.

7. The school should be involved in treatment planning, if possible. The school principal, teacher, counselor, nurse, or truant officer should be present at a treatment session to work out the mechanics of school attendance: the timing of arrival at school, strategies for containing panic, and prevention of running away.

8. If a comprehensive therapeutic program fails, the clinician may need to consider alternative placement of the child. If the parents have been cooperative and the symptom is still intractable, drug therapy might be introduced. Imipramine (Tofranil) is effective, particularly in adolescents who have accompanying depressive symptoms. The child can be started on an initial dose of 25 mg/day for three days, then 50 mg for four days. By the second week, the dose should be increased to 75 mg/day. Thereafter, the dose can be increased by 25 mg every few days until a dose of 75 to 150 mg (about 3 to 5 mg/kg) is reached. Some clinical effect is usually evident after four to six weeks although it may require two to three months in some cases. Adverse effects include dizziness, headache, insomnia, and gastrointestinal symptoms. After

complete symptom remission, imipramine can be gradually tapered over three months.[114]

12. Other Problems

Up to this point, this chapter has focused on some psychiatric conditions of childhood and adolescence that warrant emergency attention—generally aberrant or destructive behaviors such as suicidal attempts, running away, school refusal, and aggressive behaviors. Because affective states in children typically manifest as activity or behavior, it is the activity, and not necessarily the underlying affect, that prompts acute evaluation.

The activities described thus far require some degree of self-organization. Bizarre, psychotic behavior, or intractable, seemingly autonomous symptoms like head-banging, vomiting, and hicupping are patterns that develop over time and are therefore more likely to be taken first to the pediatrician or pediatric service than to the emergency psychiatrist. For those patients who present first to the psychiatric service, it is essential to rule out a medical condition initially. If the primary diagnosis is childhood psychosis, the dispositional decision should include referral for medication-evaluation and long-term therapy. If the primary diagnosis is an intractable behavioral disorder with no identifiable organic etiology, referral to a longer-term behavioral/psychotherapy treatment program is indicated. If the welfare of the child is seriously threatened by the psychotic or behavioral symptoms, if the diagnosis is uncertain, or if the parents prove uncooperative, it may be necessary to hospitalize the child until appropriate therapeutic measures have been initiated.

13. Conclusion

Childhood and adolescent emergencies are not adult crises in miniature. They are crises of their own type with courses, pathogenic influences, and treatment requisites different from those of their adult counterparts. To say that childhood is a time of unavoidable dependency underscores the vibrant links between children and their adult caretakers. A child's psychiatric crisis is profoundly affected by his interpersonal environment, and in turn can set in motion, like ripples from a single pebble, reverberating effects throughout the entire social system.

References

General Sections 1–6

1. Khan AV: Preface, in *Psychiatric Emergencies in Pediatrics*. Year Book Medical Publishers, June 1979, pp vii–viii.
2. Sandifer MG Jr: Service and set in treatment decisions. *Am J Psychiatry* 128:1140–1145, 1972.

3. Bristol JH, Giller E Jr, Docherty JP: Trends in emergency psychiatry in the last two decades. *Am J Psychiatry* 138:623–628, 1981.
4. Huffine CL, Craig TJ: Social factors in the utilization of an urban psychiatric emergency service. *Arch Gen Psychiatry* 30:249–255, 1974.
5. Tyson R, Miller S, Brown C: A study of psychiatry emergencies: Part I. Demographic data. *Psychiatry Med* 1:349–357, 1970.
6. Parad JH, Parad LG: A study of crisis oriented planned short-term treatment. *Soc Casework* 49:346–355; 418–426, 1968.
7. Glasscote RM, Fishman ME, Sonis M: *Children and Mental Health: Progress, Problems, Prospects.* Washington, Joint Information Service of the American Psychiatric Association, 1972.
8. Morrison GC, Smith WR: Emergencies in child psychiatry: A definition, in Morrison GC (ed): *Emergencies in Child Psychiatry.* Springfield, Ill, Charles C Thomas, 1975, pp 13–20.
9. Morrison GC: Therapeutic intervention in a child psychiatric emergency service. *J Am Acad Child Psychiatry* 8:542–558, 1969.
10. Morrison GC, Smith WR: Child psychiatric emergencies: A comparison of two clinic settings and socio-economic groups. in Morrison GC (ed.): *Emergencies in Child Psychiatry.* Springfield, Ill, Charles C Thomas, 1975, pp 107–114.
11. Mattson A, Hawkins JW, Seese LR: Child psychiatric emergencies: Clinical characteristics and follow-up results. *Arch Gen Psychiatry* 17:584–592, 1967.
12. Shafii M, Whittinghill R, Healy MG: The pediatric-psychiatric model for emergencies in child psychiatry: A study of 994 cases. *Am J Psychiatry* 136:1250–1601, 1979.
13. Schowalter JE, Solnit AJ: Child psychiatry consultation in a general hospital emergency room. *J Am Acad Child Psychiatry* 5:534–549, 1966.
14. Pruett KD: Home treatment for two infants who witnessed their mother's murder. *J Am Acad Child Psychiatry* 18:647–657, 1979.
15. Simmons JE: *Psychiatric Examination of Children.* Philadelphia, Lea & Febiger, 1974.
16. Goodman JD, Sours JA: *The Child Mental Status Examination.* New York, Basic Books, 1967.
17. Cohen RL: The approach to assessment, in Noshpitz JD (ed.): *Basic Handbook of Child Psychiatry*, vol I. New York, Basic Books, 1979, pp 485–551.
18. Lewis M: *Clinical Aspects of Child Development.* Philadelphia, Lea & Febiger, 1982.
19. Group for Advancement of Psychiatry, Report # 38: The Diagnostic Process in Child Psychiatry. New York, 1957, pp 313–353.

Suicide (Section 7)

20. Holinger PC: Adolescent suicide: An epidemiological study of recent trades. *Am J Psychiatry* 135:754–756, 1978.
21. Data from the Mortality Statistics Branch, National Center for Health Statistics, Department of Health, Education and Welfare, in *Children's World.* Boston, Children's Hospital, Fall 1980.
22. Khan AV: Grief, depression and suicide, in *Psychiatric Emergencies in Pediatrics.* Year Book Medical Publishers, 1979, pp 96–119.
23. McIntire MS, Angle CR: "Suicide" as seen in poison control centers. *Pediatrics* 48:914–922, 1971.
24. Lawler RH, Nakielny W, Wright N: Suicidal attempts in children. *Can Med Assoc J* 89:751, 1963.
25. Jacobziner H: Attempted suicides in adolescence. *JAMA* 191:101–105, 1965.
26. Weiner IB: *Psychological Disturbance in Adolescence.* New York, Wiley-Interscience, 1970.
27. McAnarney ER: Suicidal behavior of children and youth. *Pediatr Clin North Am* 22:595–614, 1975.
28. Tuckman J, Cannon HE: Attempted suicide in adolescents. *Am J Psychiatry* 119:228–232, 1962.

29. Teicher JD: Suicide and suicide attempts, in Noshpitz J (ed): *Basic Handbook of Child Psychiatry*, vol. II. New York, Basic Books, 1979, pp 685–697.
30. Morrison GC, Collier JG: Family treatment approaches to suicidal children and adolescents. *J Am Acad Child Psychiatry* 8:140–153, 1969.
31. Ackerly WC: Latency age children who threaten or attempt to kill themselves. *J Am Acad Child Psychiatry* 6:242–261, 1967.
32. Paulson MJ, Stone D, Sposto R: Suicide potential and behavior in children ages 4 to 12. *Suicide Life Threat Behav* 8:225–242, 1978.
33. Aleksandrowicz MK: The biological strangers. *Bull Menninger Clin* 39:163–176, 1975.
34. Haider I: Suicidal attempts in children and adolescents. *Br J Psychiatry* 114:1133–1134, 1968.
35. Otto U: Suicidal acts by children and adolescents. *Acta Psychiatr Scand Suppl* 233:5–123, 1972.
36. Green AH: Self-destructive behavior in battered children. *Am J Psychiatry* 135:579–582, 1978.
37. Schrut A: Suicidal adolescents and children. *JAMA* 188:1103–1107, 1964.
38. Schecter MD: The recognition and treatment of suicide in children, in Shneidman ES, Farberow N (eds.): *Clues to Suicide*. New York, McGraw-Hill, 1957, pp 131–143.
39. Litman RE: Sigmund Freud on suicide, in Schneidman ES (ed.): *Essays on Self Destruction*. New York, Holt, Rinehart & Winston, 1968.
40. Margolin NL, Teicher JD: Thirteen adolescent male suicide attempts. *J Am Acad Child Psychiatry* 8:296–315, 1968.
41. Toolan JM: Suicide and suicidal attempts in children and adolescents. *Am J Psychiatry* 118:719–724, 1962.
42. Mattson A, Hawkins JW, Seese LR: Suicidal behavior as a child psychiatric emergency. *Arch Gen Psychiatry* 20:100–109, 1969.
43. Teicher JD, Jacobs J: Adolescents who attempt suicide: Preliminary findings. *Am J Psychiatry* 122:1248–1257, 1966.
44. Lukianowicz N: Attempted suicide in children. *Acta Psychiatr Scand* 44:415–435, 1968.
45. Pfeffer CR, Conte HR, Plutchik R, et al: Suicidal behavior in latency age children: An outpatient population. *J Am Acad Child Psychiatry* 19:703–710, 1980.
46. Poznanski RO, Krahenbuhl V, Zrull JP: Childhood depression: A longitudinal perspective. *J Am Acad Child Psychiatry* 15:491–501, 1976.
47. Waldron S: The significance of childhood neurosis for adult mental health: A follow-up study. *Am J Psychiatry* 133:532–538, 1976.
48. Duncan W: Immediate management of suicide attempts in children and adolescents: Psychological aspects. *J Family Practice* 4:77–80, 1977.
49. Shaffer D: Suicide in childhood and early adolescence. *J Child Psychol Psychiatry* 15:275–291, 1974.
50. Petti TA: Depression in hospitalized child psychiatry patients: Approaches to measuring depression. *J Am Acad Child Psychiatry* 17:49–59, 1978.
51. Piug-Antich J, Blau S, Marx N: Prepubertal major depressive disorder: A pilot study. *J Am Acad Child Psychiatry* 17:695–707, 1978.
52. Citryn L, MckNew DH Jr, Barney WF Jr: Diagnosis of depression in children: A reassessment. *Am J Psychiatry* 137:22–25, 1980.
53. Kashani JH, Husain A, Shekim WO, et al: Current perspectives on childhood depression: An overview. *Am J Psychiatry* 138:143–152, 1981.
54. Carlson GA, Cantwell DP: Unmasking marked depression in children and adolescents. *Am J Psychiatry* 137:445–449, 1980.
55. Anthony EJ: Childhood depression, in Anthony EJ, Benedek T (eds.): *Depression and Human Existence*. Boston, Little, Brown & Co, 1975, pp 231–277.
56. Bemporad JR, Wilson A: A developmental approach to depression in childhood and adolescence. *J Am Acad Psychoanal* 6:325–352, 1978.
57. Glaser K: Marked depression in children and adolescents: Psychodynamic observations. *Am J Psychother* 21:565–574, 1967.
58. Maurer A: Motivation of concepts of death. *Br J Med Psychol* 39:35–41, 1966.

59. Pfeffer PR, Conte HR, Plutchik R, et al: Suicidal behavior in latency aged children: An empirical study. *J Am Acad Child Psychiatry* 18:679–692, 1979.
60. Toolan JM: Depression in children and adolescents. *Am J Orthopsychiatry* 32:404–414, 1962.
61. Nagy M: The child's view of death, in Feifel H (ed): *The Meaning of Death*. New York, McGraw-Hill, 1959.
62. Gould RE: Suicidal problems in children and adolescents. *Am J Psychother* 19:228–246, 1965.
63. Shaw CR, Schelkun RF: Suicidal behavior in children. *Psychiatry* 28:157–168, 1965.
64. Anthony S: *Discovery of Death in Childhood and After*. New York, Basic Books, 1972.
65. Jacobs J: *Adolescent Suicide*. New York, Wiley Interscience, 1971.
66. Laufer M: The body image, the function of masturbation, and adolescence: Problems of the ownership of the body. *Psychoanal Study Child* 23:114–137, 1968.
67. Erlich HS: Adolescent suicide. *Psychoanal Study Child* 33:261–277, 1978.

Homicide (Section 8)

68. Marohn RC: Adolescent violence: Causes and treatment. *J Am Acad Child Psychiatry* 21:354–360, 1982.
69. Hollinger P: Violent deaths among the young: Recent trends in suicide, homicide and accidents. *Am J Psychiatry* 136:1144–1147, 1979.
70. Hollinger P: Violent deaths as a leading cause of mortality: An epidemiological study of suicide, homicide and accidents. *Am J Psychiatry* 137:472–476, 1980.
71. Bender L: Children and adolescents who have killed. *Am J Psychiatry* 116:510–513, 1959.
72. Carek DJ, Watson AS: Treatment of a family involved in fratricide. *Arch Gen Psychiatry* 11:533–542, 1964.
73. Curtis GC: Violence breeds violence—perhaps? *Am J Psychiatry* 120:386–387, 1963.
74. Paluszny MD, NcNable M: Therapy of a 6-year-old who committed fratricide. *J Am Acad Child Psychiatry* 14:319–336, 1975.
75. Adelson L: The battering child. *JAMA* 22:159–161, 1972.
76. Tooley K: The small assassins. Clinical notes on a subgroup of murderous children. *J Am Acad Child Psychiatry* 14:306–318, 1975.
77. Malmquist CP: Premonitory sign of homicidal aggression in juveniles. *Am J Psychiatry* 123:461–465, 1971.
78. West DJ: *Murder Followed by Suicide*. Cambridge, Harvard University Press, 1967.
79. Burks HL, Harrison SI: Aggressive behavior as a means of avoiding depression. *Am J Orthopsychiatry* 32:416–422, 1962.
80. Macdonald JM: Homicidal threats. *Am J Psychiatry* 124:475–482, 1967.
81. Gibson E, Klein S: *Murder*. London, H. M. Stationery Office, 1961.
82. King CH: The ego and the integration of violence in homicidal youth. *Am J Orthopsychiatry* 45:134–145, 1975.
83. Hellman DS, Blackman N: Enuresis, firesetting, and cruelty to animals: A triad predictive of adult crime. *Am J Psychiatry* 122:1431–1435, 1966.
84. Justice B, Justice R, Kraft IA: Early-warning signs of violence: Is a triad enough? *Am J Psychiatry* 131:457–459, 1974.
85. Sendi IB, Blomgren PG: A comparative study of predictive criteria in the predisposition of homicidal adolescents. *Am J Psychiatry* 132:423–427, 1975.
86. Lewis DO, Pincus JH, Shanok SS, Glaser GH: Psychomotor epilepsy and violence in a group of incarcerated adolescent boys. *Am J Psychiatry* 139:882–887, 1982.
87. Robins L: *Deviant Children Grown Up*. Baltimore, Williams & Wilkins, 1966.
88. Detre TP, Kupfer DJ, Taub S: The Nosology of violence. Read at Symposium on the Neural Basis of Violence and Aggression, Houston, Tex, 1972.
89. Pincus JH, Tucker GJ: Violence in children and adults: A neurological view. *J Am Acad Child Psychiatry* 17:227–288, 1978.
90. Inamdar SC, Lewis DD, Siomopulous G, Shanok SS, Lamela M: Violent and suicidal behavior in psychotic adolescents. *Am J Psychiatry* 139:932–935, 1982.

Firesetting (Section 9)

91. Dietz J: Punishment no answer for kids who set fires, doctors say. *Boston Globe*, February 14, 1982, p 31.
92. Kaufman I, Herms LW, Reiser DE: A reevaluation of the psychodynamics of firesetting. *Am J Orthopsychiatyr* 31:123–136, 1961.
93. Vanersall TA, Weiner JM: Children who set fires. *Arch Gen Psychiatry* 22:63–71, 1970.
94. Yarnell H: Firesetting in children. *Am J Orthopsychiatry* 10:272–286, 1940.
95. Macht LB, Mack JE: The firesetter syndrome. *Psychiatry* 31:277–288, 1968.
96. Lewis NDC, Yarnell H: Pathological firesetting (pyromania). *Nerv Ment Dis Monogr* No. 82, 1951.

Runaway (Section 10)

97. Schmidt WM: Runaway children. *JAMA* 232:651–652, 1975.
98. Montgomery BJ: Teenagers trade homes for streets: Why? *JAMA* 240:16–17, 1978.
99. Shafii M, Whittinghill R, Healy MG: The pediatric psychiatric model for emergencies in child psychiatry: A study of 994 cases. *Am J Psychiatry* 136:1660–1601, 1979.
100. Stierlin H: A family perspective on adolescent runaways. Arch Gen Psychiatry 29:56–62, 1973.
101. Stierlin H, Ravenscroft K: Varieties of adolescent "separation," *Br J Med Psychol* 45:299–313, 1972.

School Refusal (Section 11)

102. Rogers K, Reese G: *Health studies. Am J Dis Child* 109:9–27, 1965.
103. Berganza CE, Anders TF: An epidemiologic approach to school absenteesm. *J Am Acad Child Psychiatry* 17:117–125, 1978.
104. Crusnley FE. A school phobia in a three-generational family conflict. *J Am Acad Child Psychiatry* 13:536–550, 1974.
105. Skynner AC: School phobia: A reappraisal. *Br J Med Psychol* 47:1–16, 1974.
106. Waldron S Jr, Shrier DK, Stone B, Tobin F: School phobia and other childhood neuroses: A systematic study of the children and their families. *Am J Psychiatry* 132:882–888, 1975.
107. Coolidge JC: School phobia, in Noshpitz JD (ed): *Basic Handbook of Child Psychiatry*, vol. II. New York, Basic Books, 1979, pp 453–463.
108. Green M, Solnit AJ: Reactions to the threatened loss of a child: A vulnerable child syndrome. Pediatrics 34:58–61, 1964.
109. Rodriguez A, Rodriguez M, Eisenberg L: The outcome of school phobia: A follow-up study based on 41 cases. *Am J Psychiatry* 116:540–544, 1959.
110. Coolidge JC, Brodie RD: Observation of mothers of 49 school phobia children evaluated in a 10-year old follow-up study. *J Am Acad Child Psychiatry* 13:275–285, 1974.
111. Waldfogel S, Tessman E, Hahn PB. A program for early intervention in school phobia. *Am J Orthopsychiatry* 29:324–352, 1959.
112. Coolidge JC, Hahn PB, Peck AL: School phobia: Neurotic crisis or way of life. *Am J Orthopsychiatry* 27:296–306, 1957.
113. Lassers E, Nordan R, Bladholm S: Steps in the return to school of children with school phobia. *Am J Psychiatry* 130:265–268, 1973.
114. Kaplan C: Pediatric psychopharmacology, in Bassuk EL, Schoonover SC, Gelenberg AJ (eds.): *The Practitioner's Guide to Psychoactive Drugs*, ed 2. New York, Plenum Publishing Corp, 1983, pp 313–352.

19

Elderly Psychiatric Emergency Patients

Sarah L. Minden, M.D.

1. Introduction

This chapter is devoted to the special problems of geriatric patients in crisis. Although traditional assessment and management techniques are generally applicable to elderly patients, the clinical problems unique to this population warrant separate treatment. This chapter presents general guidelines for working effectively with the elderly and their families in an emergency setting.

2. Overview

2.1. Extent of the Problem

In 1980 there were an estimated 25 million Americans over 65. By 2000 there will be 33 million, constituting 12–25% of the total population.[1] The elderly comprise nearly one-third of all first admissions to psychiatric hospitals.[2] Household surveys of elderly patients living in the community reveal that significant numbers are mentally ill. One study noted that 6.3% were so disordered that they met clinical criteria for involuntary mental hospital admission.[3] Other research indicates that between 10 and 20% of senior citizens have "a significant degree of memory defect, disorientation, and decline in intellectual performance."[4]

It is important to note that most geriatric patients do live in the community—only 5% are in institutions (mental hospitals, nursing homes, etc.) Yet, because community services are so limited,[5] the problems of the elderly can reach crisis proportions before adequate care is received. The problems themselves are typically complex, involving physical illness, intellectual impairment, social and economic hardships, and personal losses.

2.2. Some Facts about Aging

Some decline in intellectual ability, sensory acuity, and motor skill is an inevitable part of aging,[3] but the degree to which it is felt varies with the in-

Sarah L. Minden, M.D. • Harvard Medical School, and Brigham and Women's Hospital, Boston, Massachusetts 02115.

dividual. Some persons continue vigorous physical activity well into their 70s, while others are slowed and weakened by age 60. These individual differences reflect the intricate interplay of genetic and constitutional factors, personality, roles and relationships (work, marriage, friendships), current life situation (financial resources, available supports), and medical history. In 1955 the National Institute of Mental Health began to study healthy older people living in the community to assess the effects of aging alone, uncontaminated by illness and institutionalization. They found that "the men . . . over 65 [$N = 47$, mean age = 71] . . . [had] cerebral physiological and intellectual functions that compared favorably with a young control group," and concluded that "intellectual abilities declined not as a consequence of the mysterious process of aging, but rather as a result of specific diseases [e.g., Alzheimer's disease, cerebrovascular disease, etc.]. Therefore, senility is not an inevitable outcome of aging."[6] Slowed responses were not due to aging alone but were "statistically related to environmental deprivation and depression as well as to declining health."[6]

Many elderly persons cannot reliably retain new and complex information, although old and familiar or recent, personally significant material is well preserved. They also experience a predictable and progressive deterioration of vision and hearing.[7] Such losses can lead to anxiety, withdrawal, and distortion of meaning sometimes evolving into paranoia. These sensory and cognitive deficits, compounded by increased motor instability, contribute to the high incidence of accidents.[8]

Sleeping difficulties increase with age. The deeper phases of the sleep cycle are lost and there are more periods of brief arousal throughout the night, giving the impression of sleeplessness even though there is no real reduction of total sleep time. There is, therefore, little rational basis for prescribing hypnotics in this situation.

3. Working with the Geriatric Patient

Effective emergency work with geriatric patients requires passing beyond the stereotypes of old age to the actual person in crisis, and regarding him within the context of his life and social circumstances. Proper evaluation entails involvement with family or other persons close to the patient.

3.1. Stereotypes of the Aged

Stereotypes of the aged are prominent in our society: There is, for example, the good-natured, bespectacled grandparent, the cantankerous scrooge, the foolish old woman, or the lecherous old man, all of which portray senile incompetence. The real person is obviously not a stereotype but a human being with a unique personality and particular problems. Vigilance against the nihilism that comes from preconceived ideas and unwarranted feelings of fear, contempt, and anger results in better psychiatric care for older people.

A myth about old age is that it is a time of hopelessness and progressive disengagement from life. On the contrary, the NIMH study found that "psychological flexibility, resourcefulness, and optimism, rather than the stereotype of rigidity, characterized the group."[6] The report emphasized the stability of character over time: A person who was creative, sociable, adaptive when young would continue to make a satisfying life for himself and cope effectively with the inevitable losses of old age. It also stressed the interaction of biology and psychology in accounting for differences between those who survived and those who died during the five-year follow-up study. The nonsurvivors showed a "greater [incidence] of arteriosclerosis and chronic cigarette smoking . . . [but also they] had not adapted as well psychologically, were more likely to have lost their spouses, and had been more dissatisfied with their living situations" than their counterparts who had survived. They also had fewer clearly defined goals. The report concluded that "survival was associated with the individual's self-view and a sense of continued usefulness, in addition to good physical health. At the end of eleven years, structured and varied new contacts and self-initiated activities and involvement were also strongly associated with survival, an observation counter to the disengagement theory [of aging]."[6]

Another myth is that nothing can be done about the problems of the elderly. Gibson notes that 75% of geriatric patients in a private psychiatric hospital from 1960 to 1964 improved and went home within two months.[9] The likelihood of successful treatment is even greater today given the psychopharmacological advances in the management of depression, anxiety, and psychosis and the broader understanding of organic causes of psychiatric illness. Moreover, according to the NIMH study, the factors crucial to outcome are likely to be the malleable ones: "education, occupation, and other lifelong social factors were as critical to adaptation as was the degree of current environmental deprivation."[9] Given appropriate treatment for underlying psychiatric disorders and opportunities for enhanced social involvement, older people can improve their quality of life and consequent chances of survival; improved self-esteem and sense of purpose in turn contribute to better physical health.

In fact, there is reason for optimism. Palmore et al.[10] evaluated the impact of the major crises of aging, retirement, illness, widowhood, and the departure of the last child from home, and found that even "the most seriously ill persons manage to limit [adverse] social-psychological reactions to a short period after the illness and to return to baseline within a few months."[10] Only the cumulative effect of these events was sufficient to cause a notable degree of distress, and outcome again depended on the physical, social, and psychological resources of the individuals themselves.

3.2. Engaging the Geriatric Patient

Engaging an older person in a meaningful interaction to obtain a complete history and mental status examination can be a challenge. The suggestions that follow may seem obvious but are worth noting again: The aged patient should be seen alone first, if possible, and he should be addressed by title and surname.[11] Relatives should not be included in any interaction without the express permission of the patient, unless there is no way to communicate without them. The patient's capacity to see and hear ought to be explicitly assessed and the interview structured accordingly; patients with visual or auditory impairment can usually suggest the best way to proceed. Idiosyncratic communication patterns should be judged in context: Rambling or repetitiveness may not be signs of psychopathology but instead may reflect great loneliness or be an attempt to postpone return to an isolated setting; suspiciousness and overt hostility may be the result of living in a crime-ridden community or may indicate realistic fears of being placed in a nursing home. To clarify the situation, the interviewer should encourage the patient to talk freely about his worries, fears, and attitudes.

3.3. Talking with Persons Close to the Patient

Whether the elderly patient comes to the ER alone or is brought by others, a central part of the assessment involves evaluating his social system. In doing so, conflicting interests may emerge: The patient has his own problems while those close to him may have their own "chief complaint." Caretakers may refer to troublesome behavior—the patient is noisy, up all night, stubborn or abusive, dangerous to himself or others. Careful observation of the interaction between patient and caretakers or family members may suggest ways in which the social system has contributed to the development and maintenance of symptoms and provide a starting point for management.

If the patient comes alone, every effort should be made to locate people who know him in order to corroborate history and provide pertinent information about the current crisis. Given the high incidence of subtle cognitive dysfunction in this age group, it is essential that historical and medical data be confirmed by other sources. Since diagnosis is based in part on historical data, an accurate picture of baseline function and onset of symptoms is essential. Dementia, for example, can be distinguished from both depression and delirium on the basis of history: i.e., a gradual deterioration of short-term memory over five years signifies a disease process very different from the one that produces a sudden failure to recall recent events. Learning that a patient has "always been unhappy" may suggest a characterologic rather than a medication-responsive depression. Historical information of this sort is typically provided by persons other than the patient himself.

4. Assessment, Management, and Treatment

4.1. Triage

Because of the frequency and seriousness of medical illness, triage assumes a central place in the care of geriatric patients. The first sign of a life-threatening medical illness in an elderly person may be an abnormal mental status. Florid psychiatric symptoms can obscure a coexisting medical problem (e.g., broken hip or myocardial infarction), and an acute physical disorder can cause an aberration in mental status (e.g., subdural hematoma or pneumonia).

Assessment begins with noting the patient's level of consciousness. Unless fully alert, the patient should be evaluated immediately by medical staff. Similarly, inability to attend to and grasp the current situation may point to underlying organic problems. Because "a little disorientation" in a normal elderly patient is a meaningless concept, disorientation of any degree suggests a pathological process in the brain. While disorientation and inattention may be part of a long-standing dementing process that does not require immediate medical attention, the same symptoms may also be of relatively recent onset. A brief history from family members will usually clarify the situation. If such a history is not available, however, it is necessary to proceed with a physical examination.

Checking vital signs is imperative. Since aged persons frequently fail to produce an elevated body temperature in response to infection, other signs are important: rapid pulse, low blood pressure, subnormal temperature, cool and clammy skin. Check mucous membranes for hydration and extremities for edema.

Many old people do not complain of pain with myocardial infarction, fractured hip, or infarction of the bowel, for example. The reasons for this are complex and include acute confusion and diminished awareness, altered pain sensation because of aging, and deliberate concealment of pain to avoid hospitalization.

Historic data are also essential to triage. Medications, for example, might be the cause of an organic brain syndrome: intracranial hemorrhage with coumadin, confusion with analgesics, antidepressants, digoxin, and antihypertensives. There should be direct inquiry about recent falls, head injury, and other physical trauma. Finally, it is essential to determine if the patient is troubled by suicidal impulses.

Violence is not common in the geriatric population, but there are situations when an elderly patient is combative due perhaps to delirium or paranoid fears. Management follows the guidelines for other assaultive patients, but with some special considerations (see Chapter 6). Because it is possible that the aged patient has an organic brain syndrome, it is prudent to rely on physical restraint and avoid antipsychotic medication until a diagnosis has been made. Such medication could aggravate a drug-induced delirium, depress CNS function, and obscure essential neurologic signs. Care must be taken in using physical restraints: elderly patients have fragile bones that easily fracture. In most cases, patients respond to reassurance and another person's presence. If medication is necessary, however, haloperidol (Haldol) is the drug of choice, beginning with small doses of 0.25 mg IM, repeated every 1–2 hours, with a ceiling of 2–4 mg in 24 hours. This schedule should be sufficient to calm the patient without excessive sedation.

4.2. Mental Status Examination (MSE)

The mental status examination of the geriatric patient is the same as that for younger individuals, but it may be more difficult to administer because of frank resistance or impaired concentration. Fearing ''failure,'' the patient may refuse to answer questions by registering protest verbally or silently, changing the subject, or even experiencing a panic attack. Since many elements of the MSE are just as well evaluated informally through history-taking and conversation with the patient, it is possible (and desirable) to use examinationlike questions sparingly. When formal testing is required, the purpose should be made explicit—''I want to test your memory''—and the patient should be reassured in a general way about his performance. Testing should never proceed beyond the point where enough information has been gained to make sound clinical judgments.

The overriding purpose of the MSE in this population is to distinguish functional from organic disorders and to assess the degree of impairment. The items outlined in Table 1 have been selected for their usefulness in making these distinctions. Some familiar tests[12-17] such as subtraction of serial sevens, spelling *world* backwards, or repeating digits forward and backward have been omitted because they do not specifically differentiate between organic and functional disorders,[15-17] although they do measure attentiveness. Structured questioning may amplify, but does not replace, thoughtful observation of appearance and behavior, thought processes, mood, and attitude.

4.3. Medical Status

Organic brain syndromes, particularly delirium and dementia, occur more frequently in the elderly population than in any other. Delirium, also called acute confusional state or acute organic brain syndrome, is characterized by ''a clouded state of consciousness, that is, a reduction in the clarity of awareness of the environment. This is manifested by difficulty in sustaining attention to both external and internal stimuli, sensory misperception, and a disordered stream of thought.''[18] The sleep cycle is also disturbed, and there may be significantly increased or decreased psychomotor activity. The patient is typically disoriented, has impaired memory, and may be emotionally labile. These features develop over a short period of time, hours to days, with a striking tendency to fluctuate so that at times the patient may seem quite normal. Delirium in the geriatric patient may have some atypical features that can obscure the diagnosis: insidious onset and quiet, withdrawn, or apathetic attitude. When delirium is superimposed on other chronic disorders such as dementia or schizophrenia, alterations in mental status may be incorrectly attributed to the primary syndrome.

Delirious patients are only dimly aware of what is happening to their mental functioning; they may be frightened and paranoid as a result. Support, reassurance, reality testing, frequent repetition of instructions and explanations, and attention to physical safety (Posey® restraint, constant observation) are essential to sound management.

Table 1. Mental Status Examination Questions

Question	Function tested
1. "Where are we now?" 2. "What is the name of this place and where is it located?"	Orientation to place
3. "What is the day of the week and the date today?"	Orientation to time
4. "Who is . . . ?" Point to a familiar person, or ask for that person's name and relationship.	Orientation to person Orientation distinguishes organic and functional disorders; it should be intact with the latter. It does not test a specific cognitive function. Orientation should be exact to within a day of the actual day and to within a few dates of the actual date. Orientation to person tends to be better preserved than orientation to time.
5. "Please repeat this sentence after me; try to remember it and I will ask you to repeat it later: 'The purple fox runs.'" OR "Please repeat these items after me, and then I'd like you to remember them. I will ask you to repeat them later: Name three objects." 6. At three- and five-minute intervals ask patient to repeat items of question #5.	Immediate recall and short-term memory The true tests of memory are recall of recent and remote personal events and recent events of general interest; these are obtainable through history-taking. While the questions given here do not test such memory *per se,* they do represent a valid test for detecting organicity.
7. "Take this pencil and paper and draw a clock; make it read the time that you think it is now." 8. "Please copy this cube." 9. "Please write the sentence (or three items) I asked you to remember."	Construction, comprehension, copying, memory Construction is an important part of the MSE in geriatric patients. Errors may indicate focal brain dysfunction that needs further neurologic evaluation. Also tested are ability to comprehend and follow verbal commands, ability to write, and short-term memory.
10. To test the patient's fund of general information, ask about the names of the present and previous presidents, well-known historical events, or current affairs.	General information This is useful for differentiating functional and organic disorders; it is not a test of a specific cognitive function.
11. "Please explain this proverb: 'A rolling stone gathers no moss' or 'People in glass houses shouldn't throw stones.'"	Proverbs (concrete vs. abstract thought) Explanations of proverbs are not particularly useful for distinguishing organic from functional disorders; concrete thinking occurs in organic brain disorders and schizophrenia. However, they do indicate an ability to use abstract thought. Abstraction requires fully intact cognitive function and is suggested by such responses as "Someone on the move never establishes a stable life," or "You shouldn't criticize other people if you are vulnerable to criticism yourself." Concrete thinking is demonstrated by such responses as "When a stone moves down a hill no moss sticks to it" or "If you throw a stone through glass it will break the glass." Concrete or constricted answers suggest cognitive limitations, whereas bizarre or elaborate answers may indicate functional psychosis.

Dementia refers to "a loss of intellectual abilities of sufficient severity to interfere with social or occupational functioning." Memory, abstract thinking, judgment, and many of the higher cortical functions may be impaired. There is also a corresponding personality change.[18] While dementia technically does not involve clouding of consciousness, distinguishing it from delirium in a confused, frightened elderly person in the ER can be difficult.

The clinician should be aware of the following facts about delirium and dementia: Delirium is potentially reversible if the underlying disorder is treated effectively; without treatment, there may be a progression to dementia or even death. Dementia may be corrected and the course of the disease halted in cases such as hypothyroidism, subdural hematoma, nutritional deficiency, chronic drug intoxication, and normal pressure hydrocephalus.

Pseudodementia refers to a form of severe depression in the elderly that presents with cognitive impairment[19-22] and may be indistinguishable from true dementia. Even with sophisticated neuropsychological testing, sometimes only a trial of antidepressant medication can differentiate between the two. Patients with a major depression may complain of impaired memory or difficulty thinking and concentrating. They may be disoriented and apathetic, performing poorly or inconsistently on tests of cognitive function. An accurate history may help to clarify the diagnosis. With pseudodementia, there may be a prior depression and a clear onset of symptoms with fairly rapid intellectual deterioration. Even if the diagnosis of dementia seems clear, all patients should be referred from the emergency setting for further evaluation (see Chapter 12).

Establishing the etiology of organic mental disturbance is preliminary to effective treatment. The interview should include a detailed account of the patient's past medical and surgical experiences, present medical illnesses, review of systems, and medications taken now and in the past. A list of over-the-counter drugs should be explicitly elicited since many elderly patients use laxatives, cold medicines, tonics, and sleeping pills without considering them medication.

Because the distinction between delirium and dementia is often not clear on initial presentation, the causes of delirium and dementia have been subsumed under the general symptom-heading "confusion" in Tables 2 and 3. All patients with disturbed consciousness and impaired attention should be evaluated medically with physical examination, complete blood count, chemistries and thyroid function, electrocardiogram, urinalysis, chest X ray, and relevant special studies.[23]

4.4. Use of Medication

Medications represent an important and remediable cause of mental disorders in the elderly. Whether because of a caregiver's illness, habit, or frustrated attempts to "do something," the elderly consume more medication than younger patients.[24] Errors in dose or schedule are frequently made because the patient did not hear, remember, or understand the instructions, could not read the label, or because the directions were not sufficiently clear.

The aging body handles drugs differently from the younger one.[24] For example, impaired renal function due to aging (with a decrease often to half the normal rate of excretion) or actual disease may cause drugs that are ordinarily eliminated via the kidneys to accumulate to toxic levels. This may occur, for example, with lithium and digoxin, both of which can cause acute confusion. With normal increases in fat content accompanying aging, fat-soluble compounds like barbiturates are stored rather than eliminated. Similarly, the aging liver's reduced capacity to degrade and detoxify drugs prolongs the drug's active life. The long-acting benzodiazepines—(e.g., chlordiazepoxide [Librium] and diazepam [Valium])—are notable in this regard.

Many elderly patients take several medications at once. The drugs most commonly used in this age group can produce serious interactions when combined. Antipsychotic medications and barbiturates, for example, induce the liver enzymes responsible for degrading many drugs, which results in faster drug elimination. The patient who also takes an anticoagulant will require a larger dose to achieve a therapeutic blood level. If the psychoactive drug is stopped, however, the enzymes will not be activated to the same degree and the anticoagulant may accumulate to a dangerous level unless the dosage is adjusted. The same process occurs with anticonvulsants.

Other drug interactions should also be noted. Antipsychotics and antidepressants used together create an additive anticholinergic load, with increased risk of delirium. The problem is further compounded when antiparkinson drugs are added. Similarly, lithium can rapidly increase to toxic levels when a diuretic is given, for sodium is lost and lithium retained. The same can be true for lithium in combination with a low-sodium diet, or substantial fluid loss for any reason (e.g., diuresis, diarrhea, sweating).

Psychoactive drugs must be used cautiously in elderly patients. Orthostatic hypotension occurs with drugs such as chlorpromazine (Thorazine), thioridazine (Mellaril), amitriptyline (Elavil), and imipramine (Tofranil), potentiating the risk of serious falls, stroke, or myocardial infarction. These types of drugs have been implicated in cardiac arrhythmias and decreased cardiac output as well as acute urinary retention and glaucoma.[25–27]

Some nonpsychiatric drugs commonly taken by the elderly have adverse effects on mental status. The oral hypoglycemic chlorpropamide (Diabenase) increases the activity of antidiuretic hormone, which may in turn lead to water intoxication and hyponatremia, with resultant confusion. Psychotic behavior is not infrequent with L-dopa (and other medications used in treating Parkinsonism), indomethacin, and steroids. Many drugs can cause confusion in the elderly: diuretics (by altering fluid and electrolyte balance), anticonvulsants, narcotic and nonnarcotic analgesics, and antihypertensives whose locus of action is the central nervous system (reserpine, alpha-methyldopa).

4.5. Level of Functioning

Besides clarifying the particular features of mental and physical states, the emergency evaluator should make an overall assessment of the patient's ability

Table 2. Some Clues to Causes of Acute Confusional States Demanding Urgent Attention

Metabolic disorders
1. Hypoglycemia: history of diabetes or alcoholism; reduced level of consciousness, shaky, sweaty, perhaps combative.
2. Hyperglycemia: history of diabetes; complaints of increased thirst, urination, or "flu-like" symptoms.
3. Hyponatremia: underlying illness like lung cancer, recent stroke, chronic pulmonary infections, heart failure, cirrhosis, diuretic use.
4. Hypernatremia: dehydration from inadequate fluid intake or excessive fluid loss without replacement.
5. Hypercalcemia: underlying disorder such as cancer metastatic to bone, sarcoidosis, lung and renal cell cancer, multiple myeloma, and/or prolonged immobilization.
6. Hypoxia: inadequate oxygen supplied to the brain because of poor pulmonary or cardiac function or carbon monoxide poisoning.
7. Hypercarbia: history of chronic lung disease characterized by carbon dioxide retention; may use oxygen at home.
8. Hepatic encephalopathy: history of chronic liver disease or alcoholism; probably jaundiced; ascites.
9. Uremia: history of kidney disease, enlarged prostate, recent inability to pass urine.
10. Thiamine deficiency (Wernicke's encephalopathy): variable degrees of ophthalmoplegia, ataxia, and mental disturbance; history of nutritional deficiency secondary to alcoholism, particularly of thiamine. Since remaining thiamine in the body is rapidly utilized when the patient is given intravenous glucose, any patient with alcoholism should immediately receive intramuscular thiamine prior to glucose infusion to prevent precipitating this encephalopathy. Untreated, this disorder rapidly progresses to a permanent memory disorder (Korsakoff's syndrome) and, in some advanced cases, death.
11. Hypothyroidism: history of progressive fatigue, constipation, sensitivity to cold, weight gain, coarsening of hair and skin, mental slowing; exam shows abnormally low temperature and enlarged heart and slow pulse; may be precipitated by the effects of lithium on thyroid function.
12. Hyperthyroidism: patient may be either hyperactive or apathetic; history may reveal rapid weight loss, diarrhea, heat intolerance, and emotional instability; exam shows goiter, silky fine hair, warm moist skin, proptosis and wide-eyed stare, fine tremor, rapid or irregular pulse; in elderly patients muscle weakness and heart failure may be most apparent.

Systemic illness
1. Decreased cardiac output from various causes such as congestive heart failure, arrhythmia, pulmonary embolus, and myocardial infarction; "acute myocardial infarction presents with confusion as the major symptom in 13% of elderly patients."[20] Remember that aged patients do not complain of typical pain; often they complain of indigestion. Vital signs may be abnormal and patient may look ill (ashen coloring, weak, nauseated, sweaty) and be confused.
2. Pneumonia: recent history of a cold, becoming bedridden and aspirating; fever may not be apparent, but tachycardia or hypotension are evident on vital signs.
3. Urinary tract infection: especially in patients with indwelling urinary catheters, prostatic hypertrophy, diabetes, neurogenic bladder.
4. Anemia: especially with acute blood loss (injury, intestinal bleeding), chronic illness, occult gastrointestinal malignancy.
5. Acute surgical emergencies: infarction of the bowel, appendicitis, and volvulus are common in this age group and often present only with confusion and no other complaints.
6. Hypertension: sustained or rapid increase in blood pressure may cause encephalopathy; often has history of elevated blood pressure; may occur in patient on MAO Inhibitor antidepressants who has eaten food containing tyramine.
7. Vasculitides: e.g., systemic lupus erythematosis, confusion arises from cerebral involvement or treatment with steroids.
8. Any febrile illness and infection can cause confusion in the aged.

(Continued)

Table 2. (*Continued*)

Central nervous system disorders

1. Subdural or epidural hematoma: may or may not have history of head trauma; fluctuating mental status often present; may have no focal neurologic signs.
2. Seizure: unwitnessed seizure may be suggested if patient was found on floor with evidence of incontinence or vomiting; history of seizure disorder or alcoholism.
3. Stroke: history of transient ischemic attacks or strokes; may have no signs except confusion.
4. Infection: meningitis (bacterial, fungal, or tuberculous), viral encephalitis.
5. Tumor, primary or metastatic: with a growing mass, raised intracranial pressure may cause local compression of vital structures or herniation of the brain. In the elderly, brain atrophy allows for greater space inside the skull so that symptoms may not appear until the mass is quite large.
6. Normal pressure hydrocephalus: presents with triad of gait disturbance, incontinence, dementia; surgery may be curative.

Drugs and medication

1. Almost all drugs are capable of causing confusion in the elderly. The most commonly implicated drugs include those with strong anticholinergic effects (antidepressants, antipsychotics, and antiparkinsonian drugs, and many over-the-counter preparations), sedative-hypnotics (barbiturates, benzodiazepines), cardiac medications (digoxin, propranolol, lidocaine, quinidine), antihypertensives, anticonvulsants, cimetidene, nonnarcotic and narcotic analgesics, and corticosteroids.
2. Alcohol: intoxication and withdrawal syndromes occur as in younger patients, but poor health in the elderly may put geriatric patients at greater risk.
3. Drug abuse: far less common in elderly persons, but chronic intoxication with bromides, minor tranquilizers (especially meprobamate, barbiturates) occurs.

Table 3. Causes of Acute Confusional States Requiring Less Urgent Treatment

Malnutrition

1. Vitamin deficiencies: 10% of older people suffer from the simultaneous deficiency of at least three of the following: thiamine, riboflavin, ascorbic acid, niacin, and vitamin A.[20]
2. Vitamin B12 deficiency: commonly due to pernicious anemia or malabsorption syndromes; may not have the typical hematologic or motor system changes.
3. Combined nutritional deficiencies (vitamin, protein).

Central nervous system disease

1. Tertiary neurosyphilis: treatment with high dose penicillin will sometimes arrest its progress.
2. Parkinson's disease, multiple sclerosis, multiinfarct dementia: all three can produce dementia with acute episodes of superimposed confusion; antiparkinson medications may aggravate confusion and cause psychosis.
3. Jakob-Creutzfeldt disease, Huntington's chorea, postanoxic and posthypoglycemic states, posttraumatic dementia, and Alzheimer's disease: these disorders have no known cure, but management of symptoms and rehabilitation efforts can enhance the quality of life and minimize such sequelae as injuries.

Systemic illness

For reasons that are often unclear, improvement in a chronic disorder such as congestive heart failure, rheumatoid arthritis, or chronic lung disease can result in considerable improvement in mental status although no specific metabolic disturbance is identifiable. Similarly, cancer (apparent or undiagnosed) can cause confusion.

to maintain a safe and healthy independent living situation. A home visit or discussion with family or neighbors should indicate the patient's current level of functioning and any risks the living arrangements entail. Should the patient be unable to care adequately for himself, all effort should be made to create a safer and more manageable environment before radically altering the present living situation.

4.6. Management in the Emergency Setting

The critical tasks of an emergency intervention include (1) a detailed, accurate assessment of the total problem—psychiatric and medical symptoms, level of functioning, living conditions, and nature of the support system; (2) formulation of a realistic, concrete treatment plan, and (3) implementation of the plan to contain the current crisis and promote long-term well-being.

4.7. Treatment Planning

The goals of treatment for the elderly are similar to those for younger patients: to help the individual regain or achieve an adequate level of functioning, to enhance the quality of life, to diminish pain and distress, to slow the progression of disease, and to prevent further complications.

Resolving the current crisis *without* moving the elderly person from his home should be the central objective. Many studies have indicated that illness and death are more likely to occur when old people have been removed from their homes.[6] Adaptation to a new environment is stressful and often leads to fatigue, confusion, depression, and physical illness. Remaining at home affirms one's identity and sense of autonomy. The evaluator must consider carefully the conditions under which home is, or can be made to be, a viable place to live.

4.7.1. Services

Depending on the elderly patient's disability, a number of mechanical and human services are available to make life safer and more comfortable. A patient may require a walker or wheelchair, a hospital bed, TV, radio, newspaper, calendar. Handrails, nonskid rugs, adequate lighting, emergency phone numbers by the telephone, medical alert devices may all reduce the risk of serious accidents. A homemaker to clean, cook, and shop or a mobile meal service offer companionship to a lonely shut-in, while a visiting nurse administers medication and monitors medical status and treatment. Information regarding the range of services available to the elderly may be obtained from the Department of Health and Human Services, Administration on Aging, in Washington, D.C. Local governmental and private agencies are good resources for information on social and leisure-time activities, transportation, and paid or volunteer work for senior citizens.

4.7.2. Outpatient Treatment

Most psychiatric treatment modalities are appropriate for geriatric patients, including individual psychotherapy, group therapy, family or couple therapy, medication or electroconvulsive therapy, day or partial hospitalization. Insight-oriented psychotherapy for the older patient[28–30] stresses the value of establishing relationships, reviewing one's life, and resolving intrapsychic conflicts. Transgenerational family work can be useful for clarifying even longstanding differences and bringing family members closer together at a time when they need mutual support. Therapy groups promote resocialization and offer support during the difficult process of reinvestment in life.[31]

While psychoactive medication may be indicated in the overall treatment plan, it should not be initiated in the emergency room except in a few situations. For example, a patient who has improved on haloperidol (Haldol), 1 mg at bedtime, but is still somewhat agitated may benefit from increasing the dose to 2mg. The regular physician should be notified about the change. A patient who is acutely anxious because of the recent death of a spouse may be helped through the crisis period with oxazepam (Serax), 10 mg once or twice daily, and a follow-up appointment or referral for short-term outpatient work. A patient with a history of psychosis treated with thioridazine (Mellaril) who is becoming psychotic again may benefit from the same prescription. It is unwise to begin antidepressants in the emergency room because of the difficulties of diagnosis and the need for comprehensive treatment that includes establishing a supportive, therapeutic relationship. Adequate supervision and follow-up are necessary in all cases where medication is prescribed.

4.7.3. Inpatient Treatment

A patient should be hospitalized if he is suicidal or dangerous to others, if he cannot adequately care for himself, or if further diagnostic work is indicated. Admission to a medical unit should be arranged if there is evidence of an organic condition. Hospitalization can occur directly from the emergency room if the situation is urgent; if not, the patient and family may benefit from a few days to prepare for, and adjust to, hospitalization. Sensitivity to both the elderly person's and his family's fears is necessary to effect the transition.

5. Clinical Presentations

5.1. Depression

Depression is probably the most common disorder in the aged. Authors have estimated that it ranges from 37 to 52% of elderly patients admitted to a psychiatric hospital or seen as outpatients.[32] This increased frequency likely reflects both age-related changes in neurotransmitters and the impact of multiple losses. It is often extremely difficult to distinguish depression from dementia, physical illness, and grief. A definitive diagnosis in the emergency room is almost impossible; instead, the major work in the emergency setting should be to rule out life-threatening illness, contain the crisis, begin the evaluation process, and ensure appropriate disposition and follow-up.

> Mrs. A., a 71-year-old widowed woman, came with her daughter to the emergency room because of depression and suicidal ideas. She had been well until 6 years earlier, when she was attacked and robbed while walking to her car from her home of 40 years. Following the incident she became depressed and experienced sleep and appetite disturbances, agoraphobia, and chronic and panic anxiety. She sought treatment, was placed in a group, but quit after three months with no symptom relief. She felt unable to carry on her job as a nurse and retired. Although she gradually improved over the next four years, she never felt "back to her old self," spent most of her time at home alone, and lost most of her work and social relationships. A year before the ER visit, her sister died of the same type of cancer that claimed their mother when Mrs. A. was 12, her daughter and son-in-law separated, her son began to drink heavily just as her husband had done, and she learned that by retiring a few months before her 65th birthday she had forfeited several thousand dollars in benefits. She again became very depressed, had trouble falling asleep, would awaken at 3:00 a.m., lost 35 pounds over six months, and could not maintain a hygienic living situation. She felt helpless, hopeless, and worthless, castigating herself for her perceived failures as a wife, mother, and nurse. She found no pleasure in life and no relief even though attention from her family increased. When she began to contemplate suicide, she became alarmed enough to seek emergency help.
>
> The emergency assessment included a complete medical evaluation: review of systems, physical examination, blood work (complete blood count, thyroid studies, serum electrolytes), and ECG, all of which were negative. Mental status examination revealed no psychosis; her suicidal ideas were vague, unformed, and centered on wanting relief from her pain rather than dying. Psychiatric history was positive for a previous depression and family depression. Mrs. A. had sustained various acute losses, but the severity and length of the current episode, together with her history and family history indicated a depressive illness consistent with DSM III criteria and not a typical grief reaction.[18]

While the clinical picture of acute grief may be very close to that of a major depressive syndrome, a grieving patient usually does not experience persistent feelings of worthlessness, or marked functional impairment beyond several months. "Guilt, if present, is chiefly about things done or not done at the time of the death by the survivor; thoughts of death are usually limited to the individual's thinking that he or she would be better off dead or that he or she should have died. . . . "[18] Acute grief usually lasts from a few months to a year. If depressive symptoms persist for more than a year or if psychotic symptoms appear, a diagnosis of a major depressive disorder should be considered.

On the one hand, depression may be the presenting symptom of a variety of physical disorders—e.g., hypothyroidism, chronic infection, brain tumor—

while, on the other hand, somatic complaints like fatigue or chronic pain may be symptoms of depression.

In Mrs. A.'s case, it was decided that she could remain in her home with the support of her family and receive treatment for her depressive illness on an outpatient basis. She was referred for outpatient psychotherapy and was ultimately started on desipramine because of its minimal anticholinergic and cardiovascular effects. Psychotherapy helped her to grieve her many losses—mother, husband, sister—and in reviewing the course of her life to gain a sense of accomplishment and satisfaction.

5.2. Suicide

> Mr. B. was found dead, hanging from his belt in the garage. The history was obtained from his son, who lived in another city. Mr. B. was 81 years old; his wife had died four months earlier from a sudden heart attack. After her death, he began to deteriorate. Following his wife's funeral, at which it was noted that he was "remarkably stoical, didn't shed a tear," he refused to leave his home, sat staring blankly at the wall, and ate and went to bed only when forced to do so by the housekeeper. He developed pneumonia, was hospitalized for a week, and seemed to recover adequately. His son became concerned about his repetitive talk of death and took him to the emergency room three days before the suicide. Father and son were told by emergency personnel that it would take a while for the father to get over his wife's death, and that he could be given sleeping medication if he wished. Three days later, the father committed suicide, and the son discovered that his father had updated his will, had organized all of his personal effects, and had left a note. Given the premonitory signs and the father's age and bereavement, an extremely high level of suicidal risk should have been ascribed to the patient's situation.

While the suicide rate for the population as a whole in 1973 was 12 per 100,000, for men over 65 it was 36 per 100,000 and for those over 85, 45 per 100,000.[33] "White males over 65 commit suicide three times more often than do white males aged 20–24, and their suicide rate is four times greater than the overall rate for the United States. White females over 65 commit suicide twice as often as white females aged 20–24, although (for women) the highest rate occurs earlier, between the ages of 45 and 54."[34] Suicide threats and attempts are rare in elderly people; instead, they choose violent methods, plan carefully, and generally succeed.

Prediction of suicide is notoriously unreliable, but there are statistical profiles of those at increased risk: white, elderly men who live alone, lack social supports, and suffer poor physical health.[34] In fact, 85% of patients over 60 who committed suicide had a serious illness at the time of death. There is often a history of psychiatric illness and/or previous attempt(s) of high lethality. The clinical presentation includes symptoms of depression, a history of alcohol abuse, and frequently a recent loss or disappointment (see Chapter 7). Most elderly patients do not seek medical or psychiatric help for suicidal ideas, so that when such a patient does appear, the seriousness of the situation must not

be underestimated. Furthermore, the elderly are more likely to develop disorders (paranoid psychoses, delirium, dementia) that undermine their capacity
to control impulsive behavior or estimate the dangerousness of their actions.[34]
In addition, a nonlethal method may prove fatal to an elderly person, who is
naturally more sensitive to the effects of medication or toxic substances, or
who may be more seriously injured by a fall or a brief period of anoxia than
a younger person. Finally, covert suicidal behaviors are often seen in the geriatric population: slow starvation, self-neglect, especially in the face of serious
medical illness, refusal to follow important medical advice, progressive withdrawal, and isolation.

5.3. Confusion

Mr. C., a 78-year-old man, was found unconscious on the floor of his apartment. The EMTs who brought him to the emergency room commented that
the place was littered with junk, looking "like the home of a crazy person."
By the time of his arrival in the ER, Mr. C. was awake and thrashing around;
his agitation alternated with drowsiness and incoherent mumbling. The
triage officer noted his abnormal mental status, saw no obvious signs of
injury, found a blood pressure of 90/60 and a temperature of 97°, and called
for immediate medical evaluation. Mr. C. was suffering from bilateral pneumonia with significant hypoxia, dehydration, and hypernatremia. He was
started on antibiotics, oxygen, and fluid replacement, admitted to the medical service, and seen by a staff psychiatrist.

Mental status examination revealed a fluctuating level of consciousness, ranging from alertness to drowsiness. He was inattentive and easily
distractible and could not attend to many of the questions asked. He was
disoriented to time and place but knew his own name. He was unable to
repeat a sentence said to him and had no memory for recent events, although
he knew his date of birth and the name of his high school. He appeared to
comprehend only the simplest commands. His speech was not dysarthric
but was so cluttered with nonsense words and irrelevant phrases that he
was virtually unintelligible. He appeared to be talking to persons who wer-
en't there and seeing invisible objects.

A longtime friend of Mr. C. was located, and he described Mr. C. as
a pleasant man who had never married, lived alone, and had worked past
retirement age as a salesman. He was an active member of a stamp-col-
lecting group and was considered to be "pretty sharp" despite his years.
The friend knew of no psychiatric history but did mention that "he collects
a lot of junk; he keeps everything he's ever had and also gets intrigued with
things he finds. He's done that for years and it reminds him of his youth.
Don't worry, he takes perfectly good care of himself."

From the friend's account and the clinical evidence, it became clear
that Mr. C. had become acutely confused from a combination of hypoxia,
dehydration, and sodium imbalance secondary to the bilateral pneumonia.
The encephalopathic picture cleared over the next two weeks as the medical
condition improved. It was later discovered that Mr. C. had gone to his
local clinic two days before he was found by the EMTs. There, he had
complained of trouble sleeping and had seemed "a little confused." He was

given flurazepam (Dalmane) 30 mg and sent home. Since he appeared disheveled and had loose mental associations, the clinic felt he was probably a chronic schizophrenic and referred him to the local mental health clinic.

5.4. Dementia

Mrs. D. was brought to the ER by her daughter because she was becoming confused and somewhat agitated at night. When first seen, Mrs. D. was sitting calmly, staring vacantly into space. Mental status examination revealed that she was disoriented to time and place, spoke spontaneously about wanting to go home, and answered most questions with only a yes or no. She could follow simple commands, but her attempt to draw a clock resulted only in a circle; she could not name the president nor explain why she was in the emergency room. Her daughter was tearful and anxious. Mrs. D. had been living with her for the past five years, and over this time the mother's mental functioning had gradually deteriorated. She spent her days watching television, fed herself, but had recently become incontinent. She had begun to wander away from the apartment, and the daughter feared that she might fall or walk into the street.

Mrs. D.'s history and mental status suggested dementia. In her present situation, she was in danger of harming herself, and her daughter could not provide adequate supervision. Although feeling sad and guilty, Mrs. D.'s daughter agreed with the evaluator that a nursing home placement seemed necessary. With support, she was able to make a suitable plan: to contact the social service staff for help in finding a nursing home and to continue caring for her mother until placement could be arranged. Mrs. D. was started on haloperidol 0.5 mg at bedtime to calm her nocturnal agitation, and a follow-up appointment was made with her family physician.

6. Conclusion

Elderly patients present various challenging clinical problems to the emergency worker. The direct physiological effects of aging may render them vulnerable to serious psychiatric and medical disorders and sensitive to the effects of medication. The socioeconomic and interpersonal consequences of growing older often lead to an impoverished and lonely existence, which contributes both to physical and mental illness and to failures in treatment. The problems of the geriatric patient in crisis are not insurmountable; rather, if they are given thoughtful, compassionate, and consistent attention, rewarding and sometimes dramatic changes can be effected.

References

1. Bellak L, Karasu T: *Geriatric Psychiatry, A Handbook for Psychiatrists and Primary Care Physicians.* New York, Grune and Stratton, 1976.
2. Bozzetti LP, MacMurray JP: Contemporary concepts of aging: An overview. *Psychiatr Ann* 7:117–127, 1977.

3. Group for the Advancement of Psychiatry: *Psychiatry and the Aged: An Introductory Approach.* New York, Group for the Advancement of Psychiatry, 1965, p 541.

4. Pollack ES, Locke BZ, Kramer M: Trends in the hospitalization and patterns of care of the aged mentally ill, in Hoch PH, Zubin J: *Psychopathology of Aging.* New York, Grune and Stratton, 1965, pp 21–56.

5. Schwab JJ: Depression among the aged. *South Med J* 69:1039–1041, 1976.

6. Butler RN: Psychiatry and the elderly: An overview. *Am J Psychiatry* 132:893–900, 1975.

7. Rossman I: *Clinical Geriatrics.* Philadelphia, JB Lippincott Co, 1971.

8. Rodstein M: Accidents among the aged: Incidence, cause and prevention. *J Chron Dis* 17:515–526, 1964.

9. Gibson RW: Medicare and the psychiatric patient. *Psychiatr Opinion* 7:17–22, 1970.

10. Palmore E, Cleveland WP, Nowlin JB, et al: Stress and adaptation in later life. *J Gerontol* 34:841–851, 1979.

11. Goodstein R: The diagnosis and treatment of elderly patients: Some practical guidelines. *Hos Community Psychiatry* 31:19–24, 1980.

12. Kahn RL, Goldfarb AI, Pollack M, et al: Brief objective measures for the determination of mental status in the aged. *Am J Psychiatry* 117:326–380, 1960.

13. Silver CP: Tests for assessment of mental function. *Age Aging* 7(Suppl):12–16, 1978.

14. Folstein MF, Rostein SE, McHugh PR: "Mini-mental state"—A practical method for grading the cognitive state of patients for the clinician. *J Psychiatr Res* 12:189–198, 1975.

15. Goldfarb AI: The aged in crisis. In Glick RA, Meyerson AT, Robbins E, et al (eds): *Psychiatric Emergencies.* New York, Grune and Stratton, 1976, pp 241–257.

16. Shapiro MB, Post F, Lofving B, et al: Memory function in psychiatric patients over sixty, some methodological and diagnostic implications. *J Ment Sci* 102:233–246, 1956.

17. Strub RL, Black FW: *The Mental Status Examination in Neurology.* Philadelphia, FA Davis Co, 1979.

18. American Psychiatric Association: *Diagnostic and Statistical Manual of Mental Disorders,* ed 3. Washington, American Psychiatric Association, 1980.

19. Wells CE: Geriatric organic psychoses. *Psychiatr Ann* 8:57–73, 1978.

20. Libow LS: Pseudosenility: Acute and reversible organic brain syndromes. *J Am Geriatr Soc* 21:112–120, 1973.

21. Post F: Dementia, depression and pseudodementia. In Beason DF, Blumer D (eds): *Psychiatric Aspects of Neurologic Diseases.* New York, Grune and Stratton, 1975, pp 99–120.

22. Folstein MR, McHugh RR: Dementia syndrome of depression, in Katzman R, Terry RD, Bick KL (eds): *Alzheimer's Disease: Senile Dementia and Related Disorders* (Aging, vol. 7). New York, Raven Press, 1978, pp 87–92.

23. Bassuk EL, Minden SL, Apsler R: Geriatric emergencies: Medical or psychiatric? *Am J Psychiatry,* 140:539–543, 1983.

24. Lamy PP, Vestal RE: Drug prescribing in the elderly. *Hosp Pract* January 1976, pp 111–118.

25. Van Praag HM: Psychotropic drugs in the aged. *Compr Psychiatry* 18:429–442, 1977.

26. Salzman C, Hoffman SA, Schoonover SC: Geriatric psychopharmacology, in Bassuk EL, Schoonover SC, Gelenberg AJ (eds): *The Practictioner's Guide to Psychoactive Drugs,* ed 2. New York, Plenum Publishing Corp, 1983, pp 293–311.

27. Gulevich G: Psychopharmacological treatment of the aged, in Barchas JO, Berger PA, Ciaranello RD, et al (eds): *Psychopharmacology from Theory to Practice.* New York, Oxford University Press, 1977, pp 448–465.

28. Ross M: A review of some recent treatment methods for elderly psychiatric patients. *Arch Gen Psychiatry* 1:578–592, 1959.

29. Rechtschaffen A: Psychotherapy with geriatric patients: A review of the literature. *J Gerontol* 14:73–84, 1959.

30. Butler RN: The life review: An interpretation of reminiscence in the aged. *Psychiatry* 26:65–76, 1963.

31. Palmore E: Predictions of successful aging. *Gerontologist* 19:427–431, 1979.
32. Busse EW, Pfeiffer E: *Mental Illness in Later Life*. Washington, American Psychiatric Association, 1973.
33. Kopell B: Treating the suicidal patient. *Geriatrics* 32:65–67, 1977.
34. Resnik HLP, Cantor JM: Suicide and aging. *J Am Geriatric Soc* 18:152–158, 1970.

VIII

Special Settings, Circumstances, and Approaches

20

Managing Emergencies in the Practice of Psychotherapy

Lee Birk, M.D., and Ann W. Birk, Ph.D.

1. Introduction

Psychiatric emergencies that occur in the context of ongoing psychotherapy can share many of the features of crises that present to the emergency room: manifest symptomatology, etiology, diagnostic labels, and course. There is a notable difference, however, that strictly distinguishes the focus and orientation of intervention in these two settings.

For the emergency room physician, the typical patient is a stranger in crisis, one on whom there is little or no retrospective information, no medical, family, or psychosocial history, and no baseline of usual behavior. The patient may be psychotic, violent, uncommunicative, confused, or overwhelmingly distressed, unable to contribute to the critically urgent process of evaluating and diagnosing the roots of his psychiatric disturbance. In this context, the primary focus of management is diagnosis, and ultimately the identification of pathogenic influences or factors responsible for the immediate crisis. When the causal chain has been at least presumptively determined, treatment decisions can begin to take shape, tailored to individualized diagnostic findings, patient variables, and resource availability. Within the brief interval thus defined as emergency intervention in a time-limited setting, the major clinical task is two-phased: data acquisition and evaluation first, with symptom abatement/crisis containment second. Referral for longer-term treatment usually marks the end point of emergency care in this context.

For crises occurring within the practice of outpatient psychotherapy, the focus and orientation of management differ. From the single point-in-time perspective of the emergency room, the reference points and periods of contact between patient and therapist expand to encompass wide and complex bands of association that may include direct interaction with members of the patient's family or ongoing involvement with the patient in a therapy group. In this context, the acute crisis of a patient forms one atypical episode among many other episodes from which the therapist has already derived information about the patient: medical history, family background, and baseline functioning. Be-

Lee Birk, M.D. • Harvard Medical School, Boston, Massachusetts 02115.   *Ann W. Birk, Ph.D.* • Learning Therapies, Inc., Newton, Massachusetts 02163.

yond this, the therapist has usually developed a clinical sense of how the patient's developmental history, personality and life experiences have combined to vitalize particular psychological issues and conflicts, and to activate transference distortions and defensive postures. From such a broad-based clinical perspective, crisis points within ongoing psychotherapy cease to be absolute diagnostic puzzles but may in fact be readily intelligible in context, if not in some cases almost predictable. Without the need for extensive data collection and evaluation, the primary focus of the emergency intervention can be the "reason" for the crisis, and the orientation of management can be the integration of established goals with short-term measures taken to protect the patient at risk. The challenge here—unlike emergency room practice where diagnosis is inevitably in the forefront—is to find ways of managing the crisis that protect the patient from undue risk yet do not infantilize him, encourage dependency, or otherwise set back the goals of his ongoing psychotherapy.

The reasons for crisis in psychotherapy are multiply determined: They may arise spontaneously from unanticipated occurrences in the patient's life; they may result from family or marital discord, psychiatric illness, or medical conditions; or they may reflect trouble in the psychotherapeutic relationship. Crises may relate to the actual severity of a patient's symptoms, to his subjective distress, to the objective risk of the situation, to the intensity of his feelings about the therapist, or to his wishes for a different reality in his life. Whatever the reasons for trouble, when the alarm is sounded, it is the therapist's responsibility to discriminate between genuinely urgent circumstances and nonurgent distress, covert cries for help or support, patient manipulations, exaggerated assignment of risk or seriousness. Each emergency must be evaluated in its own right, for to adopt in advance a rigid limit-setting therapeutic stance or to offer unthinking accessibility may equally prejudice a patient's ultimate well-being.

2. Types of Genuine Emergencies

2.1. External Stresses

Psychotherapy patients, like everyone else, are subject to the whims of fortune. Children drown or die from debilitating disease, parents are weakened by old age and depressed by the loss of spouse, health, and vitality, grandchildren develop drug addictions and abusive habits. The patients themselves become ill, sometimes seriously, require surgery, lose their jobs, fail to achieve lifetime goals, and suffer loss of stature in their own eyes. All these life crises can produce acutely turbulent, even dangerous, emotional states and carry the risk of chronically troublesome sequelae.

The prominence of discord in a couple or a family system is hard to overrate as a source of rage, despair, suicidal preoccupation, or violence. Explosive symptomatic patterns that develop acutely can frequently be traced to events that throw the individual out of synchrony with his spouse or family: Abruptly discovered (or revealed) extramarital affairs constitute one of the most extreme and severe stresses to a person's adaptation. Even an ostensibly amicable, mutual decision to divorce can be powerfully disorganizing. Mild disharmony within the couple or the family system can be pushed to a dangerous point by unempolyment, sudden illness, or alcoholism on the part of a spouse, or by delinquency, accident, or illness in the children.

The death of family members, especially of one's young children, probably causes the worst and most prolonged grief reaction, but the death of a parent who was held in unusually strong ambivalence is also among the most potent causes of intensely guilty suffering and depression.

2.2. Internal Crises

Psychotic breaks, manic episodes, and acutely distressing periods of endogenous depression are classified as internal, although in fact they are probably the manifest correlates of a complex interactive mixture of external precipitating stresses and psychophysiological processes. Internal crises differ from external crises insofar as they reflect the course of an ongoing psychiatric disturbance, whereas traumatic life events do not necessarily correspond to a previously extant disorder.

2.3. Drug-Linked Emergencies

Another large class of psychiatric emergencies arise from the action (or interaction) of biological interventions; a psychotic patient abruptly switched from chlorpromazine alone to chlorpromazine plus fluphenazine or perphenazine or haloperidol to reduce sedation may develop akathisia or acute dystonia. Simiarly, a lithium patient who experiences sudden dehydration because of illness or prescribed diuretics may suffer severe, possibly lethal electrolyte imbalance.

In addition to the effects of polypharmacy and drug toxicity are the cases of pharmacological factors combining destructively with known depressive or aggressive tendencies. A depressed patient may become acutely suicidal following the use of alcohol or marijuana, for example, or as the result of cumulatively retained sleeping pills. Rage attacks are not uncommon in aggressive patients following benzodiazepine-induced disinhibitory reactions in the central nervous system.

2.4. Drug Stoppage

One of the most common psychiatric emergencies is precipitated by the abrupt cessation of psychoactive medication. When drugs that have been central to the maintanence of a patient's adaptation are discontinued for whatever reason, overt brain dysfunction and massive social decompensation typically ensue. Clinical examples abound of ambulatory psychotic patients who create acute emergencies by stopping or "running out" of their medication, or of mania-prone individuals who "forget" to take their lithium or deliberately abandon medication because it is thought to "inhibit creativity," block their best ideas, sap their energy, and even spoil their sex life.

2.5. Medical Emergencies

It is not unusual for a patient to use his regular psychotherapist as an informal triage consultant for medical symptoms; in the course of reviewing problems in the patient's life, medical symptoms or disorders are almost universally presented. Most of these medical symptoms are transient and benign, and the patient can be referred in a timely way to the appropriate specialist if necessary; occasionally, however, they are not benign. Patients who repeatedly complain about irregular bleeding, skin lesions that do not go away, lumps, unusual fatigue, chronic coughing, or indigestion should be urged to consult a specialist without delay. Other conditions such as stomach upset with pain or numbness in the arms or chest, severe leg cramps or pleuritic pain, abdominal pain with nausea, unusually high fever with abrupt onset should be considered indications for immediate referral.

2.6. Crises Arising out of Psychotherapy

Psychotherapy of any kind is in itself a stress, and so it should not be surprising that serious disturbances result as the clinical process reaches critical turning points, internal and external. An internal turning point occurs in psychotherapy, for example, when unconscious rage erupts into consciousness accompanied by either premonitory panic or hyperaggressive behavior, or both. External crises may be generated as the therapy shifts to accommodate termination, emerging new needs of the patient, demise of a marriage, crucial involvement in the therapy of other family members. Family meetings, particularly when they occur as dreaded but necessary adjuncts to a long and intense therapy process, can precipitate anxiety atacks and/or behavioral symptoms.

Disruption of the patient–therapist relationship itself presents a powerful stimulus for patient distress. Unusual dependency that is fostered and then abruptly threatened by the real or imagined loss of the therapist can pose potential dangers for the patient. Similarly, a patient so intensely involved in the therapeutic relationship that he employs or threatens self-destructive or overtly aggressive behavior to manipulate the therapist's responses can unwittingly become a victim of his own actions. Anger at the therapist—real, transferred, or paranoid—that is persistent and uncorrecting can result in violence directed against the therapist. Any disruption of the therapy relationship due to the therapist's illness, pregnancy, retirement, or vacation or to the patient's intensification of ambivalence can precipitate a serious crisis.

3. Pseudoemergencies

In a few cases, pseudoemergencies occur because a patient becomes needlessly alarmed about something that, if he possessed more information, would not seriously concern him. Routine adverse effects of newly prescribed medication are an example of this type of problem. For example, a dry mouth sensation and unusual lethargy during the first few days of a tricyclic antidepressant trial might trigger alarm unless the patient has been adequately prepared to anticipate drug side effects.

Other types of pseudoemergencies are precipitated when a patient wishes to prove a point to spouse, family, therapist, or others, or to objectify his distress externally. While it is true to say of these pseudoemergencies, in general, that they reflect an enormous gap between an objective reality that is not particularly urgent and the patient's subjective experience of that reality, it would be a mistake to dismiss entirely the cry for help in any expression of urgency. The ostensible reason for a crisis may be trivial, repetitive, unalterable, or blatantly manipulative, but the covert communication to the therapist must be acknowledged nevertheless.

Finally, as every therapist knows, there is the type of pseudoemergency that in some patients evolves into a regular, serious pattern of maladaptive behavior. Without proper management, these repetitive cries for help can easily escalate to the point of real risk to the patient or, with hyperaggressive patients, to the therapist or others. The earliest "emergencies" may harbor no underlying threat to the well-being of the patient, but over time the need to demonstrate real urgency can intensify; the patient may in fact "make good" on his threats to demonstrate that his distress is real.

4. Management

4.1. Preventive Measures

Orientation. During the initial phases of therapy, as the therapist is beginning to structure the patient's expectations, focus, and goals, it should be clear that scheduled face-to-face sessions are the place where, and the way in which, the work of therapy is accomplished. It should be emphasized that the therapist is available for real emergencies, that he and the patient will work together to forestall the emergence of crisis conditions, but that in general he would like to reserve the use of the telephone and extra sessions for genuinely urgent situations, and not for obtaining extra measures of moral support, advice, interpretation, and additional contact from the therapist.

Increase appropriate help-seeking behavior while decreasing "wolf-calling" activity by the use of discriminatory learning. If a good foundation has been laid during the initial phase of orientation to psychotherapy, it is a natural next step to continue helping patients to refine, and be alert to, vulnerable points or distortions in the way each reacts to life experiences. Sensitized to these weak links in the chain of experience, interpretation, and response, a patient can gradually learn to modify his interaction with the object world. A patient with hyperaggressive tendencies, for example, can learn to check his heightened impulse to act, while a depressed individual may learn to circumvent a chronically nihilistic attitude by substituting appropriate self-protective action. Patients prone to psychotic episodes can learn to discern the early warning stages of incipient psychosis, thus forestalling the emergence of full-blown symptoms. To help with this discriminatory process, the therapist might say, "I would like you to let me know as soon as possible if you begin to develop the symptoms we have been talking about. If you think that people you see on the street are looking at you strangely, or if you feel special messages are coming to you from books, TV, or strangers, I would like you to call me." Or a patient on lithium might be told: "If you should notice an unusual amount of thirst or loss of appetite, you should take this very seriously and call me right away."

In behavioral terms, the therapist is indicating to the patient his investment in helping the patient to manage potentially serious symptoms by employing positive discriminative stimuli. In the first case, the verbal stimuli are directed to ideas of reference as an early threshold-level psychotic symptom, and the second case to early physical signs of lithium toxicity.

On the other hand, a patient who calls frequently for advice or support, but does so seemingly from a geniune confusion about the appropriate boundaries of the psychotherapeutic relationship, might be told: "If you have a real emergency, I want to hear from you right away. I will help you deal with the upsets in your life, if you and I can weed out the calls that are not genuinely urgent. If you are calling me just for support or because it seems hard to wait until the next appointment, I won't welcome your call, and will probably tell you that I cannot talk until we see each other at the next scheduled session. We need to work together to figure out what the real problems are, and why some of these other things seem compelling enough at the time for you to call me." This example shows the use of a negative discriminative stimulus that signals to the patient the therapist's intention to disregard nonurgent calls for help or requests for increased contact.

It is important for the therapist to be consistent in his use of discriminative stimuli and in his response to actual calls from patients regardless of his own circumstances or mood at the time. If ideas of reference are first reported at 3:00 a.m., the response should be to reinforce the report, and conversely, calls stemming from a clingy, dependent attachment to the therapist should be disregarded irrespective of their potential to gratify him in some way. This type of consistency, however, should not be adhered to slavishly without regard for the patient or a change in circumstances. Occasionally, true emergencies lurk beneath the seemingly inconsequential call, so that the therapist should try to cultivate a suspended judgment/fact-gathering approach to emergency calls in order to classify these calls accurately before responding to them.

Anticipating trouble when possible. Scheduling interim appointments is one of the most effective safety measures for patients who are subject to unusually high levels of stress, are reacting poorly to it, or are reporting shaky adaptations. Anticipating surgery, stressful family visits, birth of a child, financial difficulties, or other foreseeable highly unsettling circumstances with the enhanced security of additional therapy sessions could make the difference between mastery of the crisis points and unmanageable levels of distress.

Checking on missed, canceled, and "postponed" appointments and especially ambiguous telephone messages can be important in the preventive management of crises. If a patient in known crisis misses a scheduled appointment without warning or explanation, it is virtually always prudent to call him for an explanation. If a patient not known to be in crisis calls to cancel an appointment and does not yet have another appointment, it may still be important to check directly with the patient for covert signs of trouble in the therapeutic alliance, or worse, of suicidal intent. When patients are known to be in emotional distress or in the midst of highly stressful life situations, it is advisable for the therapist to pay very close attention to the pattern of attendance at therapy sessions, most especially group therapy sessions, and to telephone messages with seemingly innocuous content. Patients in known crises should not leave any therapy session within explicit agreement on the next appointment.

Using the telephone electively is a vastly underutilized strategy in the preventive management of genuinely urgent psychiatric crises. Not only can this vehicle be highly efficient and effective in providing support in times of high stress, and in gaining information about potentially emergent situations, but a series of scheduled telephone calls can provide an enormously beneficial sense of anticipatory relief as the patient prepares for a difficult event. An appointment to call the therapist at a particular time and place is preferable to a vague request to "call me over the weekend," because it commits the patient to a mutually agreed schedule and procedure in the management of his stress.

Shifting gears within the therapy session itself may be required if the therapist senses a crisis brewing. It is critical to sound management that the therapist not dismiss his clinical perceptions, but react quickly to explore with the patient his premonitory feelings. For patients in group therapy it may be necessary to suggest an individual meeting for the patient in crisis, or to devote a substantial portion of a regular session to his needs. In individual therapy, adjunctive meetings with family or spouse might have to be arranged, or more intensive work with the therapist scheduled, depending on the combination of factors underlying the immediate crisis. In any case, if the first signs of heightened stress, suicidal rumination, rage reaction, significant confusion, or incipient psychosis become evident during any regular therapy hour, it is absolutely imperative for the therapist to take seriously his clinical impressions, communicate them to the patient, and begin to develop a collaborative plan for managing the acute situation.

4.2. Management Techniques

When anticipating crisis points in a patient's life and therapy are insufficient, or when traumatic or internally disruptive situations develop from sudden and unanticipated causes, it becomes necessary for the therapist to act rapidly and effectively. While he is spared the burden of extensive history-taking and information-gathering because of his prior association with the patient, the therapist does bear responsibility for integrating the patient's acute needs with the overall treatment objectives.

Face-to-face interactions. Patients who are in extreme distress or who have experienced sudden trauma where the psychological consequences could be, but are not yet, severe, patients who are evincing early psychotic symptoms, hypomania, or despair, or those caught in volatile social systems should be seen as soon as possible. The focus of the emergency intervention should be the crisis at hand, regardless of the regular focus, content, and style of previous therapy sessions, and the goal should be twofold: moderation of the symptoms and longer-term planning.

Anxiety, panic attacks, grief, and disappointment, while subjectively distressing to the patient, may require no dramatic intervention technique beyond careful examination of the sources of the stress, and planning for either the alteration of stressful conditions in the patient's life or evaluation for biochemical aids to the management of chronic or episodic anxiety or panic attacks, depression, or mania. Calming the patient with reassurance, appropriate information, and counsel, and providing the opportunity for extended review of the stressful experience may be sufficient to restore equilibrium. Patients in deep distress should be asked to call at a certain time to let the therapist know how they are, and should not leave the office after the emergency session without a clear understanding of the next step and exactly when it will occur.

Psychopharmacology. Biochemical therapy is necessary for individuals in psychotherapy who begin to manifest incipient psychotic signs, hypomanic symptoms, deep depression with severe insomnia, and other somatic correlates. Severe anxiety, especially together with spontaneous panic attacks, also calls for drug treatment. Patients with these presenting symptoms should be given a prescription at the time of the emergency visit, and should be informed at the same time about adverse effects, dosage schedules, and benefits of the drug. If the patient is so disorganized, stressed, or agitated during the office visit that he is clearly evincing psychotic signs, or is a threat to himself or others, appropriate doses of a high-potency neuroleptic should be administered at once. In that case, the patient should be asked to remain in the office or waiting room until the acute symptoms have subsided and the effects of the neuroleptic can be safely monitored. Adequate supervision for these patients is a must, and follow-up in all cases where medication is prescribed or administered should be arranged within 12 to 18 hours.

Hospitalization. Patients should *not* be managed outside the hospital if the clinical evidence suggests a substantial risk of violence, suicide, or rapid decompensation. If, however, frequent appointments, telephone support, family consultation, environmental alterations, and/or medication can be used in combination to avert a potentially serious, regressive event like hospitalization, they should be tried first. Under no circumstances should a patient at risk be allowed to leave the office unaccompanied. If necessary, family members, taxi, or police should be called. Involuntary hospitalization may be indicated for the high-risk uncooperative patient.

Patients who require some structured supervision, monitoring of medication, and an intensive program of rehabilitative therapy should be referred to day or partial hospitalization programs, which are both less regressive and less expensive. The chief criterion to be considered in these situations is the need, dictated by safety and practicality, for totally versus partially supervised management.

Violence management. Immediate chemical restraint of a violent or extremely agiated patient is necessary when the patient is clearly out of control and cannot be calmed by ordinary measures. If the violence is directed against a specific victim, the therapist should alert the victim and the police. If the violence is directed against the therapist, chemical restraint may be impossible, and the therapist should take steps to avoid antagonizing or bullying the patient. Continuing to talk to the patient, attempting to disarm him or physically restrain him may not be advisable for the solo practitioner unless he is quite sure that his strategies will work. Otherwise, he should get outside help immediately, call the police, and protect himself by whatever means he can.

Medical management. When a patient mistakes somatic complaints for a severe psychological reaction, he may present at an emergency therapy meeting with an acute, serious medical condition such as myocardial infarction, thrombophlebitis, or psychomotor seizure. The therapist should be prepared to provide assistance for an emergency of this sort. Arranging for an ambulance or medical support is mandatory, followed by making the patient comfortable and not leaving him unattended. If breathing stops, CPR should be administered immediately.

If a patient shows up at an emergency session dangerously intoxicated, or has taken an overdose of drugs, medical assistance should be requested immediately. No procedure should be attempted by the therapist, such as gastric lavage or the administration of ipecac, unless there is no chance at all that the patient can be moved rapidly to a hospital for treatment.

Managing crisis in the patient–therapist relationship. Transference distortions, realistic elements of incompatibility, persistent disagreements about the focus, course, or goals of therapy, displacement, poor therapeutic management, and countertransference issues can cause mild to serious disruption in the therapeutic process. Disruption or trouble in the relationship is not necessarily cause for alarm at all, and may indeed signal that the patient and the therapist are "on the right track." But when the relationship degenerates to the point where the patient is dangerously regressed, angry, or self-destructive, or the work of therapy has ceased altogether, it is time to call the disruption a crisis. The following are guidelines for resolving the crisis:

- Identify the crisis—discuss with the patient as openly as possible his feelings about the therapy, about the origin of the problems, and his impression of the possibility for resolution.
- Arrange for a consultation with an independent therapist to evaluate the situation and to provide strategies for resolution.
- In some cases, referring the patient for adjunctive therapy can break an impasse. The two therapists must be aware of the possibility of object-

splitting as a pitfall of this strategy, however. But the added perspective of work in a different therapeutic modality and with a different therapist can help to deflate transference distortions or refocus displaced anger, and thus benefit the original therapeutic alliance.

- Under rare circumstances it may be necessary to terminate entirely with a patient rather than run the risk of exacerbating an already serious pattern of violent anger, suicidal dependency or self-destructive activity. In those cases, termination should be handled nonjudgmentally and decisively. Referral to another therapist would be appropriate if acceptable by the patient, but the stressed therapeutic relationship may deteriorate still further if insistent attempts to effect such a transition are made. In some cases, the patient may need to put distance between himself and the terminating therapist by selecting his own new consultant.

5. Conclusion

Psychotherapy, like the rest of life, is subject to fluctuations in quality and benefit—sometimes at the whim of events external to itself and, at other times, as the victim of its own process. But when psychotherapy helps a person to do and enjoy things that he could not previously, or helps him to see himself in new ways, and to integrate the ordinary ups and downs of experience into a personally enriching existence, then it has done its work well. Perhaps only under crisis conditions, however, does that work encounter its most revealing challenge.

Postscript

In place of the usual long list of references that might typically be appended to a chapter of this kind, the authors felt that it would be more honest as well as more useful simply to say that in our thinking and in our craft as we practice it day to day, we freely acknowledge our enormous debt to many disciplines, many diverse streams of thought, research, and practice, and many, many people, from Pavlov to Freud, Sullivan to Skinner, Ackerman to Schildkraut.

On the other hand, in writing *this chapter*, what we have essentially done is to try to produce a faithful distillation of our own accumulated clinical experience over the last two decades, in managing emergencies occurring in patients who are in ongoing psychotherapy. For such an enterprise the only honest reference would have to be the experience itself.

General Hospital Psychiatric Emergency Services

Ellen L. Bassuk, M.D.

1. Introduction

> From humble origins in the occasional consultations provided by general hospital psychiatric departments for problems encountered in hospital wards, "acute psychiatric services," "walk-in clinics"—call them what you will—have mushroomed in the past decade partly as a response to a growing need for emergency care and partly under the stimulus of the community movement. At the same time, the case load of these facilities has grown at a phenomenal pace . . . and those responsible for running psychiatric units have sometimes felt as if they were fighting the battle of the bulge as they have poured staff and residents into the breach to stem the onslaught.[1]

Written more than a decade ago, this editorial comment still captures the prevailing mood surrounding the astounding growth in utilization of psychiatric emergency services in general hospitals. If the expected rate of increase of total emergency room (ER) visits continues at 11% per year, then the patient volume will double every year.[2–4] These trends cannot be accounted for by the increase in population and far exceed the growth in inpatient or outpatient facilities.

Factors contributing to increased utilization are the growing "ghettoization of inner city populations," increasing medical specialization, and the flight of general practitioners away from the city, thus "creating a medical care vacuum for the slum poor."[4–7] Now more than 80% of emergency patients are from the two lowest socioeconomic classes.[8] Because of these trends and because the ER is open 24 hours and every patient is seen without an appointment, it has slowly been transformed into a family drop-in clinic, where primary medical and psychiatric care can be obtained without the usual difficulties experienced in the private sector of the general hospital.[9,10] Instead of life-and-death problems, the ER now manages predominantly nonemergency patients from "economically deprived, socially isolated, minority populations." Most often, these

This chapter was condensed from Bassuk E, Gerson S: Into the breach: Emergency psychiatry in the general hospital. *Gen Hosp Psychiatry* 1:31–45, 1979.

Ellen L. Bassuk, M.D. • Harvard Medical School, Boston, Massachusetts 02115.

patients have chronic illnesses superimposed on complex psychosocial problems.[7,11]

Another significant trend has been the progression of deinstitutionalization and the partial shift in responsibility for the chronic mentally ill from state mental hospitals to community mental health centers and general hospitals. Since many of these patients were not adequately followed or even given basic guidance in the mechanics of daily living, they frequently made a poor readjustment in the community and have turned to the general hospital ER for a solution to their problems. However, since the general hospital lacks comprehensive services for the severely disturbed individual (e.g., partial hospitalization, psychosocial rehabilitation programs) and the community does not have a full range of treatment alternatives, the emergency setting has been converted into a "revolving door." Patients with chronic problems repeatedly return for help only to be referred to unavailable or inadequate dispositional alternatives. The burden of the chronic mentally ill will be increasingly felt in general hospitals as states continue to withdraw from the business of directly providing inpatient care. Some authors have speculated that just as the decade of the 1970s witnessed the transformation of the general hospital ER into a family drop-in clinic, the 1980s will witness its further evolution into an aftercare clinic.[12-15] This chapter describes how the general hospital has responded to the rapid growth in psychiatric emergency utilization and focuses on organization of services, staffing patterns, and emerging clinical issues.

2. Organization of Services

Of nonfederal general hospitals with one or more psychiatric services (inpatient, outpatient, day treatment, or other partial hospitalization program), approximately 50% surveyed by the National Institute of Mental Health (NIMH) provide emergency psychiatric care. Virtually all these services are walk-in and are available 24 hours per day, 7 days per week. Around-the-clock suicide prevention services are offered by 10%, telephone hotlines by 12%, and home visits by 13%.[16]

The relationships of emergency services to the psychiatry department, to other general hospital services, and to the community are intricate and varied. Figure 1 shows the potential routing of patients through the general hospital psychiatric emergency network, the relationships of facilities within this setting, and their interface with other psychiatric service modes.

Despite the impressive growth of services, psychiatric emergency facilities are at times viewed as "unwanted stepchildren with neither parity or autonomy from the other major services."[17] Several authors have commented on the low status accorded psychiatric emergencies both by the medical-surgical staff and the psychiatry department.[17,18] Despite this low status and the resistance toward indigent and chronic community patients, many hospitals are beginning to recognize the necessity of caring for these patients and the value of this setting for teaching general hospital psychiatry.

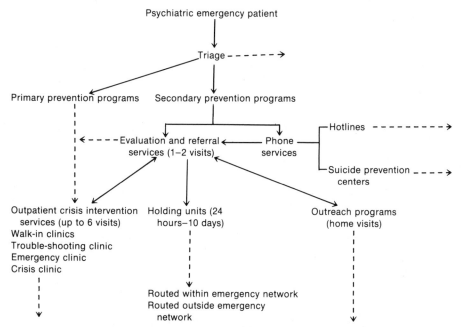

Figure 1. Psychiatric emergency network in a general hospital: potential routing of patients through the general hospital psychiatric emergency network, the relationships of facilities within this setting, and their interface with other psychiatric service modes.

2.1. Triage

In general hospital ERs, the care of the psychiatric patient has often caused tension among the traditional medical model, systems and network approach, and patient expectations. The primary objective of triage in medical settings is to assist patients with "nonurgent conditions to make proper use of regular available community resources and to protect the 'readiness-to-serve' capacity of the emergency station."[19] Implicit in this approach is that the nonemergent patient should be screened out and sent to an outpatient department. In a medical ER, psychiatric problems are often therefore a low priority and a nonurgent condition. From the patient's standpoint, a psychiatric problem may be subjectively unbearable and therefore of the highest priority—a truly urgent situation.

To align the broad scope of psychiatric presentations with the capabilities of emergency services, a number of authors have defined psychiatric emergencies according to a severity-based triage model.[5,20] However, in a survey of 89 ER services, Glasscote et al. found that only two staff groups decided whether or not a patient was an emergency.[21] Operationally, then, what constitutes a psychiatric emergency is determined by the wishes of patients, relatives, and/or friends rather than by the staff or structure of the service.

The discrepancy between the staff's and the patient's view of a psychiatric emergency is that many general hospital ERs are ill-equipped to respond to the demands of those it serves.[22] Typically, a patient using the ER because of convenience, insurance reimbursements, rapid treatment, and anonymity runs into a triage system that refers him to another service or agency that offers few of these attractions.[11] It should be no surprise when follow-up reveals that the patient either has not completed the referral or has returned to the ER. Silbert, studying the process of triage of psychiatric patients by medical interns, also found that only those who asked to see a mental health worker or who presented with obviously bizarre behavior or symptomatology were referred to a psychiatrist.[23]

The combination of adherence to a medical triage model and lack of development of a full range of accessible and unrestricted in-house services has had the paradoxical effect of increasing the influx of emergency patients while further alienating the core urban community.[24,25] Blane et al. have suggested that perhaps the hospital should accept the influx of nonemergent patients "as a permanent part of institutional practice . . . stop trying to exclude a patient group . . . and plan for appropriate services, within the general hospital emergency ward."[26]

On the more positive side, it has been shown that in the general hospital, patients presenting with combined medical and psychological disease seem to be the rule rather than the exception. Browning et al. found that the total medical admission rate for patients with psychiatric problems was 128% higher than the published figure for all patients admitted for any reason, including psychiatric, to an accredited hospital.[27] Despite the tendency of physicians to compartmentalize organic and psychological problems, the patient in a general hospital ER is more likely to have his medical needs met.

2.2. Primary Prevention Programs

The concept of primary prevention implies that when a patient is faced with a situational or developmental crisis, intervention will reduce the incidence of mental disorders by helping the patient develop new problem-solving techniques. Because of the pressured atmosphere of the ER and its emphasis on the needs of the "true" emergency patient, it has not been viewed as an ideal setting for the development of primary prevention programs. Despite this viewpoint, however, clinicians have developed innovative programs.

Hankoff described a crisis intervention program staffed by ER nurses with psychiatric consultation that primarily serves relatives of patients who are *in extremis* or deceased.[28] They found that although their aim was the rapid resolution of the immediate crisis, their program crossed into the area of secondary prevention; many of those newly identified as patients had prior psychopathology. The crisis was used to motivate the patient to obtain definitive psychiatric treatment.

Another area of burgeoning interest has been the crisis provoked by rape. Rape crisis centers have been established in the general hospital medical ER.[29,30] The choice of this setting was based on the recognition of the victim's varied needs, including immediate gynecological care and treatment of possible injury, management of the "rape trauma syndrome," and the need for legal intervention and collection of evidence. The staff, however, sometimes views rape as a questionable health priority in a medical setting, and this resistance must be worked through. Recently, the American College of Obstetrics and Gynecology acknowledged the need for emergency care of all rape victims and published a set of objectives, including "protection against disease, pregnancy, and psychic trauma."[31] In the experience of one program, women who chose to remain in treatment were self-selected and included a large percentage with preexisting psychiatric difficulties. As in Hankoff's experience, the crisis was used as an opportunity to engage patients in ongoing treatment.

2.3. Secondary Prevention Programs

The majority of psychiatric emergency services adhere to a traditional medical model and follow the principles of secondary prevention.[10,32] These services offer "first aid" aimed at reducing the patient's current stress rather than attempting to work through the crisis definitively.[33] This is accomplished by rapid clinical evaluation, emphasizing a functional assessment, and focusing on the availability of the support network.[10] An initial priority is to determine the need for hospitalization and to rule out organic problems. This is followed by administering "psychological, social and/or pharmacologic first aid" and, lastly, by planning a disposition—a process generally requiring one and occasionally two patient visits.[33]

Because of the disproportionately large numbers of psychiatric patients who present to the ER with chronic illness and psychosocial problems, many general hospitals have established walk-in clinics that are part of either the ER or the outpatient department.[34–38] The crisis intervention model of the walk-in clinic goes beyond the first-aid function of the evaluation and referral service. Its goal is the resolution of the crisis through a variety of short-term psychotherapeutic modalities, including individual, couple, family, and group. Other interventions consist of the use of drugs and the mobilization of environmental resources.

Organizationally, the basic model consists of a 24-hour evaluation and referral service located in the ER and an auxiliary 9:00 a.m. to 5:00 p.m. walk-in clinic providing brief psychotherapy for up to six sessions. Patients present for unscheduled visits at either facility or are triaged to the walk-in clinic from the ER. Structurally, these psychiatric emergency services consist of a common triage reception area, one or two interview rooms, and possibly a seclusion room and overnight beds.[4,22]

In addition to the outpatient crisis intervention clinics, many general hospitals established holding units that were utilized for overnight observation or for inpatient crisis intervention.[39–42] Similar to the model of the walk-in clinic, these units are integrated into the psychiatric ER or inpatient setting. Patients are triaged to these units either solely from the ER or from other referral sources. They generally consist of 2–11 beds and are staffed by multidisciplinary teams, which usually include a psychiatric resident on rotational assignment.

A psychiatric emergency overnight ward at one general hospital is used as an adjunct to the evaluation and referral service and not as a primary treatment center. It serves two functions: to assess more acutely disturbed patients and to hold a patient until a disposition is made. Patients are generally observed for less than 24 hours.[39]

An intermediate 72-hour service model provides brief intensive hospitalization that minimizes the secondary gain, infantilization, and dependency that sometimes accompany longer inpatient stays.[38,40,42] Generally, patients admitted to these units are psychotic, suicidal, or severely depressed.[42] A time-limited treatment contract is negotiated that minimizes regression and accelerates treatment planning. Crisis intervention is offered and consists of the same treatment modalities described for the walk-in clinic. Emphasis is on the resolution of the current stress with rapid involvement and mobilization of the support system.

A more extensive undertaking is the establishment of a "crisis ward" located in the inpatient unit but administratively integrated into the psychiatric emergency service. There is no absolute time limitation for hospitalization, but generally the mean length of stay is 7.5 days, of which roughly half consists of partial hospitalization. Admission is viewed as the first step in the treatment process and the beginning of crisis therapy. The only patients not consistently benefiting from this setting are those diagnosed as psychotically depressed. A one-year postdischarge follow-up study revealed that 30% of these patients were either transferred for longer inpatient care or were rehospitalized.[41]

2.4. Tertiary Prevention Programs

Before the effects of deinstitutionalization were felt, the general hospital ER functioned comfortably as an evaluation and referral unit. Patients were seen briefly and then sent to the catchment area CMHC for their care. There they were accepted for treatment, often an inpatient stay. In essence, the ER had merely acted as a conduit or a referral agency. But now, with the changes brought about by the closing of state hospitals and the patients' rights movement, responsibility for these patients has shifted, in part, to the general hospital. The chronic deinstitutionalized patient began to arrive in their ERs in significant numbers in 1976—13 years after President John F. Kennedy mandated a "bold new approach" to the care of the mentally ill. This lag period may reflect the time required to saturate community services and to overwhelm the individual's support networks.[15,43]

Although many general hospitals have developed innovative program models and crisis intervention psychotherapies, few have specifically attended to the needs of the chronic mentally ill. This requires a further shift in orientation—from primary and secondary prevention programs to tertiary prevention programs that are based on principles of psychosocial rehabilitation.[43,44] In addition to their psychiatric and medical problems, the ER must develop resources to help these patients by attending to their immediate social, housing, and financial problems. This may require not only developing new programs in the general hospital but establishing affiliations with various community services. This is a jarring prospect for those general hospitals that have maintained an insular stance by avoiding any real involvement with the community system. Despite the reality, they have tried to guard against the further onslaught of these troublesome patients. Most important in this context is the development of training programs that address both the clinicians' attitudes and the clinical needs of the chronic patient.[45] General hospitals can no longer afford to limit themselves to models of care that only apply to the acutely ill.

3. Staffing Patterns

In past years, most emergency services were primarily service-oriented. More recently, however, many training programs in general hospitals have recognized that the ER is an optimal setting for the teaching of general hospital psychiatry. Attention has been focused increasingly on the issues underlying the choice of staffing patterns.[40,46] In many settings, direct service is still provided by psychiatric residents who rotate through the ER for different periods of time and in combination with other responsibilities.[22,33,37,38] Numerous authors have noted that residents typically experience their emergency work as an unwanted and distressing intrusion on their usual activities and have responded with anxiety, poor performance, and even phobic avoidance.[18,19,47] The many factors contributing to these strong responses include overwhelming service demands, inexperience of the staff, anxiety and helplessness experienced by the trainee in managing difficult patients, "social distance" between staff and patient, difficulties with referral institutions, and necessary emphasis on rapid, concrete decision-making and brief intervention, rather than on elaborate psychodynamic formulations.[1,6,18]

Controversy continues about the necessary level of training of the ER house officer. Many programs have changed from first-year to second-year resident coverage and third-year supervisory and teaching support.[22] In addition, staff consultation is offered and formalized didactic and supervisory conferences are usually available.

In addition, nonphysicians have a special set of problems and training needs in a medical milieu. Barlow described a program for psychology interns who rotated through the ER seven days a week.[48] Initially, these trainees developed moderate to severe anxiety, but by the third to sixth month, they began to experience increasing confidence. This rotation offered the opportunity to evaluate acutely disturbed patients, to make active and immediate decisions, and to improve interviewing and therapeutic skills. Other reports have focused both on the training opportunities and on the special expertise of the social worker in dealing with the wide range of dispositional alternatives in this setting.[49]

In response to the accusation that many psychiatric ERs were providing fragmented care and alienating their patients, the old system of psychiatric resident coverage has been replaced in some hospitals by a new delivery system, which in its most sophisticated from consists of complex "medico-psycho-social teams" comprising an experienced nurse, a social worker, and a psychiatrist.[10,18] Beahan describes a unique multidisciplinary team that follows the patient from admission through inpatient stay and outpatient treatment.[34] Many authors agree to the necessity of hiring a permanent staff, including a psychiatrist, to ensure continuity of care.[10,18,28] Spitz has emphasized the effectiveness of teams comprising permanent medical and nonmedical personnel working together as equals; all members have similar responsibilities for the evaluation and referral of patients.[18] Zusman discusses an interesting alternative to these mental health teams particularly suitable for general hospitals without a large psychiatric presence.[50] A part-time psychiatrist was added to the medical-surgical ER staff in a 600-bed general hospital without an inpatient psychiatric unit. This psychiatrist provided evaluation and referral, five sessions of crisis-oriented treatment, and teaching for the entire range of ER personnel. At the end of one year, the psychiatrist concluded that the ER personnel had become more skilled at identifying and managing patients with emotional difficulties.

4. Conclusion

The psychiatric ER in the general hospital occupies a unique position. It faces the difficult task of reconciling community needs with traditional organizational structures. The community, seeking solutions to both chronic problems and acute situational crises, encounters a medical model of emergency treatment that is generally unresponsive to these needs. Rather than specifically defining the patient's request and engaging him in treatment, the emphasis in the majority of ERs has been on evaluation and referral. This model would be adequate if most patients complied with referral recommendations, and if community alternatives were available. Poor compliance is more often attributed to poor patient motivation than to unresponsive programs. As a result, more adaptive service-delivery models generally have not evolved.

Model programs and outcome research in a few facilities provide a direction for innovative ER care. The thrust of these programs is basically threefold. First, there is an attempt to provide continuity of care through extended crisis intervention in the emergency setting. This is particularly useful for patients whose orientation toward help or whose current condition militates against transfer of care to another service. Second, when referral outside of the ER is necessary, procedures have been modified in a manner that significantly improves the rate of completion. Third, there are efforts to identify subgroups of patients with special needs for whom specific techniques of intervention can be developed. Services incorporating these innovations will aid in meeting the challenges facing the general hospital psychiatric ER. Continued research in delineating patient needs, treatment models, and intervention strategies can better integrate the services of the general hospital with the needs of the community.

References

1. Nemiah J: Help! *Am J Psychiatry* 124:1698–1699, 1968.
2. Shortliffe E, Hamilton T, Noroian E: Emergency room and changing patterns of medical care. *N Engl J Med* 258:20–25, 1958.
3. Zonana H, Henisz J, Levine M: Psychiatric emergency services a decade later. *Psychiatry Med* 3:273–290, 1973.
4. Satloff A, Worby C: The psychiatric emergency service: Mirror of change. *Am J Psychiatry* 126:1628–1632, 1970.
5. Chafetz M, Blane H, Muller J: Acute psychiatric services in the general hospital: Implications for psychiatry in emergency admissions. *Am J Psychiatry* 123:664–670, 1966.
6. Coleman J: Research in walk-in psychiatric services in general hospitals. *Am J Psychiatry* 124:1668–1673, 1968.
7. Coleman J, Errera P: The general hospital emergency room and its psychiatric problems. *Am J Public Health* 53:1294–1301, 1963.
8. Errera P, Wyshak G, Jarecki H: Psychiatric care in a general hospital emergency room. *Arch Gen Psychiatry* 9:105–112, 1963.
9. Huffine C, Craig T: Social factors in the utilization of an urban psychiatric emergency service. *Arch Gen Psychiatry* 30:249–255, 1974.
10. Bartolucci G, Drayer C: An overview of crisis intervention in the emergency rooms of general hospitals. *Am J Psychiatry* 130:953–960, 1973.
11. Chafetz M: The effect of a psychiatric emergency service on motivation for psychiatric treatment. *J Nerv Ment Dis* 140:442–448, 1965.
12. Bassuk E, Gerson S: Deinstitutionalization and mental health services. *Sci Am* 238:46–53, 1978.
13. Weisz A, Houts P, Straight D: Effects of increased therapist commitment on emergency psychiatric evaluations. *Am J Psychiatry* 127:237–241, 1970.
14. Bassuk EL, Schoonover SC: The private general hospital's psychiatric emergency service in a decade of transition. *Hosp Community Psychiatry* 32:181–185, 1981.
15. Bassuk EL, Apsler R: Managing the chronic patient in an acute care setting. *Psychosoc Rehab J* 6:20–26, 1982.
16. Witkin M: Emergency Services in Psychiatric Facilities in the United States, NIMH Mental Health Statistical Note #136, July 1977.
17. Jacobson G: Emergency services in community mental health—Problems and promises. *Am J Public Health* 64:124–128, 1974.
18. Spitz L: The evolution of a psychiatric emergency crisis intervention service in a medical emergency room setting. *Compr Psychiatry* 17:99–113, 1976.
19. Weinerman E, Rutzen S, Pearson D: Yale studies in ambulatory medical care: II. Effects of medical triage in hospital emergency service. *Public Health Rep* 80:389–399, 1965.
20. Schwartz D, Weiss A, Miner J: Community psychiatry and emergency service. *Am J Psychiatry* 129:710–715, 1972.
21. Glasscote RM, Cumming E, Hammersley D, et al: *The Psychiatric Emergency—A Study of Patterns of Service*. Washington, Joint Information Service, 1966.
22. Atkins R: Psychiatric emergency service. *Arch Gen Psychiatry* 17:176–182, 1967.
23. Silbert R: Psychiatric patients in the admitting emergency room. *Arch Gen Psychiatry* 11:24–30, 1964.
24. Craig T, Huffine C, Brooks M: Completion of referral to psychiatric services by inner city residents. *Arch Gen Psychiatry* 31:353–357, 1974.
25. Kaufman E, Klagsbrun S: An emergency room changes. *Dis Nerv Syst* 33:241–234, 1972.

26. Blane H, Muller J, Chafetz M: Acute psychiatric services in the general hospital: II. Current status of emergency psychiatric services. *Am J Psychiatry* 124:37–45, 1967.
27. Browning C, Miller S, Tyson R: The psychiatric emergency: A high risk medical patient. *Compr Psychiatry* 15:153–156, 1974.
28. Hankoff L, Mischorr M, Tomlinson D, et al: A program of crisis intervention in the emergency medical setting. *Am J Psychiatry* 131:47–50, 1974.
29. Bassuk E, Savitz R, McCombie S, et al: Organizing a rape crisis program in a general hospital. *J Am Med Wom Assoc* 30:486–490, 1975.
30. McCombie S, Bassuk E, Savitz R, et al: Development of a medical center rape crisis intervention program. *Am J Psychiatry* 133:418–421, 1976.
31. ACOG: Technical Bulletin Number 14, The American College of Obstetricians and Gynecologists, July 1970.
32. Caplan G, Grunebaum H: Perspectives on primary prevention—A review. *Arch Gen Psychiatry* 17:331–356, 1967.
33. Frankel F, Chafetz M, Blane H: Treatment of psychosocial crises in the emergency service of a general hospital. *JAMA* 195:626–628, 1966.
34. Beahan L, Dumain H, and Resnik H: The evolution of a coordinated emergency service. *Hosp Community Psychiatry* 22:214–216, 1971.
35. Bellak L: A general hospital as a focus of community psychiatry. *JAMA* 174:2214–2217, 1960.
36. Coleman M, Zwerling I: Psychiatric emergency clinic, flexible way of meeting community mental health needs. *Am J Psychiatry* 115:980–984, 1959.
37. Wilder J, Coleman M: The "walk-in" psychiatric clinic: Some observations and follow-up. *Int J Soc Psychiatry* 9:192–199, 1964.
38. Straker M, Yung C, Weiss L: A comprehensive psychiatric service in a general hospital. *Can Psychiatr Assoc J* 16:137–139, 1971.
39. Daggett L, O'Connor G: The psychiatric emergency room of the Johns Hopkins Hospital. Is it meeting the needs? *Johns Hopkins Med J* 129:304–310, 1971.
40. Guido J, Payne P: 72-hour psychiatric detention. *Arch Gen Psychiatry* 16:223–238, 1967.
41. Rhine R, Mayerson P: Crisis hospitalization within a psychiatric emergency service. *Am J Psychiatry* 127:1386–1391, 1971.
42. Weisman G, Feirstein A, Thomas C: Three day hospitalization—A model for intensive intervention. *Arch Gen Psychiatry* 21:620–629, 1969.
43. Bassuk E: The impact of deinstitutionalization on the general hospital psychiatric emergency ward. *Hosp Community Psychiatry* 31:623–627, 1980.
44. Anthony W, Cohen MR, Vitalo R: Measurement of rehabilitation outcome. *Schizophr Bull* 4:365–383, 1978.
45. Rusk T: Psychiatric education in the emergency room setting. *Can Psychiatr Assoc J* 16:111–120, 1971.
46. Kritzer H, Langsley D: Training for emergency psychiatric services. *J Med Educ* 42:1111–1115, 1967.
47. Beahan L: Emergency mental health services in a general hospital. *Hosp Community Psychiatry* 21:81–84, 1970.
48. Barlow D: Psychologists in the emergency room. *Prof Psychol* 5:251–256, 1974.
49. Nash K: Social work in a university hospital. *Arch Gen Psychiatry* 22:332–337, 1970.
50. Zusman J: The psychiatrist as a member of the emergency room team. *Am J Psychiatry* 123:1394–1401, 1967.

Psychiatric Emergency Care in Resource-Poor Areas

W. R. Cote, R.M.C., C.A.C.

1. Introduction

Much of the literature on psychiatric emergencies is based on the experiences of established treatment facilities such as emergency rooms, crisis clinics, or psychiatric units. Thus, standard emergency protocols tend to overlook the problems of resource-poor areas such as limited manpower, inaccessibility of inpatient and outpatient facilities, and the economic, social, and political realities of various localities. Persons in rural regions generally live in numerous small villages (pop. 50–700) surrounded by vast expanses of agricultural lands, forests, or deserts. These communities receive social, commercial, and medical services from larger surrounding towns (pop. 2500–7500). Delivery of health care may be hampered by sheer distance, difficult to sparse road systems, and challenging climatic conditions. Since rural patients in crisis cannot easily be treated in standard settings, the concept of emergency care must be considerably broadened. It must comprise interventions that begin outside traditional treatment settings and may, for economic, geographic or social reasons, remain outside. Table 1 describes these settings.

In addition to the settings and interventions, the economics, low population density, and large distances influence also the structure and staffing of rural mental health services. In resource-poor areas, nonmental health professionals and nonprofessionals link the community service network. For some (townspeople, friends, neighbors) this function may be unfamiliar, while for others it is ancillary to their primary professional roles. The police and clergy, for example, often provide immediate aid in emergencies until responsibility is transferred to designated mental health crisis teams. These latter individuals are frequently outpatient clinicians who provide this service in addition to their regular duties. They have broad general skills and are recruited for their willingness and ability to manage difficult clinical situations flexibly and with minimal administrative support and supervision. Often, they do not have ready access to a psychiatrist and must rely on their own staff or local family practice physicians for medical backup. Differences from an urban treatment model

W. R. Cote, R.N.C., C.A.C. ● Northeast Kingdom Mental Health Services, St. Johnsbury, Vermont 05819.

Table 1. Psychiatric Emergencies Settings in Low-Resource Areas

	Description
1. Client's home	Crises may evolve entirely in the patient's residence. Often involves the aid of persons other than the designated crisis team. Intervention must take place here because of logistical limitations and/or patient's refusal or inability to leave the premises.
2. Health centers, physicians' offices, prescreening clinics, etc.	The patient/family may have sought crisis services through channels normally used for medical emergencies. The crisis worker may have to use these resources to assist in assessing and managing the situation.
3. Social service agencies, schools	Crises occur in the normal course of activity in these institutions. Personnel will usually become involved in attempts to assess/resolve the crisis. The mental health clinician may be called when the situation is perceived as escalating past the point of their ability/willingness to cope.
4. Police stations, jails	Law enforcement officials are often the first on the scene in emotional/psychiatric crises. Many times the officer may want mental health personnel to assist in decision-making and in providing less intrusive care; "talking someone down" versus physical restraint.
5. Other/field	Crises occasionally occur and must be dealt with in various field settings. These include locations such as saloons, state forests, farms, roadside rest areas, and radar traps. The response must be tailored to the particular situation.

also are reflected in the intervention process itself. This chapter focuses on the salient differences between standard emergency psychiatric care and rural care, and on those clinical issues that are essential for providing high-quality patient care in resource-poor areas.

2. The Intervention

The objectives of emergency care outside a traditional setting are necessarily limited in scope and include containment of the crisis within its present boundaries and maximal utilization of available resources. This should ensure the engagement of the patient in the treatment process and provide opportunities for longer-term crisis resolution. The intervention process consists of three phases that may be sequential, concurrent, or overlapping. They include (1) gathering data for preliminary assessment, (2) determining and initiating the most appropriate immediate response, and (3) treatment planning: coordinating and brokering necessary resources. Figure 1 summarizes various pathways of emergency interventions outside traditional settings.

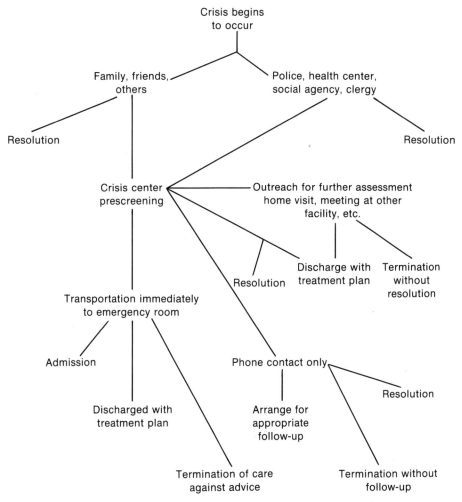

Figure 1. The emergency intervention outside of traditional settings.

2.1. Gathering Data for Preliminary Assessment

The immediate objective is to determine whether or not a crisis involves an immediate life-threatening problem such as severe medical disorder, serious overdose, or self-injury; dangerous or potentially dangerous behavior (e.g., a person who is intoxicated and intending to operate a motor vehicle or other piece of machinery such as a chain saw or farm equipment); and violent, potentially violent, or extremely agitated behavior. Situations involving any of these conditions should be managed immediately. If the crisis contains elements that threaten to erupt or escalate, plans should be made to provide protection, further observation, confinement, medication, or a combination of approaches. In addition to identifying risk factors, the clinical should gather other information as rapidly and accurately as possible. He should elicit information about the presenting problem, current level of functioning, available resources, and recent past history. It may be necessary to talk with persons other than the patient. Besides obtaining essential information from them, the caretaker can begin to shape their roles within the support system. Positive rapport established initially with family, friends, or other participants can facilitate longer-range crisis resolution and involvement in an effective treatment program.

> For example, a crisis teamworker was called by the sister (Mrs. F.) of a former patient (D.). The sister insisted that someone come to her house immediately and "do something" because she was convinced that D. was deteriorating and no one "knows what she will do." The worker obtained information from the old records and called a clinician who had worked with the client. He reported that although the patient often manifested a serious thought disorder, she usually became quietly withdrawn. He then went to Mrs. F.'s house. According to Mrs. F., D. had refused her efforts to help and was not eating properly or tending to matters of personal hygiene. Mrs. F.'s husband remained in another room during the interview, and it became clear that Mrs. F. was responding to pressure from him to have D. removed from the house. On examination, D. was slightly delusional and possibly hallucinating. She admitted not taking her haloperidol (Haldol) for several weeks. There was no evidence of acute suicidal or homicidal behavior from the history, the patient's statement, or information given by Mrs. F. Although D. was disheveled and dressed inappropriately, she did not appear to be dehydrated or to have any obvious medical problem. The emergency worker concluded that the current crisis resulted from Mr. and Mrs. F.'s frustrations about D., who had a long history of acute exacerbations usually following her discontinuation of antipsychotic medications. They had cared for her for many years. In the past, they had agreed "to take her back, but only after a period of rest from her constant demands." In this case, however, D. refused hospitalization and was not regarded as committable. The F.'s agreed to care for her until the following day, when placement could be arranged at a transitional care facility. The emergency evaluator also encouraged Mr. and Mrs. F's continued participation in longer-term dispositional planning.

2.2. Determining and Initiating an Immediate Response

The emergency worker should develop a step-by-step plan for managing and containing the crisis. The problem should be formulated hierarchically by degree of severity (life-threatening, high risk, or potentially life-threatening, low risk), by immediacy, and by ease of solubility. Must the patient be treated on the scene or can he be transported? Is there a need for assistance from law enforcement personnel or emergency medical technicians? (See Table 2 for a description of common clinical presentations and various management approaches.)

The protection of the person in crisis and those around him must always be considered in determining the initial intervention. Issues of safety for the

Table 2. Clinical Presentations and Management Approaches

Presentation	Action
1. Potential for violence	1. Initiate a response in the field by appropriate personnel. Physical intervention/restraint may be required.
2. Suicidal threat or action	2. Mobilize resources for medical assistance. Provide means for next therapeutic action (such as voluntary or involuntary admission to a psychiatric unit, use of emergency bed in the community, arranging for client to stay with friends/relatives for the night, etc.).
3. Physical problems—adverse drug reaction, symptoms of withdrawal	3. Depending on the clinician's background, a decision must be made as to the most appropriate mode of assessment.
4. Social needs—housing, food, companionship, transportation	4. Arrange contact between the patient and the agency/individual responsible for providing services. In some communities the mental health agency is the only after-hours broker of any social service.
5. Need to talk with someone immediately about intense feelings	5. Use telephone interventions when possible. Arrange for face-to-face contact either immediately or during the next working day.
6. Request for information	6. Provide it, or arrange for contact with the appropriate person.

crisis personnel and the patient often dictate where and under what conditions an emergency intervention should occur. In rural areas, it is also frequently necessary to attend to basic survival needs such as shelter, food, and clothing, as well as child care requirements. The clinician must often develop creative approaches that include mobilizing many nontraditional resources. It cannot be emphasized too strongly that using available resources—nonprofessional care providers, the telephone, family networks, and nonhospital housing—is the key to developing a workable management and treatment plan. To ignore the realistic sources of help in favor of optimal resources may result in a further escalation of the crisis, an unsuccessful treatment plan, and a waste of available assets. In fact, in some situations the support network that exists at the time of crisis may be the only resource available.

The emergency clinician in a rural community endeavors to accomplish as much as possible with the smallest output of resources. Intervention becomes a matter of compromise and accommodation, not maximal response.

> For example, a call on a wintry Saturday evening was received by the crisis worker from the chief of police of a town 35 miles away. The chief had been called by Mr. L., the father of a retarded adult woman, Ann. Ann had been kept at home with her parents for the past 20 years since she had been released from a special school. The L.s, in their 70s, found themselves

increasingly unable to care for Ann, until a heated argument prompted Mr.
L. to call the police chief, demanding that "something be done NOW!"
The crisis worker called Mr. L., assessed the situation by phone, and discussed alternative care modes (respite care, home health aides, advocacy,
senior companion programs, sheltered workshops) that might help maintain
Ann at home. It was arranged for Ann to stay with her brother until she
could be seen by an agency social worker the next day. The brother agreed
to call the crisis worker if problems developed. The settlement, reached by
telephone, relieved the L.s, involved the reluctant brother, and pleased
Ann, who was eager to be away from home for a weekend.

In short, the hallmark of emergency care in a nontraditional setting is
flexibility—the capacity to take a limited, concrete, problem-solving approach
to the crisis situation—and creativity—the capacity to make use of any available resources and design innovative, workable treatment plans. It is neither
necessary nor desirable to attend to longer-term issues unless the patient's
motivation, resources, and condition, as well as the accessibility and feasibility
of treatment possibilities, warrant such planning.

2.3. Treatment Planning/Coordinating and Brokering Resources

It should be borne in mind that most often the options for treatment and
crisis resolution are not ideal; the objective is to manage and contain the crisis
and provide follow-up according to the limitations imposed by the economics,
geography, and resources of the setting and the patient's wishes. It is imperative, therefore, to design a treatment plan that takes into account the actual
features of the patient's everyday life, such as finances and availability of
transportation to and from established care centers. Treatment plans based on
an unrealistic assessment of available resources, or of the patient's requests,
have a low likelihood of working.

It falls to the prescreening clinician to take responsibility for directing the
immediate plan. Field intervention almost invariably involves other individuals,
including friends, family, police, clergy, and other community providers. They
are important elements in this phase of the crisis management process. The
primary caretaker and person or agencies who will be involved in the patient's
continued care should also be considered. The emergency clinician often must
take the role of negotiator and mediator in obtaining the needed consent to a
specific plan. Although other people serve as clinical links in the treatment
planning phases, it is ultimately the crisis worker who must effect the transfer
of patient care to the treatment team or support network. This can be as simple
as arranging for a follow-up phone call; it could involve more complex interventions such as coordinating diagnostic work. The crisis clinician is responsible for getting the patient beyond the crisis and into follow-up.

3. Conclusion

The emergency clinician in a resource-poor area is not unlike his counterparts in urban settings. Each must use rapid assessment techniques, and

engage the patient in the process of resolving the crisis, planning treatment, and facilitating the transfer of responsibility to the appropriate system. However, there is a major difference. The urban emergency clinician can base his intervention more fully on clinical parameters: the nature and severity of the crisis and the patient's psychological status and resources. The rural emergency worker also must orient his intervention to the specific crisis but more often must allow it to be shaped by factors independent of the clinical presentation.

Bibliography

1. Ames DA: Developing a psychiatric inpatient service in a rural area. *Hosp Community Psychiatry* 29:787–791, 1978.
2. Berry B, Davis AE: Community mental health ideology: A problematic model for rural areas. *Am J Orthopsychiatry* 48:673–679, 1978.
3. Carter AP: Rural emergency psychiatric services. *Am J Nursing* 73:868–869, 1973.
4. Cesnik BI, Pierce N, Puls M: Law enforcement and crisis intervention services: A critical relationship. *Suicide Life-Threatening Behav* 7:211–215, 1977.
5. Daniels DN: The community mental health center in the rural area: Is the present model appropriate? *Am J Psychiatry* 124 (Suppl):32–37, 1967.
6. Duran FA: The Northeast Kingdom: Developing a mental health nursing service in rural America. *Nursing Clin N Am* 5:669–676, 1970.
7. Eisdorfer C, Altrocchi J, Young RF: Principles of community mental health in a rural setting: The Halifax County program. *Community Ment Health J* 4:211–220, 1968.
8. Everstine DS, Bodin AM, Everstine L: Emergency psychology: A mobile service for police crisis calls. *Fam Proc* 16:281–292, 1977.
9. Gertz B, Meider J, Pluckham MA: A survey of rural community mental health needs and resources. *Hosp Community Psychiatry* 26:816–819, 1975.
10. Herbert GK, Chevaliet MC, Meyers CL: Factors contributing to the successful use of indigenous mental health workers. *Hosp Community Psychiatry* 25:308–310, 1974.
11. Husaini BA, Neff JA: Characteristics of life events and psychiatric impairment in rural communities. *J Nerv Ment Dis* 168:159–166, 1980.
12. Jeffrey MJ, Reeve RE: Community mental health services in rural areas: Some practical issues. *Community Ment Health J* 14:54–62, 1978.
13. Jones JD, Robin SS, Wagenfeld MD: Rural mental health centers: Are they different? *Int J Ment Health* 3:77–92, 1974.
14. Jones JD, Wagenfeld MD, Robin, SS: A profile of the rural community mental health center. *Community Ment Health J* 12:176–181, 1976.
15. Lee SH, Gianturco DT, and Eisdorfer C: Community mental health accessibility: A survey of the rural poor. *Arch Gen Psychiatry* 31:335–339, 1974.
16. Levenson AI, Reff SR: Community mental health centers staffing patterns. *Community Ment Health J* 6:118–125, 1970.
17. Marshall CD: The indigenous nurse as community crisis intervener. *Semin Psychiatry* 3:264–270, 1971.
18. Porritt D: Social support in crisis: Quantity or quality? *Soc Sci Med* 13:715–721, 1979.
19. Segal J (ed.): *The Mental Health of Rural America.* Washington, Department of Health, Education and Welfare, 1973.
20. Stobie EG, Hopkins DHG: Crisis intervention 1 and 2: A psychiatric community nurse in a rural area. *Nursing Times* 68:165–172, 1972.
21. Walfish S, Tulkin SR, Tapp JT, et al: Crisis clinic. *Community Ment Health J* 12:89–94, 1976.

Psychiatric Home Visiting Services

Steven E. Samuel, M.Ed., Iris Lee Bagwell, M.Ed., and James P. Jones, Ph.D.

1. Introduction

To reduce the need for in-hospital care, psychiatric home treatment services were first promoted in Amsterdam in the 1930s. Emergency personnel, organized into multidisciplinary teams, made on-site visits to patients in crisis. These teams conducted brief emergency evaluations to determine whether or not continued home treatment—with medication and also with some counseling—could prevent hospitalization. These early services successfully minimized hospitalizations and demonstrated their utility as emergency care services in their own right. Today, home visiting is an integral part of the community mental health network, extending psychiatric care to those who either cannot or will not use established hospital or office-based services.

2. Function, Composition, and Structure

Services provided by mobile crisis units or home visiting teams have grown to fit the needs of the community. Although originally designed to evaluate on site the need for psychiatric hospitalization, crisis teams now may act as primary providers for families and individuals who reject other caregivers, refuse hospitalization, or seek care only during episodes of violence, disruption, or psychiatric decompensation. Crisis teams may, therefore, be the only liaison between individuals or families in crisis and the community mental health system. These individuals or families are not necessarily the same as outpatient or emergency department populations. They include persons experiencing a situational crisis that demands on-the-scene intervention; chronically ill, deinstitutionalized patients who are dangerous, bizarre, psychotic, and not treatable in established settings; and individuals who refuse established psychiatric outpatient care, yet need continuing treatment. Whatever the type of patient or

Steven E. Samuel, M.Ed., Iris Lee Bagwell, M.Ed., and James P. Jones, Ph.D. • West-Ros-Park Mental Health Center, Roslindale, Massachusetts 02131. Present address for Steven E. Samuel is Counseling Psychology Department, Temple University, Philadelphia, Pennsylvania 19122. Present address for James P. Jones is Department of Mental Health, Cape Ann Area Office, Beverley, Massachusetts 01919.

family, home visiting has proved to be an effective alternative to hospitalization and outpatient psychiatric care. When the crisis team decides that it cannot substitute for hospitalization or established forms of outpatient treatment, it acts as a facilitator among, and coordinator of, other branches of the mental health system.

The essence of home visiting is mobility and teamwork. The team delivers services outside the usual office structure—most often in the home, but frequently in police stations, schools, social agencies, anywhere emergency psychiatric care is needed. To maximize the immediate benefits of on-site care and to minimize the danger to emergency personnel working by themselves, mobile crisis units should be staffed by multidisciplinary teams. They are traditionally composed of psychiatrists, psychologists, social workers, psychiatric nurses, paramedics with mental health training, and trained volunteers or nonprofessionals. A team, consisting of two people, often is needed to evaluate the complex factors operating in a crisis situation: the crisis itself and its impact on the patient and his family; the need for hospitalization, medication, medical treatment, and protective measures; the resources available; the patient's and the family's personal/interpersonal dynamics. Adequate assessment must be completed on the spot and, if necessary, active intervention planned and implemented. Although personnel with different training tend to focus their attention on different aspects of the crisis situation, a successful home visiting team must be flexible, switch roles and functions when warranted, and coordinate team efforts.

The benefits of a multidisciplinary approach are obvious—at least theoretically. However, if the team members have difficulty working across interdisciplinary boundaries, developing a cooperative mode of interaction, or resolving intrastaff conflict smoothly, the benefits of a team approach are lost. Basic to the process of weaving a cohesive team out of individual members is mutual respect, a clear understanding of the team's assets and weaknesses, and a regular forum for handling disagreements and grievances.

To ensure mobility while maintaining continued accessibility, the home visiting team staff must keep communication channels open and have transportation readily available. The team should also have a "portable office" that contains essential information and equipment. These include resource lists (shelters, nursing homes, drug and alcohol programs, inpatient units, ambulances, physicians, therapists, etc.); intake and evaluation forms, involuntary commitment forms, consent and release forms; standard medical equipment to be used only by appropriate personnel. Practical necessities include such equipment as flashlights and batteries, handbooks, and maps, and should become part of a standard kit.

3. Intervention Techniques

Because mobile crisis units do more than evaluate the need for hospitalization, their ability to facilitate the resolution of a crisis depends in large measure on establishing an alliance with the patient or family. Sometimes the mere fact of the team's availability and willingness to make a home visit is sufficient to form a working alliance. In general, however, the team should anticipate some resistance to the emergency intervention. Entry to the house may be refused; the fact of the crisis may be denied; transportation to a mental health facility may be resisted. In short, the team may find itself faced with the decision to initiate involuntary procedures; or the team may decide to abandon efforts altogether. The legal, clinical, and ethical implications of this type of impasse are felt by emergency teams who specialize in on-site care (see Chapter 3).

Once the request for help is initiated, usually with a preliminary telephone call, the crisis team should consider various intervention options. A home visit is not always required. The telephone may be used for crisis management without necessitating an in-person consultation. In cases where the potential for violence is great, a home visit may be contraindicated; removal of persons at risk or transportation of the potentially violent patient may have to be considered before a face-to-face intervention can safely occur. In either case, assessment of immediate risk to the identified patient or to family members must begin at the first point of contact and must continue throughout the intervention. Steps should be taken immediately to protect persons at risk. If restraint is necessary, only those persons authorized to restrain people against their will should be involved. If safety factors warrant changing the intervention site, removing the patient or other people, or even beginning involuntary procedures for dangerous individuals, those decisions should be made and implemented at once. In lower-risk situations, home visiting can follow a typical course as follows.

Responding to the emergency call promptly allows the clinical team access to the patient and family in crisis at the point where the greatest impact can be made. Since home visiting provides an opportunity to evaluate persons and families in crisis in the context of their own environment, the resultant assessment has an unusual degree of detail, accuracy, and depth. Recommendations based on home evaluations have a high likelihood of working since they must account for factors such as family dynamics, patient resistance, or quality of life—factors that might not otherwise be obvious during off-site evaluations.

As in other types of crisis intervention programs, home visiting teams selectively evaluate the current situation, its immediate precipitants, and environmental, interpersonal, and psychologic factors maintaining it. The team also needs to know about past crises, how they were managed, and the nature and extent of personal and/or social resources available to the patient or family. It is essential, although not always easy, to clarify the factors contributing to the crisis, whether they are indigenous to the individual or the social system of which he is a part, whether they are medical in origin or reflect a functional psychiatric disorder. If drugs, alcohol, or other substances are involved, it is important to ascertain type, usual amount consumed or used, and the patient's reaction to them. As the nature of the crisis becomes clear to the emergency team, and its course amenable to intervention, the risk of future problems such as suicide, homicide, domestic violence, and psychotic decompensation can be assessed.

Pharmacologic management of the patient should not be considered unless there is frank psychosis with accompanying thought disorder, major depression with vegetative symptoms, or severe anxiety or insomnia. In these cases, the patient should be advised of the risks and benefits of the medication, the right not to take medication, and the need to follow a responsible, supervised regimen. If there is any question about the latter, a maintenance regimen should not be administered. Treatment strategies should be designed to ensure safety, accomodate and contain the crisis, prevent hospitalization if possible, and encourage new, problem-solving patterns of behavior for the persons in crisis. Deep-seated conflict and life-long psychological problems are not an appropriate focus for crisis intervention except as they conspicuously affect the current situation.

Referral should be made to other clinical services in the community mental health system. It is the responsibility of the clinical team to tailor the referral to the needs and resources of the patient or family in crisis, and to follow through with the referral. The differences between getting the patient or family into treatment and their dropping out is often determined by how active the team is with the patient, family, and various referral networks. Continuity of care necessitates that the team stay in touch with the patient—bridging the gap until the clinician responsible for ongoing treatment has made personal contact with the patient or family. The transfer of responsibility from emergency team to treatment facility is far easier if rapport with the patient and family has been established at the outset, and if the patient and/or family in crisis understand the rationale for further treatment. The team's findings should be shared with the patient as matter of factly and simply as possible. Aftercare plans should be clarified, questions answered honestly, and decisions to report specific findings discussed. For example, it is a law in some states that child abuse be reported to the appropriate state department. The decision to take such a step must be discussed with the family. Regardless of the specific laws of any state, however, the home visiting team has an ethical obligation to intervene immediately in any situation thought to involve child abuse, or indeed any other form of abuse (see Chapter 17).

Referral to an agency, private therapist, or outpatient clinic may be appropriate if the patient and/or family are cooperative and have resources (transportation, finances, or insurance) available to them. Scheduling a series of follow-up home visits is also a possibility when patient resistance, resources, and/or problems militate against referral to an established facility. Hospitalization should be recommended if the crisis cannot be contained, a serious medical disorder is present, or there is real danger of suicide, homicide, or uncontrolled violence. Involuntary hospitalization may be necessary when danger is likely and the patient uncooperative. Because various treatment options are usually available to the team, assessment should be undertaken with an eye to treatment planning.

4. Conclusion

Home visiting services have made psychiatric care available to a patient population otherwise unreachable within the established mental health framework. For chronically ill, deinstitutionalized patients, persons or families in crisis too disruptive for off-site intervention, and individuals resistant to standard treatment formats, mobile crisis units provide essential, stabilizing services: crisis management, evaluation for hospitalization and/or subsequent outpatient treatment, follow-up care and consultation to support groups—families, friends, police, etc. Without these emergency teams, many patients in crisis would have literally no access to psychiatric care; with them, the network of emergency mental health services is more extensive and manages to cover a critical subgroup of the patient population.

Bibliography

1. Bochar JA: *Primer for the Nonmedical Psychotherapist.* New York, SP Medical and Scientific Books, 1976.
2. Edelwich J (ed): *Burn Out: Stages of Disillusionment in the Helping Professions.* New York, Human Sciences Press, 1980.
3. DiMascio A, Goldberg H: *Emotional Disorders: An Outline Guide to Diagnosis and Pharmacological Treatment,* ed 3. Oradell, NJ, Medical Economics Co, Book Division, 1976.
4. Herbert C, Cross T: A psychiatric emergency kit for use by clinicians in emergency services. *Hosp Community Psychiatry* 32:726–727, 1981.
5. Becker A, Goldberg H: Home treatment services, in Grunebaum H (ed): *The Practice of Community Mental Health.* Boston, Little, Brown, and Co, 1970, pp 277–296.
6. Satir V: *Conjoint Family Therapy.* New York, Science and Behavior Books, 1964.
7. West L, Oberlander M: Emergency psychiatric home visiting: Report of four years experience. *J Clin Psychiatry* 41:113–118, 1980.
8. Woodbury M, Woodbury M: Community-centered psychiatric intervention: A pilot project in 13th Arrondissement, Paris. *Am J Psychiatry* 126:619–625, 1969.

The Telephone in Psychiatric Emergencies

Barbara Schuler Gilmore, R.N., M.S.N., C.S.

1. Introduction

The human voice was first conveyed electronically through space in March 1876, when Alexander Graham Bell summoned his assistant with the memorable words "Mr. Watson, come here. I want you."[1] Since that time, the telephone has evolved from a costly luxury to an essential part of life. The telephone has made immediate communication possible, even over vast distances. For medicine, in particular, the telephone has had an enormous impact on the availability of health care; it is literally a "physician extender" and can be used for diagnostic purposes (e.g., electrocardiogram transmissions), medical arrangements (e.g., admission to the hospital), and consultation.[2–7] The telephone, however, is no substitute for face-to-face contact. Especially in psychiatry, the lack of visual cues presents a decided handicap in evaluating a patient's behavioral and emotional symptoms. For accurate assessment and management, it is generally not enough to hear what the patient says about himself; at times, however, the telephone may be the first and only link with the patient in crisis.[8–10]

2. Hotlines

The telephone entered a new era of service in the 1950s with the birth of the Samaritans. Supervised volunteers provided instantaneous telephone contact for persons in crisis.[11] Under a cloak of anonymity, callers could share even their most painful problems with open, nonjudgmental listeners. Once contact was made by telephone, the caller's increasing isolation and loneliness had been interrupted, at least for the moment, and desperate impulses were weakened.

Originally aimed at suicide prevention, telephone hotlines were extended to crises of different sorts: rape, domestic violence, alcohol and drug abuse, and runaway children.[12–16] Social service agencies and clinics currently rely

Barbara Schuler Gilmore, R.N., M.S.N., C.S. • Newton-Wellesley Hospital, Newton Lower Falls, Massachusetts 02162.

heavily on telephone interventions. By now, the use of the telephone for crisis intervention and referral is commonplace. There may be differences in style and approach, but the link among hotlines is 24-hour telephone service.[17] One type is that of the Los Angeles Suicide Prevention Center, where available professionals or trained secretaries answer the telephone during the day. After hours, volunteers staff the telephone—often graduate or medical students trained and supervised by professionals.[18] If there is a common denominator among the diverse approaches to telephone counseling, it is to focus on the caller's potential for effective coping, to mobilize available personal resources, to encourage realistic problem-solving, and to provide reassurance, not to dwell on personal psychopathology. In addition to supportive counseling, hotlines now offer the following services: giving information; providing referrals to hospitals, private therapists, or agencies; contacting relatives or friends if the caller permits; involving police or ambulance with the caller's consent; and arranging follow-up calls to persons considered at risk (e.g., suicide).

The vast majority of telephone calls made to hotlines are help-seeking, but some are problem callers. These include the obscene caller, the chronic caller, the one-counselor caller, and the fearful caller who either by silence, need for total anonymity, or the "calling for a friend" routine expresses extreme difficulty in asking for help.[19] Although responses to each call should be individualized, it is generally agreed that the counselor should respect the *fact* of the call over its content and maneuver the caller toward a more therapeutic form of interaction.

3. Crisis Centers and Other Emergency Facilities

Unlike hotlines, crisis centers and other emergency care facilities provide more than telephone capability; they offer in-person emergency counseling and referral services. Telephone contact with a crisis center can be the initial phase of an ongoing process that includes emergency evaluation, treatment, and referral. Similar to the hotline, the immediate goal of the telephone interviewer may be to establish an alliance with the caller, but the focus is on in-person arrangements rather than one-time telephone crisis management.

4. Personnel

Controversy surrounds the staffing of hotlines and crisis centers.[20] Volunteers have played a critical role in telephone counseling since the program was conceived in the 1950s, but, as mental health professionals have been quick to point out, volunteers are by definition nonprofessionals. However, they provide a decided economic advantage to the sponsors of the hotline or crisis center; beyond that, they bring an enthusiasm and fresh perspective to their work.[21] For social or ethnic reasons, they may provide strong links between the neighborhood or community and the mental health system that they serve.

Although they require training and ongoing supervision by professionals, they are indispensable to the hotline or crisis center organization.[22-25]

5. The Emergency Call

The emergency telephone call must be handled differently from an in-person interview. In the latter, assessment can be more thorough and treatment more immediate. Over the telephone, the rules change. The caller is in control. He initiates the call and can terminate it at will. He can remain a voice with no identifying features. The counselor has only that voice with which to work.

Interviewing by means of the telephone necessitates a very active therapeutic stance. It is essential to assess the situation, manage the crisis, and formulate an ongoing treatment plan while keeping the caller on the line and establishing rapport.[10,26] There are no discrete steps; the counselor must weave back and forth among these tasks while trying to build a relationship with the caller.

5.1. Keeping the Caller on the Line

Keeping the caller on the line is critical, but not always easy. The caller may break the connection for a number of reasons: If intoxicated or disorganized, he may be too confused or panicky to continue. Shame, embarrassment, and intense conflict about asking for help are common reasons for terminating a call. The usual psychotherapeutic techniques for building rapport are used, but they must be converted to audible cues. Actively encouraging the caller to tell his story, acknowledging his pain, and offering help are signs that the counselor is interested and supportive.

In general, it is useful to ask for, and expect to have, some identifying information early in the call. When that is not forthcoming, it is better to continue talking in an anonymous fashion rather than struggling with the caller. The longer the telephone relationship continues, the greater the likelihood that useful information will be offered.

When the caller abuses the telephone intervention with obscenity, multiple calls, or active hostility, limits need to be set. The caller, however, should always be told he can call again. The following is an example from the Samaritans*:

VOLUNTEER: Samaritans. Can I help you?
CALLER: Who's this?
VOLUNTEER: It's Pat. (recognizing the voice) Hello, Stuart.
CALLER: Oh no. Are you the———who hung up on me a minute ago?
VOLUNTEER: I had to. We can only give you one call a day and you talked to Kay this morning.

* Adapted from Casper S: Unpublished training materials. Boston Office of the Samaritans, 1981.

CALLER: How do you know? Do you write everything down?
VOLUNTEER: We keep track of some things.
CALLER: That's against my constitutional rights. I'm going to report you.
VOLUNTEER: What would you like me to do?
CALLER: Talk to me. That's what you people are there for.
VOLUNTEER: Kay talked to you this morning.
CALLER: Not long enough. She put me on hold three times. What kind of help is that?
VOLUNTEER: A lot of people need to talk. That's why we can't talk to you more than once a day. I have to go now. You can call again tomorrow.
CALLER: What is this, Nazi Germany?
VOLUNTEER: (Hangs up—Click—Ring) Samaritans. Can I help you?
SAME CALLER: I thought you said you were busy!
VOLUNTEER: (Hangs up—Click—Ring) Samaritans, can I help you?
CALLER: If you won't talk to me I'll kill myself!
VOLUNTEER: (Hangs up—Click—Ring) Samaritans. Can I help you?

5.2. Assessing the Crisis and the Caller

Assessment begins with understanding the reasons for the call, including the person's covert expectations. These vary from the hope for a massive intervention to the wish for simple reassurance. Some callers can only feel close at a safe distance, others call out of loneliness; some merely call to test the counselor's sincerity. Some call to say good-bye, but all call for a reason.[27]

The first call from a distressed individual is generally the most difficult; there is no previous baseline from which to assess the crisis. The caller may be confused, psychotic, and desperate, or lucid and cooperative. In any case, the work of assessment is essentially information-gathering. What is the caller experiencing currently? What led up to the crisis? What would the caller like to have happen—or not happen? Who can help? Is anyone in danger? Calls from known persons who have established a telephone alliance with a hotline or a particular counselor are easier to handle. A relationship exists and the counselor is somewhat familiar with the crisis and the caller's coping skills.

> For example, a 32-year-old single, chronically depressed woman calls her therapist at home saying that she feels suicidal and frightened. Tonight is Halloween, and the prospect of adolescent boys "trick or treating" at her door has made her so anxious that she is considering an overdose. She has been known to the clinic for seven years and has been in supportive treatment with the same therapist for three years. She only occasionally calls between appointments and seems to want her therapist to listen supportively. The therapist thinks that she can help the patient deal with her feelings over the phone. She reviews the patient's options: She could buy candy and hand it out, but is frightened to open the door; she could turn out the lights and pretend she is not at home, but the boys might know she is hiding and still ring the bell. In response to a question about where her father will be that evening, she reports that he is going to the movies. Could she go with him? She seizes on this option and at last feels she can avoid the dilemma by being out of the house completely. She no longer feels as if an overdose is her only way of dealing with the situation. Thanking the ther-

apist, she says she will fill her in next week about the outcome at their usual appointment. For her the perceived crisis has become manageable.

If the caller is a third party, the same information should be gathered, although the counselor should bear in mind that not all calls from self-identified third parties are actually so. The following case example illustrates a call from a legitimate third party.

Mrs. S., formerly a patient at the clinic, had called repeatedly about her husband of 44 years.

Mrs. S.: He can't hear me; if he does he gets so mad. What can I do?

Clinician: Where are you?

Mrs. S.: I'm at home, like always.

Clinician: Can you come in, Mrs. S.? Can I give you an appointment?

Mrs. S.: I can't get there (crying); he won't let me out of his sight. He was never like this before.

Clinician: It's been difficult for you. What happened?

Mrs. S.: Sometimes he's fine, just like he used to be. Then other times he gets like this.

Clinician: What's "this" like?

Mrs. S.: Angry, yelling at me, accusing me of running around; me, an old woman. What can I do?

Clinician: Has he hurt you? Are you scared?

Mrs. S.: I can't talk anymore. Here he comes again (crying).

Clinician: Can I call you? Give me your telephone number. . . (Mrs. S. hangs up.)

Later that morning Mrs. S. calls back:

Clinician: I'm glad you called back. Are things better now?

Mrs. S.: No better, but he's in the bathroom now and can't hear me.

Clinician: Who else is around who can help you?

Mrs. S.: Nobody—just my son, still at home, but he's no help. He yells at me too (crying). He won't help me to get him to come in and he needs help.

Clinician: Are you okay? Are you safe there?

Mrs. S.: Yes, he needs help. I'm okay, he just yells and watches me all the time. The medicine doesn't work.

Clinician: What medicine?

Mrs. S.: Haldol. Our family doctor gives it to him.

Clinician: How much does he take?

Mrs. S.: He won't take it. Sometimes he doesn't sleep all night, up roaming around and yelling. I worry about him so.

Clinician: You sound like it might be helpful for you to come in; things are so hard for you.

Mrs. S.: Maybe so, but he needs help.

Clinician: We'd like to help him. Can you bring him in? If you can't make an appointment, you could bring him to the emergency room whenever you can. We always have somebody available for emergencies.

Mrs. S.: Maybe I can, I'll see. I've got to go before he comes out of the bathroom. Thank you.

The format in Table 1 is useful for organizing and documenting emergency telephone calls. It should serve as a guide for the type of information needed by the interviewer, but not as a rigid protocol.

Table 1. Protocol for Documenting Emergency Calls

Caller:	Age:	Date and time call received:
Home address:	Sex:	Telephone worker:
Number calling from[a]:		

Address calling from (if different from home):
Living arrangements:
Problem (in caller's own words):
Significant losses:
Lethality assessment (include previous suicidal behaviors):
Symptoms (include use of alcohol and drugs):
Support system:
Formulation:
Management plan:
Others notified:

[a] This is important. If the call is placed from a phone booth and the caller is out of change, the therapist can call back and continue the intervention. The number is also a method for determining where the person is if he cannot give an address.

5.3. Intervening with Specific Suggestions and Advice

When the interviewer feels there is risk to the caller he should offer specific advice. These callers should be urged to go to an emergency facility either on their own or via police or ambulance. Those who admit to overdosing should be asked specifically about the type(s) of drugs (including nonprescription drugs like aspirin and Sominex), when and how many they ingested, and in combination with what else (alcohol, prescribed medications). Do not assume that only one drug was taken or that the caller can wait until he has reached the emergency facility to provide this information. Similarly, specific details should be obtained about lacerations and other self-inflicted injuries. Give simple instructions to dress the wound or stop the bleeding and refer the patient to an emergency facility. The caller may be unwilling to volunteer necessary information; if that is the case, do not struggle. Instead keep the line open, work to engage the caller, and obtain the one vital piece of information—the address and/or phone number of the person at risk.

5.4. Managing the Caller in Crisis

This begins at the start of the conversation. For some, the mere act of talking will suffice. Meeting the caller's temporary needs for reassurance and contact may reduce the crisis anxiety and restore a sense of identify and self-worth. Other simple, direct suggestions may address the physical well-being of the caller: "Lie down, take it easy until. . . .""Call a baby-sitter to come and stay with the children until you calm down. . . ." When it is appropriate, callers may be instructed to regulate the use of drugs already prescribed. For example, callers who admit to stopping a prescribed drug regimen (especially antipsychotics) should be instructed to take an appropriate initial dose and to call their regular therapist. In other situations a more specific plan of action requiring the collaboration of caller and counselor might be needed.

For example, Ann, a 19-year-old junior college student, daughter of a local physician, called the rape crisis center at 1:00 a.m. She had just been raped in her own apartment by a friend of her absent roommate. She was terrified, panicky, and worried that he would return. She was unwilling to give her full name or address, call the police, or go to the hospital because she was worried about confidentiality. She was not physically injured or worried about pregnancy risk because she was on the pill. Her primary worry was that he would return. The therapist acknowledged her immediate concern, and together they explored which friends might be available to help. She thought of one she could trust with the information. The therapist suggested that Ann call her friend and then contact the therapist to let her know if the plan was workable. Twenty minutes later Ann called from the friend's apartment already somewhat relieved.

Further discussion centered on her physical health and immediate medical needs. Since she refused police involvement, the therapist suggested that a bath or shower might be comforting and relaxing. She was exhausted and felt that she would be able to sleep after the bath. She was offered an appointment at the center for counseling, but declined, saying that she would think about it and call if she changed her mind.

The uncooperative caller who indicates his intent to die requires an aggressive intervention. If the caller's location is known, transportation to a hospital either by police or ambulance should be arranged immediately. If possible, the original counselor should stay on the phone while a second person calls the police or rescue squad. When a second person is not available, the counselor should inform the caller that he is going to take action and that the person should remain where he is and open the door for police or ambulance personnel. After notifying police and the receiving facility, the counselor should reestablish phone contact with the person at risk and remain on the line until help arrives. If information about the location or number of the high-risk caller cannot be obtained, there may be identifiable background sounds or other distinguishing clues in the conversation.

For example, a 48-year-old man, well-known to the mental health system, called and identified himself, saying that he had taken rat poison from his brother's garage. He added that he was not at home, but at a motel. Ostensibly he had called to say good-bye. He refused to give the motel address but said that he could see the stadium from his room. Police went to every motel near the stadium until they located him and brought him to the hospital. When he regained consciousness at the hospital later, he acknowledged that he had partly hoped to be found and rescued.

5.5. Urging Follow-Up Consultation

If the counselor feels that the telephone contact is insufficient for the needs of the caller, for the severity or chronicity of the crisis, or for evaluating the general well-being of the caller, follow-up should be encouraged. At the very least, the counselor may want to invite the caller to telephone again. Most often, the caller should be referred for outpatient consultation.

5.6. Documenting the Call

This is the final step in the intervention. Details about the caller, the situation, and the interviewer's recommendations supply valuable introductory material for the agency, therapist, or crisis center to which the caller is referred (see Table 1).

6. Conclusion

For individuals in crisis, the telephone provides instantaneous contact with helping persons. Regardless of the overt content of the call, the stubbornness or provocation of the caller, and the obliqueness of the request, every call must be seen as a "cry for help." By acknowledging the pain of the caller, respecting his need for control, and being willing to work within the limits of the medium, the telephone counselor can significantly influence the course of a crisis.

References

1. Hyde JE: *The Phone Book: What the Telephone Company Would Rather You Not Know.* Chicago, Henry Regneri, 1976.
2. Grumet GW: Telephone therapy: A review and case report. *Am J Orthopsychiatry* 49:574–584, 1979.
3. Levy JC, Rosenkrans J, Lamb, G, et al: Development and field testing of protocols for the management of pediatric telephone calls: Protocols for pediatric telephone calls. *Pediatrics* 64:558–563, 1979.
4. Strain J, Miller J: The preparation, utilization and evaluation of a registered nurse trained to give telephone advice in a private pediatric office. *Pediatrics* 17:1051–1055, 1971.
5. Perrin EC, Goodman HC: Telephone management of acute pediatric illnesses. *N Engl J Med* 298:130–135, 1978.
6. Moore GT, Wilhemain TR, Bonanno R, et al: Comparison of television and telephone for remote medical consultation. *N Engl J Med* 292:729–732, 1975.
7. Glazer E, Marshall C, Cunningham N: Remote pediatric consultation in the inner city: Television or telephone? *Am J Public Health* 68:1133–1135, 1978.
8. Rosenbaum A, Calhoun JF: The use of the telephone hotline in crisis intervention: A review. *J Community Psychol* 5:325–339, 1977.
9. Rosenbaum M: Premature interruption of psychotherapy: Continuation of contact by telephone and correspondence. *Am J Psychiatry* 134:200–202, 1977.
10. Williams T, Douds J: The unique contribution of telephone therapy, in Lester D, Brockopp G (eds): *Crisis Intervention and Counseling by Telephone.* Springfield, Ill, Charles C Thomas, 1973, pp 80–88.
11. Fox R: Help for the despairing: The work of the Samaritans. *Lancet* 2:1102–1105, 1962.
12. Burgess A, Holmstrom L: Telephone counseling, in *Rape: Victims of Crisis.* Robert J. Brady Co, 1974, pp 163–177.
13. Gilmore BS, Evans JW: Nursing care of rape victims, in McCombie SL (ed): *Rape Crisis Intervention Handbook.* New York, Plenum Press, 1980, pp 43–58.
14. Koumans AJR, Muller JJ, Miller CF Use of telephone calls to increase motivation for treatment in alcoholics. *Psychol Rep* 21:327–328, 1967.
15. Catanzaro RJ, Green WG: WATS telephone therapy: New follow-up technique for alcoholics. *Am J Psychiatry* 126:1024–1027, 1970.
16. Finkelman AW: The nurse therapist: Out-patient crisis intervention with the chronic psychiatric patient. *J Psychiatr Nursing Ment Health Serv* 15:27–32, 1977.

17. Bleach G, Claiborn W: Initial evaluation of hot-line telephone crisis center. *Community Ment Health J* 10:387–394, 1974.
18. Litman RE, Farbrow NL, Shneidman ES, et al: Suicide-prevention telephone service. *JAMA* 192:107–111, 1964.
19. Lester D, Brockopp GW (eds): *Crisis Intervention and Counseling by Telephone.* Springfield, Ill, Charles C Thomas, 1973.
20. McCloski AS: The use of the professional in telephone counseling, in Lester D, Brockopp G (eds): *Crisis Intervention and Counseling by Telephone.* Springfield, Ill, Charles C. Thomas, 1973, pp 238–251.
21. O'Donnell JM, George K: The use of volunteers in a community mental health center emergency and reception service: A comparative study of professional and lay telephone counseling. *Community Ment Health J* 13:3–12, 1977.
22. McGee RK, Jennings B: Ascending to "lower" levels: The case for nonprofessional crisis workers, in Lester D, Brockopp G (eds): *Crisis Intervention and Counseling by Telephone.* Springfield, Ill, Charles C Thomas, 1973, pp 223–237.
23. Hart LE, King GD: Selection versus training in the development of paraprofessionals. *J Counsel Psychol* 26:235–241, 1979.
24. Steele RL: A manpower resource for community mental health centers. *J Community Psychol* 2:104–107, 1974.
25. Dixon MC, Burns JL: Crisis theory, active learning and the training of telephone crisis volunteers. *J Community Psychol* 2:120–125, 1974.
26. MacKinnon RA, Michaels R: The role of the telephone in the psychiatric interview, in *The Psychiatric Interview in Clinical Practice.* Philadelphia, W B Saunders Co, 1971, pp 430–450.
27. Miller WB: The telephone in out-patient psychiatry. *Am J Psychother* 27:15–26, 1973.

Role of Family and Networks in Emergency Psychotherapy

Helene W. Kress, A.C.S.W.

1. Introduction

In an emergency, clinicians must make important assessment and management decisions, within a restrictive time frame and often on the basis of limited information. Persons close to the patient frequently are an essential resource. Not only can they provide important data about the patient, but they may also play a central role in both the genesis and the resolution of the crisis. This section discusses various levels of involvement significant others may have in emergency evaluation and treatment.

2. Who Are the Significant Others?

"Significant others" include family members as well as individuals not related by blood or legal bonds who have meaningful ties to the patient. These persons constitute the individual's support network. Effective networks maintain affective and instrumental ties. That is, the members have positive or negative feelings about each other that underlie the network's system of supports or sanctions; the members also count on each other to do certain things and perform in certain ways. An active support network provides regular and direct contact among its members.

Whenever possible, individuals seek out and create interpersonal systems. Studies have indicated that isolated families and individuals often construct an extended "family" out of interactive, supportive people who are otherwise not related. In rural areas and inner-city neighborhoods, members of the extended support network may replace the traditional family.[1-4]

The "healthy person has 20 to 30 people in this psychosocial network."[4] Speck and Rueveni suggest that "decreased rates of mental illness and juvenile delinquency result when a person has a large social network which is actively functioning and intervening in one's life."[5] Neurotic individuals demonstrate a different pattern, however. "They have 10 to 12 people in their social network, often including significant people who are dead or far away." Psychotic in-

Helene W. Kress, A.C.S.W. • Framingham Hospital, Framingham, Massachusetts 01701.

dividuals only have 4 or 5 people in their network and are therefore more vulnerable to stress.[5]

Generally, individuals turn to informal support systems before contacting professional health care providers. By the time a mental health clinician encounters the patient, he may have discussed his problem with several members of his own informal network. It is often very helpful to know about that prior help-seeking activity.

3. Assessment

3.1. Family as Source of Information

In order to gain sufficient information about patients in crisis, it is necessary to supplement and verify the history taken from the patient with data from, and about, the patient's social system. These data are available from significant people in the patient's life and can help to determine not only the quality of the patient's attachments but whether they play a supportive or antagonistic role in the patient's life.

Because of nature or training, the practitioner may hesitate to involve family members or other significant people in the evaluation and treatment planning. When a clinician feels comfortable in a one-to-one situation, he is more likely to use that modality in an emergency. He may have heard negative material from the patient about the family or may be influenced by the relationship with his own family and his own stage of development.

The family and other important members of the patient's social milieu can be used to verify aspects of the patient's account. For example, Schless and Mendels found frequent disagreements between the patient and persons close to him about the significance of various life stresses.[6] Patients often "forgot" or distorted the timing of important events. Braden et al. found that family members sometimes provided crucial historical material about patients presenting with psychotic symptomatology that helped in the differential diagnosis of mania. Carlson and Goodwin described 14 patients "who at the peak of their manic episode were panicky, dysphoric, and incoherent, with bizarre delusions and sometimes hallucinations. It was possible for them to identify this state as part of a manic episode because they had had the opportunity to observe the episode in a longitudinal fashion. For a psychiatrist to do this who is meeting the patient for the first time, a history of the development of the episode would be essential. We suggest that interviewing the patient alone is not always adequate to obtain such a history and we recommend interviewing the family for optimal diagnostic accuracy."[7]

The evaluator's first task is to identify and assess the members of the social network and their relationship to the patient. Who accompanied the patient to the emergency room? Who was with the patient at the time of the emergency? Are there conspicuous absences? It is customary to meet with whoever accompanies the patient. Their perspective, strengths, vulnerabilities, and sense of what is needed to manage the crisis are important data because the expectations, wishes, and involvement of the patient's network will often affect the outcome. As alliances emerge, the picture of the family as a system becomes clearer.

The following case illustrates the importance of the psychosocial network in the assessment process.

> Ms. R., a 55-year-old widow, was carried into the emergency department one morning by her son and a taxi driver. She had been maintained on chronic hemodialysis for almost one year. Initially Ms. R. had made a good adjustment and lived independently in her own apartment enjoying family life with her married children and grandchildren, who lived nearby. The taxi driver, who regularly picked her up for dialysis, reported that in recent times she often was not ready when he came, seemed confused, and insisted that she no longer needed treatment. When she did arrive for dialysis, she was irritable and restless. According to notes in the medical chart, she had tried to pull her needles out on several occasions. On the day of the emergency visit, the evaluator reported that Ms. R.'s speech was incoherent and rambling. She could not, or would not, say where she was, although she knew who she was.
>
> The son was a willing historian. He found his mother's recent behavior perplexing. She had made telephone calls around the world, asking whoever answered the phone to donate a kidney to her for transplant. She had purchased a car she couldn't afford and had written checks without sufficient funds. Prolonged discussion with the son revealed a history of affective cycles predating dialysis therapy. The family had ignored these episodes, stating that "mother's a character." Intermittently she refused to get dressed or go out, and at other times would go on eating or buying binges. She also kept the grandchildren amused by seeing how much they could eat in the supermarket before arriving at the checkout counter. Her inappropriate behavior was episodic. The history from the son and the taxi driver supplied the essential information about both the past history and the genesis of the current episode. Although much of the incipient symptomatology was documented in the medical record, it did not contain the essential information that the son and the regular taxi driver provided.

3.2. Family as the Patient

Often an emergency is triggered by a family event or may continue uncontained because the family's dysfunctional dynamic exacerbates individual psychopathology. For example, the identified patient may be acting-out for the family, or the family exerts such a negative influence that there may be some risk in sending the patient home. Alternative support systems can make the difference in deciding whether or not to hospitalize the patient.

The following is an example of a crisis precipitated by family dynamics.

> A 17-year-old girl, Leah, was brought into the emergency department of a general hospital by her mother, father, and maternal grandmother. She had

walked into her parents' bedroom earlier in the morning and announced that she had swallowed all her mother's pills. The parents had brought their daughter for emergency medical treatment and were enraged when a psychiatrist was called. The history was obtained from mother, since Leah said little, and mother answered every question. During the interview, father paced in and out of the room, repeatedly declaring that he was taking his daughter home. He aggressively asked each person who entered the room "What do you want?" but each time left before a response was possible. Grandmother sat in the room, announcing from time to time, "That girl always makes trouble."

Leah was the oldest of three children. None of them attended school. According to mother, she tutored them at home. Mother also worked outside of the home and complained about how much she had to do. Leah "won't even go to the store alone, so I must accompany her everywhere." Mother said that her husband had told her not to bother with Leah, who would only get married and leave them anyway. But she (mother) had to "bother" because Leah could not go out alone in their neighborhood.

When asked about the suicide attempt, Leah said she would "do it again" if she went home. She wanted to talk to someone about the fights with mother that made her so angry she wanted to die. Mother said it was father's fault. He worked erratically, drank heavily, and made them live in a bad house in a poor neighborhood. They had terrible neighbors who were "nosey" and bothered them.

Since Leah had indicated she still had suicidal intentions and the family conflict continued unabated, hospitalization was recommended. In response, Leah immediately announced she was better and would go home. She said she would *not* stay in the hospital. Her mother said she could never persuade her to stay and the family gathered itself up to leave.

This family is both the arena of pathology for the identified patient and her only existing source of support. The family is isolated from other sources of support and experiences its social environment as hostile. Because the patient's suicidal potential is entwined with family dynamics, the entire system requires treatment.

4. Management

The psychosocial network is a crucial factor in the management and disposition of patients in crisis. Its role as mediator or instigator and its availability or unavailability must be considered by the clinician. The lack of an effective support system is often a major reason for hospitalization. By mobilizing family or network cooperation, crisis intervention can offer an alternative to hospitalization.

Family or network members who accompany the patient should be seen during the initial contact with the patient. This serves two purposes: It provides the clinician with additional data sources, as mentioned above, and it promotes their involvement in the resolution of the crisis. If other important persons are not present, they should be contacted. Depending on the assessed dynamics of the system, the clinician must decide how aggressively to pursue the family and how to deal with the patient's resistances to their involvement. Because emergency caretakers are usually not involved in ongoing therapeutic systems, they are forced to work without an established alliance and with the situational risks and opportunities inherent in a crisis. Emergency clinicians, therefore, must be more active in engaging the patient, contacting others, and mobilizing environmental resources than their counterparts. A meeting of people identified as potential members of the patient's support system should be scheduled for the earliest possible time. If the group is large (greater than four) it is helpful to have a cotherapist available. The dynamics of the group will reveal the strengths and supports available to the patient.

The family group may meet at the time of the emergency visit or shortly thereafter. In either case, providing the opportunity for persons close to the patient to ventilate, ask questions, and voice concerns can lower the stress level in the network and release energy and resources to resolve the crisis constructively. The therapist can clarify the crisis dynamics and assure group members of the short-term nature of the current state of disequilibrium. Any attempts to scapegoat or project on the part of a group members can be addressed and reframed. The role of the patient's interpersonal system in exacerbating or checking the crisis should be stressed so that the individuals involved understand the broader effects of their interactions within the whole group.

Roles, responsibilities, and expectations during this critical period should be made explicit. All members of the group must be aware of treatment goals and the means of accomplishing them. The therapist or case manager/organizer should clarify what help is available and how to mobilize it. Subsequent meetings should be scheduled. A sense of control and containment in the patient's interpersonal milieu enhances his coping abilities and self-control.

Contacts among network members can be maintained throughout the crisis or until an appropriate referral for follow-up can be effected. In some situations, working within the support network may be the treatment of choice and not just a means to manage the crisis. When the entire family is in crisis, the system should be the focus of therapy, even if it is an individual who appears to need treatment. There are several approaches to systems therapy. In one approach, each family member is assigned a task, all social agencies involved with the patient are contacted, and an appointment is made for a home visit within 24 hours. Generally, six home and office visits are made over a period of three weeks, with phone calls when necessary. In this case, the major ongoing task of therapy is the renegotiation of family role assignments and relationships.[8-11]

Weakland et al. describe another family approach limited to a maximum of 10 hourly sessions in which both acute and chronic issues are addressed. This approach uses systems, behavioral, and crisis intervention techniques in order to elicit typical interactional patterns, then to interrupt maladaptive sequences by using direct behavioral interventions and "negotiations of conflict."

Insight-oriented explanation is viewed as generally counterproductive to the modification of interpersonal behavior. At three months the treatment is reviewed and suggestions are made about further intervention.[12]

Applying clinical behavior therapy techniques to family-oriented crisis intervention is described by Eisler and Heisen. The objectives include completing a formal behavioral assessment, defining mutually reinforcing family behavior, expressing feelings appropriate to the intensity of the stimulus, and generalizing newly acquired coping mechanisms to the patient's environment. New patterns of interaction are outlined by the use of instructional and behavioral contracts and are more specifically reinforced by direct feedback, modeling, role-playing, and rehearsing behaviors.[13]

Another outpatient family approach called multiple impact therapy was originally developed in remote rural areas to treat adolescents in crisis with their families. A guidance clinic team sees the entire family for two days in combined individual and joint sessions. The objectives are both diagnostic and therapeutic. In this model, follow-up sessions planned at least bimonthly are part of the treatment process.[14]

The above studies show that mobilizing family support during a crisis or involving the family/system in treatment makes immediate crisis management more effective and provides an alternative to hospitalization. The patient's chances of remaining out of the hospital, or, if hospitalized, of having a shorter stay, are enhanced if he has a generally supportive interpersonal milieu. Where positive supports are lacking, it is possible to create a support network for an individual or a family in crisis, thus reducing conflict and stress. This support network can consist of volunteers or professionals from community agencies, extended family, church, or work. Cutler and Madore describe a "network organizer" who recruits members and ensures that cohesion and communication exist among network components.[15] The model, which is applicable to both rural and urban settings, often involves a case manager. In rural settings where social agencies may be relatively inaccessible, structured networks are constructed out of informal associations. The network model also provides a resource for supportive community care when the family is absent, fragmented, noncohesive, or uncooperative.

5. Conclusion

Family and other members of the psychological network play a crucial role for the patient in crisis. The psychosocial milieu can be the provocateur or the healer; it can be a source of information that lends insight to diagnostic thinking and extends the reach of the caretakers. If the social system exerts a powerful negative influence in a patient, no intervention can turn the patient around without breaking the destructive interactional patterns. And if the social system has a positive influence, it can be a potent ally in the process of crisis intervention. For all these reasons, in emergencies, when the stakes are high and time is critical, the clinician cannot afford to ignore significant members of the social environment in the evaluation and treatment planning process.

References

1. Bott E: *Family and Social Network.* London, Tavistock Publications, 1957.
2. Sussman MB: The help pattern in the middle class family. *Am Sociol Rev* 18:22–28, 1953.
3. Gans HJ: *The Levittowners.* New York, Pantheon Books, 1967.
4. Pattison EM, DeFrancisco D, Wood P, et al: A psychosocial kinship model for family therapy. *Am J Psychiatry* 132:1246–1250, 1975.
5. Speck RV, Rueveni U: Network therapy—A developing concept. *Fam Proc* 8:182–191, 1969.
6. Schless AP, Mendels J: The value of interviewing family and friends in assessing life stressors. *Arch Gen Psychiatry* 35:565–567, 1978.
7. Braden W, Bannasch PR, Fink EB: Diagnosing mania: The use of family informants. *J Clin Psychiatry* 41:7, 1980.
8. Langsley D, Machotka P, Flomenhaft K: Avoiding mental hospital admission: A follow-up study. *Am J Psychiatry* 127:1391, 1971.
9. Langsley D, Pittman F, Machotka P, Flomenhaft K: Family crisis therapy—Results and implications. *Fam Proc* 7:145, 1968.
10. Langsley D, Flomenhaft K, Machotka P: Followup evaluation of family crisis therapy. *Am J Orthopsychiatry* 39:753, 1969.
11. Pittman F, DeYoung C, Flomenhaft K, et al: Techniques of crisis family therapy, in Masserman J (ed): *Current Psychiatric Therapies*, vol. 6. New York, Grune and Stratton, 1966, p 187.
12. Weakland J, Fisch R, Watzlawick P, et al: Brief therapy: Focused problem resolution. *Fam Proc* 13:141, 1974.
13. Eisler R, Heisen P: Behavioral techniques in family-oriented crisis intervention. *Arch Gen Psychiatry* 28:111, 1973.
14. Ritchie A: Multiple impact therapy. *Soc Work* 5:168, 1960.
15. Cutler DL, Madore E: Community-family network therapy in rural settings. *Community Ment Health* 16:2, Summer, 1980.

Crisis Groups

Michael J. Bennett, M.D., and James M. Donovan, Ph.D.

1. Introduction

In response to severe environmental or personal stress, some individuals feel overwhelmed and unable to cope, and develop an acute emotional crisis. At such times, customary defenses and usual social resources may be ineffectual. Adaptive mechanisms may fail to modify or decrease symptom formation and social supports may be inadequate in the face of the person's overwhelming distress.

Many who require help for an acute crisis have either exhausted their usual resources or found them scarce or inaccessible. Some people turn to medical providers for relief, requesting medication or other symptom-alleviating measures, such as advice and reassurance. In addition, some form of ongoing crisis intervention is almost always required. The objective of focused crisis work is to modify the circumstances that brought about the stress and to develop new and improved strategies for dealing with similar problems in the future. One such approach is a crisis group.

This chapter describes an eight-session group for patients in acute distress, distinct in concept and function from other types of group therapy practiced in the same medical setting.* In general, therapy groups antedate the 1971 appearance of this particular crisis group, but they share conceptual foundations and principles of operation. What distinguishes this particular group, however, is its context and combined medical/psychiatric format.

---

* The group was developed within a general medical setting in response to the many patients in acute crisis who required immediate treatment but not necessarily extensive work. Since many patients were referred from the walk-in (triage) unit staffed by medical nurses, a crisis group was formed as a joint project of the mental health department and the triage nursing staff. The original intent was to design a service capable of meeting patient needs and serving a training function as well. Since that time in 1971, crisis groups have been integral to the concept of emergency care at the Kenmore Center of the Harvard Community Health Plan (HCHP) in Boston. The HCHP is a federally certified, prepaid group practice (HMO) serving a population of approximately 140,000 members. Unlike many other HMOs, HCHP provides care for patients with chronic as well as acute psychiatric problems. The program is described more fully elsewhere.[1,2]

Michael J. Bennett, M.D. • Harvard Community Health Plan, Boston, Massachusetts 02215. *James M. Donavan, Ph.D.* • Harvard Medical School, Boston, Massachusetts 02115, and Harvard Community Health Plan, Boston, Massachusetts 02215.

2. Why a Group?

In Caplan's excellent review of the psychosocial aspects of stress mastery, he emphasized the importance of social support systems.[3] Effective support groups can stabilize severely disturbed persons, provide concrete assistance in dealing with precipitating factors, aid in developing and implementing a plan of corrective action, and buttress an individual's threatened, weakened, or ineffective ego resources. Many individuals lack such resources or, for various reasons, are unable or unwilling to mobilize them. These persons may be new to the geographical area, separated from family, friends, or groups of reference, and lacking spiritual, ethnic, or religious ties. Others may have exhausted their resources or eroded their support. In times of acute stress, these individuals may turn to the health care system. When group treatment is used as an interim social resource, it helps to alleviate the immediate stress and encourage patients to develop or to mobilize continuing social networks.

In addition to providing a support system, the group offers other advantages as well: First, an open group in which members can be added continuously cuts waiting time to a minimum. Second, the cost of services is reduced by the larger patient–provider ratio of a group, which in an HMO directly affects the premium and therefore the competitive status and economic viability of the organization. Third, because the crisis group can be jointly led (e.g., medical personnel or the triage unit and mental health staff), the number of professional perspectives is automatically increased.

3. Review of the Literature

In the sparse literature on short-term group therapy, crisis groups are only occasionally discussed. Strickler and Allgeyer have described five-session groups for patients in crisis, emphasizing the value of such treatment for the poor or disadvantaged.[4-6] Their innovative work at the Benjamin Rush Center in Los Angeles, where such groups have been used as a major treatment mode since the late 1960s, was further elaborated by Morley and Brown. The latter stressed the group's usefulness for walk-in patients from low socioeconomic groups.[7] According to this model, open groups of five to six patients met for six two-hour sessions. Exclusion criteria were serious suicidal or homicidal risks that could not be controlled in a group, psychotic states severe enough to disrupt the group's work, and inability to speak English. Twenty-five of 30 patients treated with this model were rated "improved," and at termination, a majority of those were considered "maximally improved."[3] No follow-up was reported. The model emphasized a specific situational focus, active therapeutic stance, and group support.

Trakos and Lloyd have described a crisis group at the Illinois State Psychiatric Institute for patients who could not wait for, or tolerate, other forms of therapy.[8] The authors emphasized an active therapeutic stance and prompt definition of goals, and rapid admission to the group. However, unlike the HMO group, they used medication frequently and often involved the patient with family and outside agencies. Of those patients who attended two or more sessions, 83% reported symptom improvement at least as great as that for control subjects. There was no follow-up. Sadock and associates used a similar group format to evaluate and treat socially deprived patients.[9] The group included unreliable, possibly frightened or poorly motivated patients, but the authors did not specifically define a clinical population. Voltolina et al. began a crisis group at a military hospital where a sparse and minimally trained staff served a large number of patients.[10]

With the exception of Chen's[11] and Bloch's[12] work, most crisis groups emphasize problem resolution and a here-and-now focus, with little attention to group process. Chen, however, capitalized on the curative elements usually associated with longer-term groups but, at the same time, defined realistic, finite, personalized goals.[13] Individual contracts were made with members who have either acute situational problems or more chronic ones. Tenure in the group ranged from 8 to 16 weeks. To facilitate their work in the group, some severely disturbed patients were seen concurrently in individual therapy. Treatment objectives varied: The group might serve as trial treatment or as preparation for longer-term groups. The groups were heterogeneous, but new members were selected on the basis of their "fit" with the existing quorum, thus de-emphasizing the usual exclusion or inclusion criteria. Only adolescents, actively psychotic patients, or drug addicts were excluded. Although the author does not provide outcome data, she contends that even more severely disturbed patients (e.g., suicidal, highly narcissistic, schizoid, or hypochondriacal) are treatable through this combined approach.

Bloch developed an open-ended group for poor, chronically ill, or crisis-prone patients presenting to the walk-in service of an urban community mental health center. The therapist's approach was less structured and directive than is typical for crisis work, and the group process was used to alter behavioral patterns. Referrals were accepted on the basis of two criteria: need for immediate treatment and lower socioeconomic status. Although the group's ostensible focus was each member's crisis situation, patients were allowed to remain in the group to work on underlying or chronic problems. The core group consisted of regular attenders, any combination of whom might be present at a given meeting. Bloch did not emphasize selection, pregroup preparation, goal formation, or a strict here-and-now focus, but allowed members to use the group as they needed—for crisis resolution, intermittent support, or longer-term goals.

Satterfield adopted operational criteria for his group: The prospective member must have the "ability to handle the group process"[14] (p. 539). The groups met twice weekly (with a renegotiable contract) for four two-hour sessions. Unlike Chen or Bloch, Satterfield worked with one group member at a time, depending little on group process to help the patient. Objectives were limited and treatment brief.

Short-term groups have also been used to treat specific populations reacting to similar types of crisis. Chrisula and Asimos began an open-ended, loosely structured group for suicidal patients employing peer pressure and support and encouraging members to assist each other both in and out of the therapy setting.[15] Motto described a similar approach in a suicide prevention telephone center using a group for high-risk callers who would otherwise have been referred elsewhere.[16] The author reported poor patient compliance and speculated that patients who initially sought help via the telephone might be resistant to face-to-face contact.

Crisis groups have also been used for persons who are not defined as psychiatrically ill but are experiencing major life stresses. For example, Ross developed a closed six-session group for the parents of children with cancer,[17] while Bloom and Lynch described a waiting room group for families of patients in a surgical intensive care unit.[18] In both groups, ventilation, sharing, and support were felt to facilitate the families' ability to manage stress.

At the other end of the psychiatric spectrum, inpatient groups have been used as an adjunct to other forms of treatment. Crary described an open group for severely disturbed patients; it facilitated adjustment to the ward and prepared some of the patients for long-term group psychotherapy.[19] This group was seen as a limited form of crisis intervention, the crisis being the severe illness and the need for psychiatric hospitalization.

Dibner et al.[20] and Peck[21] have described the use of groups for evaluating and guiding patients to other forms of treatment. While this may not be crisis intervention *per se*, it is a type of focused, short-term work addressing target symptoms, treatment goals, and orientation to therapy.

Certain facts emerge from this brief review. First, wide variation in the use of the term *crisis* makes it difficult to compare the effectiveness of various interventions. Second, standardized outcome criteria are generally not linked to treatment objectives. Although most authors conclude that the intervention was helpful, the evidence tends to be anecdotal and usually rests on therapists' observations. Third, the particular treatment model is largely determined by the context in which it evolved. Thus, settings with large service demands and/ or few treatment resources produce groups with less structure, fewer exclusion criteria, and less specific treatment objectives than settings with high research or training priorities and less extensive service demands. Finally, the studies fail to mention treatment casualties although theoretical contraindications to crisis therapy have usually been specified. Although this last point may relate more to lack of follow-up than to risk factors, it seems that this form of treatment is unlikely to be hazardous if it is used responsibly by qualified personnel.

4. Patient Evaluation and Selection

HCHP crisis group candidates are adults over 16 years of age whose experience of acute stress or trauma has led to severe emotional disturbance and/ or functional impairment. Although such states are usually of recent onset, they may reflect the worsening of a chronic problem.

For example, June was a 40-year-old social worker whose on-again, off-again relationship with her boyfriend masked a failure to grieve her previous marriage and the death of her ambivalently valued father. When her boyfriend abruptly left, she became depressed over her inability to "hold onto" a man. The current crisis seemed to be an unconscious repetition of earlier events and had reactivated her old sense of worthlessness and self-blame.

Patients should be motivated to work in a short-term group. Psychiatric diagnosis is less relevant to a patient's treatability in a group than the ability to develop a working alliance around a specific situational stress. The group can contain strong emotions and tolerate aberrant behavior patterns, but grossly disruptive or bizarre behavior is countertherapeutic, and patients who cannot or will not control their behavior in the group make poor candidates. Active psychosis, threat of harm to self or others, and current alcohol or drug abuse are absolute contraindications to this treatment format. Although a broad range of patients with preexisting character problems (including some borderline and narcissistic disorders) can be treated in a group, the participant must be able to relate to others without being too withdrawn or preoccupied, or relying on primitive defenses such as projection, distortion, denial, splitting, or acting-out. Although screening usually identifies high-risk patients, it may sometimes be necessary to remove a patient from the group after a few sessions. A trial of crisis group treatment is reasonably safe for most patients who elect to join, since those truly at risk are likely to refuse.

Prospective members should be evaluated by the group therapists prior to beginning group. The assessment helps patients to frame the presenting symptoms or complaints in understandable terms, linking the precipitating events with the feelings and reactions evoked. The therapist should discuss the formulation with the patient to help him understand why the event is stressful. A second purpose of the assessment session is to discuss the group, to clarify its function and the new member's participation, and to elucidate realistic aims. The overall objective of the individual meeting is to forge an alliance between patient and therapist, and to foster favorable treatment expectations. As in any form of brief therapy, the participant should have clear, focused, and limited goals that are consistent with achievable ends.

5. The Open Group in General •

The crisis group meets biweekly for $1\frac{1}{2}$ hours with 8 to 10 members and two cotherapists. Members remain for eight sessions, and cotherapists rotate monthly on a staggered schedule so that both leaders do not leave at once. The fact that membership and leadership change continuously is important. For one thing, the group comes to be regarded as the essential healing element rather than either of the leaders or any specific member; it "belongs" to no one, and is in some sense bigger than its membership. Follow-up reports from group participants indicate that therapeutic efficacy is associated with the group process and structure: the opportunity to share feelings, to ventilate and feel supported, to gain advice and guidance, and to be useful to fellow members. The value of insight gained through clarification or interpretation is less consistently described as being helpful.

As therapists and patients come and go, members experience a continuous cycle of loss and replacement. Separation themes are vividly elicited but are balanced by the continuing group structure. Members at different stages in their own therapy contribute to the healing of each other: There are persons in acute distress, those in the process of mastering their problems, and those preparing to leave. Terminating with only some goals met, settling for limited gains, grieving, and leaving may be the first steps in developing a new sense of mastery and competence.

6. Technical Aspects

6.1. Relevance of Time

Time-limited treatment presents the therapist and the patient with certain existential challenges and constraints.[22] Neugarten, pointing to the "change in time perspective" in the aging person, emphasizes that the cognitive interpretation of time varies with the individual's phase of life.[23] At any time, however, the need to adjust wished for expectations and to settle for limited achievements forces confrontation with undeniable realities: finiteness, separation, imperfection in self and others. The crisis group reinforces an attitude of realism and acceptance. The time limit imposes a need for appropriate pacing and exerts a natural pressure to focus on realistic goals. The resource itself is temporary and must soon be given up. The termination, if pregroup screening and preparation are adequate, occurs as a stepping-stone to continued achievement.

6.2. Transference Issues

Unlike exploratory psychotherapy or psychoanalysis, brief treatment requires that transference not be permitted to build and intensify, or detract from the therapeutic focus. This is rarely a problem in the group. Positive transference commonly occurs early in treatment, as does easy bonding with other group members. Focusing on current life issues imparts a clarity and objectivity to relationships so that intense transference distortions are rare. If they do occur, however, the therapist must deal more directly with them.

6.3. Role of the Therapist

The therapist's role in the group is to foster cohesiveness and to maintain the group culture; this is achieved by shifting attention back and forth between individual problems and objective, shared experiences and common feelings. The therapist should attempt to engage less active members, prevent domination or distraction by others, and reinforce active involvement among the members. The following account of a typical group session illustrates these points:

> Since a number of members were new to the group, Dr. B. asked that each person say why he or she was there. Jane volunteered that her sister was dying, she was having conflicts at work, and she had recently learned that her former husband was about to have another child. She expressed little feeling. Bill stated that he had been persuaded to join the group, but had reservations. In a controlled way he described several losses, including both parents, a grandfather, and a close friend within the past year. Wanda, in her second meeting, said that she had gained from the last meeting, but things were still going poorly at home, where she was trying to salvage her marriage after learning that her husband was having an affair with her niece. She continued to be irritable with the children and felt very sad and anxious, though she was a little calmer since the last meeting. Her aim in the group was to learn to control her feelings, especially her anger at her husband's lack of guilt. Since the last meeting she had been able to talk more honestly with both her husband and her niece. Sarah, who was approaching her final sessions, said that she had joined the group because of anxiety over a career change. She was feeling better, crediting much of her improvement to the group's support and understanding. Paul, in his second session, talked about his wife's affair and their impending separation, stating that he was looking for support during this painful process. Ellen reported that she had recently separated from her husband and was feeling hurt and confused. In a flat, dispassionate way she said she wanted support and feedback about how others saw her.
>
> Dr. B. said that people had made rather general statements, but a common theme that emerged was how most people felt hurt or damaged. The group continued to share their feelings and eventually focused on Wanda's sense of hurt and rejection. Various suggestions were made about how Wanda should deal with her husband and niece. Wanda rejected these and continued to emphasize her anger and hurt at how alone she felt. Dr. B. suggested to Wanda that she did not seem willing to tell people at home to stop the behavior that was hurting her, but instead continued to emphasize her pain in the hope they would care enough to stop on their own. This led to a discussion of how group members were unable to ask for what they needed or to set limits on what was asked of them. Jane joined in the discussion, but focused on Wanda's problems rather than on her own. She seemed agitated, often turning away and withdrawing. Nurse A. asked her whether she was ready to discuss her own feelings, commenting that she looked very upset. She began to talk poignantly about her sister, whom she had helped to raise, and about her own childhood, which had been filled with disappointment and loss; she described her father's death when she was 6. She connected her concern about her sister's children, who were going to be without a mother, with her own sense of loss, and began to cry. She complained about her boyfriend's and fellow workers' lack of support and said she would like to return "home" to Scotland to be with her family. She remembered her disappointment in her mother after her father's death, but added that mother was more supportive when Jane made her needs clearer. Dr. B. pointed out that major losses involved losing part of yourself

and the wish to "go back home" was a common response. A sad discussion followed in which most members leaned forward and talked intensely about their sense of loss and their wish for solace; only Bill remained aloof. Several times he was asked about his personal responses, but his answers were evasive.

Gradually, members began to speak of "we" rather than "I." Paul talked of his wish to share his pain with his parents, but said that as the "ideal" child of elderly parents he was afraid of hurting them. He began to weep. Wanda responded by saying she had also been "the good child"; much of her current distress was that her family continued to hurt her despite her goodness and self-sacrifice. Dr. B. questioned the need to be good for others, asking whether this didn't give a special status that people found hard to give up. Several members talked about their special roles in their families and how these patterns were carried into their adult lives, but without the same rewards. Toward the end of the session several members asked about the upcoming Christmas holiday, wondering whether the group would meet. Ellen said she would be with her family and felt some conflict about missing the meetings. Nurse A. suggested that her family might be as therapeutic as the group, adding that we would miss her but understood her wish to be at home. She raised the question of exploratory therapy since she wanted to evaluate life and goals. The leaders suggested she use the group to resolve the crisis and then consider further treatment if needed.

6.4. Group Leadership

Similar to other forms of focal therapy, the crisis group requires clear and explicit formulation of limited treatment objectives and the formation of a treatment alliance based on these. The therapist must be able to assess the patient's strengths and resources as well as liabilities, and be willing to tolerate limited treatment goals. He should be comfortable maintaining an active therapeutic stance, dealing with resistances and transferences, involving reticent patients, and preventing others from dominating or monopolizing the meetings. At the same time, the therapist should be sensitive to the risks of an active stance: intrusiveness, overly confrontational or challenging attitudes, and acting out the countertransference. Tact, empathy, and concern for the individual in distress are essential personal qualities, and a problem-solving orientation is an important professional quality. It is preferable for the therapist to formulate health-promoting goals rather than overemphasizing psychopathology and the treatment of illness.

6.5. Adjunctive or Extended Treatment

As a general rule, crisis group patients do not require other therapies or medication. However, when patients are severely symptomatic, the primary care physician or group cotherapist may prescribe drugs to facilitate therapy. Or, if family, couple, or behavioral problems are identified, the patient may be referred for adjunctive work. In general, the cotherapists should not see a group patient individually except as an emergency or if the patient is likely to drop out of the group.

On some occasions, a member's group tenure should be extended by a session or two to bring an issue to closure or to forestall a premature termination. Some patients may return to the group for another eight sessions when a new crisis arises. During the group's 10-year history, however, only a few patients have had a second course of treatment in the group, and none has had a third.

6.6. Follow-Up Treatment

In the HMO setting, where health care is offered to subscribers on a continuing basis, it is assumed that treatment of an episode of illness or crisis will be focused and brief, but not necessarily final. Members may return at any time. Crisis group patients are specifically advised to be treatment-free for a period of two to three months following termination, however. At that time they can return for reevaluation. As feelings about termination subside, a more objective assessment can be made of what has been gained and what further work is required.

In a setting that is highly cost-conscious, there is a distinction between "need-for treatment" and "capacity to benefit from treatment." Many who might elect to receive more treatment are judged not to need additional therapy. Despite this orientation, follow-up studies indicated that 44% of crisis group patients received some further professional help during the ensuing year, much of it brief treatment in other groups. The goals of these groups, in contrast to those of the crisis group, involved the exploration of aspects of adult development.[24]

7. Treatment Outcome

In their paper on outcome research in crisis intervention, Auerbach and Kilmann recommended that the effectiveness of treatment be assessed according to measures of behavioral change.[25] Decrying the lack of specificity of the term *crisis*, they emphasized the need for clearly delineating the population and connecting treatment objectives with explanations for the state of distress.

To assess the impact of the crisis group, a battery of tests was administered to participants before and after treatment and again one year later. These tests included a questionnaire designed to elicit the patient's perception of his problem, expectations for treatment, and, later, assessment of the value of the group; the Zuckerman and Lubin Multiple Affect Adjective Checklist (a measure of symptomatic distress) and the Barron Ego Strength Scale (designed to assess adaptive capacity under stress) were used. Therapists were also asked to rate their patients' improvement relative to inital assessment of the problem and the psychodynamic basis for it. The results are briefly summarized here.[26,27] Eighty-six patients who completed the group and the posttreatment questionnaires were queried one year later and 43 responded. All except 2 (95%) found the group to have been helpful and a positive experience at termination; those attitudes persisted at one-year follow-up. Therapists rated 26% of patients as "maximally improved" and another 49% as "improved" at the end of treatment. At completion of therapy and one year later, anxiety and depression, the most common presenting complaints, were diminished. Further, subjective accounts and measurements of adaptive problem-solving capacity suggested that patients grew in ways not directly related to the crisis or its resolution.

Outcome assessment has reinforced the impression that the crisis group is a highly effective form of treatment for a heterogeneous mix of patients. In a clinical setting characterized by high demand for service and rapid patient turnover, such a group can serve as a readily available, relatively inexpensive resource. Waiting times can be kept to a minimum; regressive and maladaptive behaviors are consequently lessened. Treatment can be focal and brief.

From the patient's perspective, the opportunity for prompt, effective, low-cost relief at a time of maximum stress is critical to longer-range outcome. There is an added benefit in the paired medical and psychotherapeutic expertise of the group's leaders. The model of the crisis has its limits, however: it is no substitute for one-to-one care, hospitalization, or psychopharmacological medication when these are clinically indicated; nor is group treatment a realistic option for those who are unwilling or unable to relate to others or those whose level of function is too severely disrupted.

When the crisis group is utilized as one arm of an acute care service that includes other forms of crisis intervention and short-term treatment, there is a reduced likelihood that patients will be inappropriately assigned to the group. Usually, one or two diagnostic interviews will be sufficient to determine the best candidates for group treatment and to screen out those who would benefit more from other crisis therapies. Even when patients are appropriately assigned to crisis groups, the responsiveness and flexibility of the therapists can prevent many potential dropouts from occurring.

Group Leaders

As noted previously, like other forms of focal therapy, the crisis group requires concise formulation of limited treatment objectives and a directive therapeutic stance. To that end, the therapist must be able to fit his assessment of the patient and presenting problem to limited, realistic treatment goals. He must tailor his interventions to promote the achievement of these goals, and deal with the content of each patient's concerns to the extent that it pertains to treatment outcome. Simultaneously, he must nurture the group process, involve reticent patients, and prevent domination of the group by others. There is no uniform formula for therapeutic effectiveness, but in general an active, health-promoting orientation has been linked to crisis resolution far more reliably than either a passive or pathology-focused stance.

8. Summary

The crisis group as presented here is an eight session biweekly group treatment mode which has been in operation continuously at the Harvard Community Health Plan in Boston since 1971. It is one component of a comprehensive crisis management program under the general umbrella of a broad-based psychiatric service. The group serves a liaison and teaching function as well as providing a readily available, cost-effective treatment resource. The model can be amplified and refined to fit a variety of clinical settings so long as it remains an extension of, and not a replacement for, other forms of crisis management.

References

1. Bennett MJ, Wisneski MJ: Continuous psychotherapy within an HMO. *Am J Psychiatry* 136:1283–1287, 1979.
2. Budman SH, Feldman J, Bennett MJ: Adult mental health services in a health maintenance organization. *Am J Psychiatry* 135:392–395, 1979.
3. Caplan G: Mastery of stress: Psychosocial aspects. *Am J Psychiatry* 138:413–419, 1981.
4. Strickler M, Allgeyer JM: The crisis group: A new application of crisis theory. *Soc Work* 12:28–32, 1967.
5. Allgeyer JM: The crisis group: Its unique usefulness to the disadvantaged. *Int J Group Psychother* 20:235–239, 1970.
6. Allgeyer JM: Using groups in a crisis-oriented setting. *Int J Group Psychother* 23:217–222, 1973.
7. Morley W, Brown V: The crisis intervention group: A natural mating or a marriage of convenience? *Psychother Theory Res Pract* 6:30–36, 1969.
8. Trakos DA, Lloyd G: Emergency management in a short term open group. *Compr Psychiatry* 12:170–175, 1971.
9. Sadock B, Newman L, Normand WD: Short term group psychotherapy in a psychiatric walk-in clinic, in Barten L (ed): *Brief Therapies*. New York, Behavioral Publications, 1971.
10. Voltolina EJ, Moskowitz MM, Kammerer WG: The adaptation of a crisis intervention group to a navy outpatient psychiatric population. *M I Med* 136:546–548, 1971.
11. Chen M: Applying Yalom's principles to crisis work . . . some intriguing results. *J Psychiatr Nursing* 16:15–27, 1978.
12. Bloch HS: An open-ended crisis-oriented group for the poor who are sick. *Arch Gen Psychiatry* 18:178–185, 1968.
13. Yalom ID: *The Theory and Practice of Group Psychotherapy*, ed 2. New York, Basic Books, 1975.
14. Satterfield W: Short-term group therapy for people in crisis. *Hosp Community Psychiatry* 28:539–541, 1977.
15. Chrisula T, Asimos MA: Dynamic problem-solving in a group for suicidal persons. Int J Group Psychother 29:109–114, 1979.
16. Motto J: Starting a therapy group in a suicide prevention and crisis center. *Suicide Life-Threatening Behav* 9:47–56, 1979.
17. Ross J: Coping with childhood cancer: Group intervention as an aid to parents in crisis. *Soc Work Health Care* 4:381–391, 1979.
18. Bloom N, Lynch J: Group work in a hospital waiting room. *Health Soc Work* 4:48–63, 1979.
19. Crary W: Goals and techniques of transitory group therapy. *Hosp Community Psychiatry* 19:389–391, 1968.
20. Dibner AS, Palmer BC, Gefstein AH: Use of open-ended group in the intake procedure of a mental hygiene unit. *J Consult Psychol* 24:83–88, 1960.

21. Peck HB: Application of group treatment to the intake process. *Am J Orthopsychiatry* 23:338–349, 1953.
22. Mann J: *Time-Limited Psychotherapy*. Cambridge, Harvard University Press, 1973.
23. Neugarten B: Time, age and the life cycle. *Am J Psychiatry* 136:887–894, 1979.
24. Budman S, Bennett M. Wisneski MJ: An adult developmental model of short-term group psychotherapy, in Budman S (ed): *Forms of Brief Therapy*. New York, Guilford Press, 1981.
25. Auerbach S, Kilmann P: Crisis intervention: A review of outcome research. *Psychol Bull* 84:1189–1217, 1977.
26. Donovan J, Bennett M, McElroy C: The crisis group—An outcome study. *Am J Psychiatry* 136:906–910, 1979.
27. Donovan J, Bennett M, McElroy C: The crisis group: Its rationale, format and outcome, in Budman S (ed): *Forms of Brief Therapy*. New York, Guilford Press, 1981.

Index

Abnormal Involuntary Movement Scale, 189
Abortion, 281, 287
Abscess, 143, 146, 207
Abuse, *see* Battered women; Child abuse
Accidents, 243, 314, 323
Acidosis, 137, 150
Acid phosphatase, 279
Acute dystonia, 30, 65, 137, 183–184, 315
Acute grief reaction, *see* Grief
Addiction, *see* specific agents
Addington vs. Texas, 48
Adjustment disorders, 85, 233, 243–245, 249–
    250; *see also* Life-stage issues
Admission, *see* Hospitalization
Adolescent emergencies, *see* specific
    emergencies
Affect, 24, 203
Affective disorder, 63, 85, 87, 100, 101, 105,
    107, 108, 129, 160, 205, 219, 224–227, 233,
    237, 242; *see also* Bipolar disorder;
    Depression; Mania
Aggression, 83, 84, 85, 86; *see also* Violence
Agitation, 83, 85, 86, 220, 221, 224, 228
    agitated behavior, confusion—table, 26
Agoraphobia, 240, 241; *see also* Phobias
Agranulocytosis, 64
Akathisia, 184–185, 375
Akinesia, 183–186
Alcohol, 62, 70, 100, 104, 105, 122, 124, 129–
    139, 149, 150, 166, 198, 207, 221, 228, 241,
    251, 360, 361, 365; *see also* Delirium
    tremens; Korsakoff's syndrome;
    Wernicke's disease
    abuse and dependence—tables, 130
    hallucinosis, 24, 62, 133, 137, 206
    stages of intoxication—table, 132
    withdrawal, treatment—tables, 135, 136
Alcoholics Anonymous, 138, 175
Alkalosis, respiratory, 236
Alliance, *see* Therapeutic relationship
Alprazolam, 67, 246; *see also* Benzodiazepines
Alzheimer's disease, 352

Amantadine, 186, 187, 188
Amitriptyline, 32, 190, 359; *see also*
    Antidepressants
Ammonium chloride, 157, 167
Amnesia, 166, 237; *see also* Dissociative
    disorders
Amobarbital, 148; *see also* Barbiturates
Amotivational syndrome, 170, 173
Amphetamine, 26, 70, 86, 147, 154–158, 160,
    161, 165, 170, 186, 187, 188, 206, 207, 251,
    331; *see also* Dextroamphetamine;
    Methamphetamine
    psychosis, 62, 157–158, 198
Anemia, 135, 226, 251, 360
"Angel dust," *see* Phencyclidine
Anorexia nervosa, 311
Antianxiety agents, *see* specific agents
Anticholinergic effects/syndrome, 30, 62, 63,
    64, 70, 157, 186, 187, 188, 189–191, 202,
    208, 213, 251, 361, 365
Anticholinesterase therapy, *see* Anticholinergic
    effects/syndrome; Pyridostigmine;
    Physostigmine
Anticoagulants, 359, 361; *see also* specific
    agents
Anticonvulsants, 92, 135, 137, 153, 361; *see
    also* specific agents
Antidepressants, 66, 68, 70, 92, 101, 157, 189,
    190, 191, 221, 223, 227, 229, 241, 246, 247–
    248, 318, 361, 377; *see also* specific agents
Antihistamines, 92, 185, 186, 187, 189, 251; *see
    also* Diphenhydramine
Antiparkinson agents, 184, 185–188, 189, 208;
    table, 187; *see also* specific agents
Antipsychotic agents, 62, 63, 65, 69, 170, 184,
    188, 189, 211–213, 215, 221, 223, 335, 359,
    396, 412; *see also* specific agents or
    classes of drugs
    table, 64
Antisocial personality disorder, 25, 83, 85, 88,
    89, 90, 92, 336
    table, 85

437

Anxiety, 62, 65, 66, 68, 147, 152, 156, 160, 164,
    166, 185, 202, 213, 221, 224, 230, 233–260,
    268, 287, 291, 311, 312, 315, 341, 352, 376,
    380, 387, 389, 434
    physiological causes—table, 251
Arrhythmias, 29, 65, 101, 138, 156, 160, 174,
    182, 190–191, 223, 228, 253–254
Assessment, 8–11; *see also* each individual
    chapter
Asterixis, 202
Ataxia, 25, 132, 133, 148, 150, 153, 166
Attention, 25, 173, 227, 308; *see also* Mental
    status examination
Attention deficit disorder, 88, 92, 154
Autonomy, 37, 38, 46, 56, 57

"Bad Trip," 161, 163, 164, 168; *see also*
    Hallucinogens
Barbiturates, 70, 86, 92, 144, 147, 148, 149, 152,
    153–154, 155, 156, 208, 241, 251, 258, 319,
    359, 361; *see also* Amobarbital;
    Pentobarbital; Phenobarbital; Secobarbital
Battered women, 285–292
Behavior therapy, 174, 175, 223, 242, 377, 378,
    421, 422, 432
Benzene, *see* Inhalants
Benzodiazepines, 62, 65, 66, 92, 147, 148, 149,
    184, 185, 211, 213, 230, 238, 246, 248, 251,
    375, 361; *see also* specific agents
    tables 67, 68
Benztropine mesylate, 65, 137, 184, 187, 212
Bereavement, *see* Grief
Bioavailability, 71
Biperiden, 184, 187; *see also* Antiparkinson
    agents
Bipolar disorder, 25, 26, 138, 221, 224–225; *see
    also* Affective disorder; Depression; Mania
Blood alcohol concentration, 131, 132; *see also*
    Alcohol
Blood group antigens, 279
Borderline personality disorder, 14, 16, 25, 78,
    85, 88, 101, 206, 221, 229, 239, 333, 336,
    429
Bradykinesia, 185, 186
Brief psychotherapy, *see* Crisis intervention;
    Emergency psychotherapy; Short term
    psychotherapy
Briquet's syndrome, *see* Somatization disorder
Bromides, 208, 361
Butyrophenone, 64; *see also* Antipsychotic
    agents; Haloperidol

Cannabis, *see* Marijuana
Cannabis psychosis, 173; *see also* Marijuana

Carcinoma, 207, 221, 222, 225, 226, 258, 361
Cardiac disorders, 173, 226, 251, 253, 360; *see
    also* Arrhythmias; Myocardial infarction;
    Tachycardia
Cardiopulmonary resuscitation, 31, 34
Care and protection, *see* Child abuse; Child
    neglect; Child Protective Services; Legal
    issues
Case manager, 421, 422
Catalepsy, 166, 168
Catatonia, 185
Characterologic depression, 229–230; *see also*
    Depression
Chest pain, 138; *see also* Myocardial infarction
Child abuse, 83, 293–300, 304, 309, 310, 315,
    404
    indications of child abuse/neglect—table, 298
Child neglect, 262, 293–300
    indications of child abuse/neglect—table, 298
Child Protective Services, 293; *see also* Child
    abuse; Child neglect
Childhood emergencies; *see also* specific
    emergencies
    table, 311
Chloral hydrate, 70, 147, 148
Chlordiazepoxide, 32, 62, 67, 135, 136, 137,
    148; *see also* Benzodiazepines
Chlorpromazine, 34, 62, 64, 65, 133, 154, 157,
    158, 162, 168, 252, 358, 375; *see also*
    Antipsychotic agents; Phenothiazines
Cholestatic jaundice, 64
Cirrhosis, 135
Clinical hypothesis, 9–11
Clorazepate, 67; *see also* Benzodiazepines
"Clouded" consciousness, *see* Consciousness;
    Delirium
Cocaine, 26, 62, 70, 147, 158–160, 206, 208, 251
Codeine, 141
Cognitive capacity, 23, 24, 86, 198, 201, 206,
    221, 234, 308, 351, 354; *see also* Mental
    status examination
Coma, *see* Consciousness
Commitment, *see* Hospitalization
Community Mental Health Centers Act, 3
Competence, 39, 48, 51
Compliance, 110
Concurrent therapy, *see* Psychotherapies,
    concurrent
Conduct disorders, 85, 88, 299, 327, 336
Confidentiality, 44–45, 295
Confusion, 155, 156, 157, 163, 167, 172, 197,
    227, 306, 310, 358, 361, 366–7; *see also*
    Consciousness; Delirium
    acute confusional states—table, 360

Consciousness, 24, 25, 31, 61, 133, 138, 144, 151, 167, 182, 235, 238, 356; *see also* Delirium
levels of—table, 31
Consent
"implied," 42–44
informed, 38–40, 48, 50, 51, 72
oral, 41–42
substitute, 40–41, 46
written, 41–42
Conversion reactions, 236, 238–239
Convulsions, *see* Alcohol; Rum fits; Seizures; Temporal lobe epilepsy
Counseling, 275, 281–282, 290–291, 401; *see also* Psychotherapy
Counteralliance, 75, 76, 77, 78, 79; *see also* Therapeutic relationship
Countertransference, 72, 75, 77–78, 79, 276, 381; *see also* Therapeutic relationship; Transference
Couples therapy, 363, 432
CPR, *see* Cardiopulmonary resuscitation
Crashing, 155, 159; *see also* Amphetamines
Crisis, 3, 7, 12–13, 75, 77, 78, 79, 80, 91, 103–104, 229, 261–262, 309, 310, 362, 373, 378–379, 381, 387, 393, 394, 397, 398, 402–403, 407, 417, 418, 420, 421, 422, 425, 428, 433; *see also* specific crises (e.g., Domestic violence, Rape, Situational crises)
centers/units, 3, 293, 385, 387, 393, 395, 401–402, 408
emotional responses to crisis—table, 262
groups, 425–436; *see also* Support networks
intervention/management, 4–8, 11–12, 16, 106, 108, 109, 110, 223, 225, 297, 386–387, 393, 394–395, 403, 420, 421
phases, 261, 262, 265
Cruelty to animals, 84, 328, 329, 336
Cushing's syndrome, 251, 252–253

Dangerousness, 47, 48, 84, 93, 107, 108, 198; *see also* Violence
Day care, 107
Death, 311, 318, 321, 343, 375, 386
child's view, 317–319
sudden, 30
Dehydration, 135, 144, 145
Deinstitutionalization, 3–4, 13, 217, 384, 388, 401
Delirium, 24, 27, 62, 63, 70, 86, 92, 133, 134, 137, 148, 152, 153, 154, 163, 164, 165, 170, 172, 188, 197, 309, 354, 355, 356, 366; *see also* Organic disorders
Delirium tremens, 133–135, 138; *see also* Alcohol

Delusions, 24, 26, 122, 168, 196, 197, 201, 203, 204, 205, 206, 209, 212, 224, 225, 234, 239, 308, 327, 396
Dementia, 85, 92, 124, 221, 227, 354, 356, 358, 361, 364, 366, 367; *see also* Pseudodementia
Dependence, *see* specific agents
Depersonalization, 237
Depressants, CNS, 147–154; *see also* specific agents
Depression, 25, 68, 100, 101, 104, 105, 106, 122, 138, 150, 155, 156, 157, 197, 204, 219–231, 286, 289, 305, 327, 354, 358, 363, 365, 375, 404, 410, 434; *see also* Affective disorder; Bipolar disorder; Grief; Mania; Pseudodementia
in children and adolescents, 316–317
major depression, criteria—table, 220
Derealization, 237
Desipramine, 246; *see also* Antidepressants
Detoxification, 105; *see also* specific agents
Dextroamphetamine, 155, 156; *see also* Amphetamines
Diabetes mellitus, 137, 207, 213, 226, 236, 252
Diarrhea, 144, 181
Diazepam, 26, 30, 33, 62, 65, 67, 101, 135, 136, 137, 147, 148, 152, 156, 160, 163, 165, 167, 170, 184, 230, 337; *see also* Benzodiazepines
Diazoxide, 26, 167
Dibenzoxazepine (Loxapine), 64; *see also* Antipsychotic agents
Digitalis/Digoxin, 208, 361
Dihydroindolone (Molindone), 64; *see also* Antipsychotic agents
Dimethoxymethylamphetamine (DOM), *see* "STP"
Dimethyltryptamine (DMT) 161, 162; *see also* Hallucinogens
Diphenhydramine, 65, 184, 187; *see also* Antihistamines
Disasters, 262, 263–270
Disorientation, *see* Orientation
Dissociative disorders, 233, 237–239
Disulfiram, 92, 138, 175, 208; *see also* Alcohol
Diuresis, 151, 182, 359
Divorce, 243, 375, 321, 343; *see also* Life-stage issues
Domestic violence, 261, 407; *see also* Battered women
Dopamine, 161, 186, 187
Drug addiction, *see* specific agents
Drug automatism, 150
Dyskinesia, *see* Acute dystonia; Tardive dyskinesia

Dysthymic disorder, 229; *see also* Depression
Dystonia, *see* Acute dystonia

Elderly, 71, 137, 189, 351–369; *see also*
    Pseudodementia
Electrocardiogram, 64, 135, 182, 203, 234, 364
Electroencephalogram, 87, 326, 330
Electroshock therapy, 228, 363
Emergency, legal definition, 42
Emergency psychotherapy, 6, 7, 8–14; *see also*
    Crisis intervention; Short-term
    psychotherapy
Endocarditis, 143, 146, 207, 209, 226
Engagement, 76, 79, 111; *see also*
    Psychotherapy; Therapeutic relationship
Enuresis, 84, 328, 329
Epilepsy, *see* Seizures
Epinephrine, 65, 70
Episodic dyscontrol, 86, 92
Estrogen therapy, 280–281
Ethchlorvynol, 147, 149
Euphoria, 142, 145, 155, 156, 159, 162, 171
Explosive disorder, 83, 85, 92; *see also*
    Violence
Extraocular movements, 24; *see also* Pupils
Extrapyramidal effects, 64, 65, 69, 183–188,
    189, 212, 223; *see also* Acute dystonia;
    Akathisia; Parkinson's syndrome; Tardive
    dyskinesia

Family, 286, 287, 293, 300, 306, 308–309, 331,
    338–339, 340, 351, 354, 362, 374, 397, 417–
    423, 432
    therapy, 223, 293, 324, 363, 376, 432
Firesetting, 84, 303, 310, 311, 316, 326, 328,
    332–337
    behavior—table, 336
Flashbacks, 62, 162, 164, 165, 170, 172, 243,
    275
Fluphenazine, 64, 87, 212, 375; *see also*
    Antipsychotic agents; Phenothiazines
Flurazepam, 68, 367; *see also* Benzodiazepines
Framework of book—table, xii
Freebasing, 158, 159, 160; *see also* Cocaine
Fugue state, 237–238; *see also* Dissociative
    disorders
Functional psychiatric disorder, 9, 23–24, 62,
    84, 85, 87, 91, 165, 203, 206, 209, 212, 221;
    see also specific disorders

Gastric lavage, 151, 168
Gastritis, 135
General hospital, 383–392
    services—table, 385

Generalized anxiety disorder, 242, 248; *see
    also* Anxiety
Glucose, 86, 135, 143, 212, 213, 252
Glue, *see* Inhalants
Glutethimide, 147, 148–149, 151
Gonorrhea, 279, 280
"Good Samaritan" statutes, 54
Grief, 80, 221, 230–231, 262, 364, 365, 380
Group psychotherapy, 15, 223, 363, 379; *see
    also* Crisis groups
Guardianship, 40–41, 43–44, 310

Habit disorders, 299
Halazepam, 67; *see also* Benzodiazepines
Hallucinations, 25, 27, 107, 122, 131, 133, 134,
    138, 152, 156, 157, 160, 163, 164, 166, 173,
    196, 197, 201, 203, 204, 205, 206, 208, 209,
    212, 224, 228, 267, 308, 331, 396
Hallucinogens, 27, 62, 160–165, 168, 170, 202,
    206, 208, 251; *see also* d-Lysergic acid
    diethylamide (LSD); Mescaline;
    Psilocybin; "STP"
    tables, 162, 170
Haloperidol, 25, 26, 27, 29, 30, 31, 62, 64, 65,
    137, 157, 158, 165, 168, 212–213, 223, 238,
    355, 363, 375, 396, 411; *see also*
    Antipsychotic agents
Hashish, *see* Marijuana
Head injury, 257
Health Maintenance Organization (HMO), 425,
    426, 433
Help-rejection, 14–15, 76, 103, 106, 229; *see
    also* Repeaters
Hepatitis, 137, 143, 145–146
Heroin, 141, 142, 143, 144, 145, 147, 154
Histrionic personality disorder, 237
Home visiting services, 401–405; *see also*
    Outreach
Homicide, *see* Children and adolescent
    emergencies; Dangerousness; Violence
Homosexuality, 122, 295
Hopelessness scale, *see* Suicide
Hospitalization, 11, 12, 39, 46–47, 48, 50, 51,
    52, 54, 55, 57, 89, 93, 94, 107, 108, 109,
    145, 212, 215, 216, 222–223, 227–228, 229,
    246, 309, 311, 312, 323, 337, 351, 363, 380,
    387, 388, 396, 401, 402, 404, 413, 420, 422;
    see also Legal issues
Hotlines, 293, 297, 385, 407–408; *see also*
    Telephone
Hyperactivity, 88, 156, 168, 237, 299
Hyperaggressive behavior, 305, 310, 311, 316,
    327, 330, 331
Hypercarbia, 360
Hyperglycemia, 360

Hyperpyrexia, 26, 70, 156, 160, 182
Hypersomnia, 220, 221
Hypertension, 26, 134, 138, 144, 155, 160, 163, 166, 167, 209, 234, 277, 360
Hyperthermia, 134, 138, 144, 152
Hyperthyroidism, 226, 251–252, 360
Hyperventilation, 234, 235–236, 251, 256
Hypnosis, 239, 242
Hypnotics, *see* specific agents
Hypochondriasis, 63, 105, 123, 221, 224, 236, 239, 299
Hypoglycemia, 70, 137, 143, 207, 208, 212, 251, 252, 360
Hypoparathyroidism, 251, 253, 360, 365
Hypotension, 29, 30, 64, 65, 137, 138, 142, 152, 153, 157, 171, 212
Hypothermia, 137, 143, 150, 213
Hypothyroidism, 225, 226, 227, 252
Hypoxia, 360
Hysteria, 239, 274, 299, 311

Imipramine, 33, 246–247, 254, 259, 345; *see also* Antidepressants
Impact phase, 262, 264–265, 274; *see also* Crisis phases
Impulse-control disorder, 305
Infections, 207, 226, 251, 257
Informed consent, *see* Consent
Inhalants, 173–174, 331
In re Richard Roe III, 41, 42, 43, 44, 49, 52, 57
Insight, 23, 171, 173, 174; *see also* Mental status examination
Insomnia, 62, 65, 66, 68, 69, 99, 134, 145, 147, 153, 156, 168, 198, 204, 224, 227, 230, 237, 265, 299, 345, 352, 380, 404
Intellectual functioning, 23, 201–202, 203, 204, 219, 351–352; *see also* Mental status examination
Intent, suicidal, 101, 107, 108, 109, 111, 114, 116–118, 119, 120; *see also* Suicide
Ipecac, 34; *see also* Overdose
Isoproterenol, 65

Judgment, 21, 23, 122, 173, 300, 308; *see also* Mental status examination

Korsakoff's syndrome, 124, 133, 207, 226; *see also* Alcohol

Lanterman-Petris-Short Mental Health Act, 54
Laryngospasm, 30, 65, 167
Learning disorders, 299
Least restrictive alternative, 13, 49, 52, 108–109, 215–216

Legal issues, 37–59
 child abuse, 295–296
 child neglect, 295–296
 rape, 278–279
Lethality, 99, 101, 105, 107, 108, 111, 114, 119, 120, 122, 365; *see also* Suicide
Levarterenol, 65
Liability, 53, 55
Lidocaine, 191
Life-stage issues, 101, 104, 243–244; *see also* Adjustment disorder
Life stress, 242, 275, 353, 374, 428
Life-threatening problems, 21, 31, 61–63, 102, 196, 202, 271, 296, 303, 313, 354–355, 395–396
Lithium, 66, 68, 92, 181–183, 359, 375, 378
Lorazepam, 67; *see also* Benzodiazepines
Los Angeles Suicide Prevention Center Scale, 122–123
d-Lysergic acid diethylamide (LSD), 27, 161–165, 213, 251

Major abstinence syndrome, *see* Delirium tremens; specific agents
Major depressive illness, *see* Affective disorder; Depression; Pseudodementia
Malingering, 236, 239
Malnutrition, 135, 361
Mania, 63, 92, 205, 224, 225, 237, 375, 418; *see also* Affective disorder; Bipolar disorder; Depression
Mannitol, 182
Marijuana, 62, 165, 165, 166, 168–173, 206, 208, 375
 reactions—table, 164
Medical disorders, 21, 63, 65, 71, 105, 133, 135, 145–146, 202, 212, 219, 221, 222, 233, 250–258, 355, 397
Medical screening, 7, 68
Medications, medications frequently used—table, 62; *see also* specific agents and disorders
Memory, 23, 25, 150, 227, 256, 308, 351, 354, 357, 358; *see also* Mental status examination
Menopause, 253
Mental illness, legal definition, 47
Mental retardation, 85, 92, 326, 327, 336
Mental status examination, 10, 23, 25, 31, 61, 86, 200–202, 206, 209, 227, 234, 235, 266–267, 308, 340, 355, 356, 357–358, 364
 for elderly—table, 357
 tables, 24
Meprobamate, 32, 147, 149, 251, 361

Mescaline, 27, 161, 162; *see also*
    Hallucinogens
Metaraminol, 65
Methacholine, 27
Methadone, 62, 141, 145, 146, 147, 154
    detoxification—table, 146
Methamphetamine, 155, 156; *see also*
    Amphetamines
Methaqualone, 147, 148
Methylphenidate, 154, 155
Methyprylon, 147, 149
Milieu therapy, 222
Minocycline, 280
Minor abstinence syndrome, *see* specific
    agents
Mitral valve prolapse syndrome, 247, 254–
    255; *see also* Panic disorder
Mobile crisis units, *see* Crisis units; Home
    visiting services; Outreach
Monoamine oxidase inhibitors (MAOI), 66,
    221, 241, 242, 247–248, 251, 252, 254–
    255, 360
    restrictions—table, 70
Mood, 22, 24, 85, 220, 224, 316; *see also*
    Mental status examination
Morphine, 141–142, 145
Multiple personality, 237
Multiple sclerosis, 257, 361
Muscarinic blockade, 27
Myocardial infarction, 34, 355, 359, 360

Naloxone (Narcan), 34, 62, 143–144
Narcissistic personality disorder, 85, 88, 427,
    429
Narcolepsy, 154
Nausea, 134, 142, 144, 152, 162
Needle tracks, 143
Neglect, *see* Child neglect
Negligence, 38, 53, 56
Neuroleptic malignant syndrome, 64
Neuroleptization, rapid, 30, 31; *see also*
    Haloperidol
    table, 30
Neurotic depression, *see* Depression;
    Dysthymic disorder
Nightmares, 274, 275
Norepinephrine, 151, 155, 156, 161
Normal pressure hydrocephalus, 361
Nortriptyline, 246; *see also* Antidepressant
    agents
Nystagmus, 25, 26, 150, 153, 166, 182, 202

Obesity, 155
Obsession, 299, 334
Obsessive–compulsive disorder, 240

O'Connor vs. Donaldson, 49–50
Oculogyric crisis, 183; *see also* Acute
    dystonia
Operant shaping, 12, 15; *see also* Behavior
    therapy
Opiates, 62, 141–147, 143, 144, 155, 251; *see
    also* specific agents
Opisthotonus, 183; *see also* Acute dystonia
Organic causes of psychosis, 207; *see also*
    specific toxic agents
    table, 207
Organic disorders, 9, 23–24, 30, 62, 65, 84,
    85, 86, 89, 91, 197, 202, 203, 206, 209,
    220, 221, 225, 227, 234, 256, 310, 326,
    327, 355, 356–358, 387
Orientation, 23, 24, 25, 122, 133, 134, 150,
    152, 163, 166, 190, 201, 227, 256, 308,
    351, 357; *see also* Mental status
    examination
Out-of-control behavior, 21, 25, 61–63, 83, 86;
    see also Physical restraint; Violence
Outreach, 200, 395, 385; *see also* Home
    visiting services
Overdose, 34–35, 97, 109, 114, 119, 143, 149,
    151, 320, 321, 381; *see also* specific
    agents; Suicide
Oxazepam, 66, 67, 148, 363; *see also*
    Benzodiazepines

Pancreatitis, 137
Panic, 62, 68, 77, 129, 163–164, 170, 172, 203,
    224, 233, 237, 239, 240–241, 242, 245,
    246, 312, 342, 345, 364, 376, 380; *see also*
    Anxiety; Hallucinogens;
    Imipramine
Pap smear, 279
Paraldehyde, 147
Paranoia, 26, 85, 88, 100, 123, 133, 150, 160,
    162, 163, 165, 170, 172, 197, 206, 355, 366
Parens patriae, 48, 55
Parkinson's syndrome, 184, 185–188, 361; *see
    also* Bradykinesia; Rigidity; Tremor
Partial hospitalization, 109; *see also*
    Hospitalization
Penicillin, 280
Pentobarbital, 33, 62, 148, 149; *see also*
    Barbiturates
    tolerance test, 152–154
Personality disorders, 87, 88, 94, 100, 101,
    229, 233, 237; *see also* specific types
Peyote cactus, *see* Mescaline
Pharmacokinetics, *see* specific agents
Phencyclidine (PCP) 22, 25, 27, 30, 62, 161,
    165–168, 175, 197, 198, 206, 251, 331
    psychosis, 160, 206–207, 208, 213

Phenelzine, 246–247; *see also* Monoamine Oxidase inhibitors; Panic disorder
Phenobarbital, 33, 62, 148, 151, 153–154; *see also* Barbiturates
Phenothiazines, 26, 29, 34, 62, 64, 70, 137, 165, 190; *see also* Antipsychotic agents; specific agents
Phenytoin, 32, 135, 137, 154; *see also* Anticonvulsant agents
Pheochromocytoma, 251, 252
Phobias, 22, 224, 233, 240–242, 268, 274, 275, 299, 312, 334, 341, 389; *see also* specific phobias
Photosensitivity, 64
Physical abuse, *see* Child abuse; Child Neglect
Physical examination, 23, 31, 61, 63, 185, 202, 221, 235, 238, 278, 289; *see also* Vital signs
Physical neglect, *see* Child abuse; Child neglect
Physical restraint, 23, 25, 28–29, 48–49, 51, 52, 61, 63, 89, 93, 167, 196, 211
    table, 28
Physostigmine salicylate, 27, 34, 92, 190–191; *see also* Anticholinergic effects/syndrome
Pilocarpine, 27
Play therapy, 307–308
Pneumonia, 135, 150, 226, 360
Polypharmacy, 69
Post-traumatic stress disorder, 233, 237, 240, 242–243, 248–249, 265, 267, 268–269; *see also* Disasters
Postural hypotension, *see* Hypotension
Post-Vietnam syndrome, *see* Post-traumatic stress disorder
Prazepam, 67; *see also* Benzodiazepines
Pregnancy, 280, 287, 322, 329, 376, 387
Premarin, 281
Presuicidal syndrome, 103, 107, 108; *see also* Suicide
Primary prevention programs, 385, 386–387
Privacy, 37, 38, 40, 46, 56
Privilege, 45
Problem-solving, 11, 12, 268
Prochlorperazine, 183; *see also* Antipsychotic agents; Phenothiazines
Propranolol, 160, 191, 208, 226, 247, 254–255, 361
Proverbs, 357; *see also* Mental status examination
Pseudodementia, 25, 221, 227–228, 358
Pseudoemergencies, 311, 376–377; *see also* Depression; Elderly

Psilocybin, 27, 161, 162; *see also* Hallucinogens
Psychological testing, 227
Psychoses, 303, 304, 305, 311, 328, 330, 333, 336, 338, 346, 373, 375, 378, 401, 404, 417–418, 429; *see also* Depression; Mania; Schizoaffective disorder; Schizophrenia; specific drugs for toxic psychoses
    acute, 62, 63, 66, 77, 85, 92
    atypical, 26, 205–206
    brief reactive, 26, 63, 100, 205–206
    chronic, 62, 85, 92, 195–218
    functional, 21–22
    organic, 21–22, 26, 87, 89, 93, 106, 108, 162, 165, 172, 207, 228, 234, 236–237, 242
Psychosocial network, *see* Support network
Psychosocial stressor, 65, 88, 89
Psychotherapies, 3, 4–8, 11, 12, 14, 15–16, 72, 76, 79, 91, 94–95, 107, 138, 146, 175, 223, 229, 239, 242, 246, 248, 249, 324, 363, 365; *see also* Counseling; Crisis intervention; Emergency psychotherapy; Short-term psychotherapy
    concurrent, 14, 15–16, 72, 76, 79
    crisis, 373–382
Psychotomimetics, *see* Hallucinogens
Pulmonary edema, 143, 150
    emboli, 256, 360
Pupils, 23, 24, 26, 27, 61, 142, 143, 149, 150, 162, 166, 190, 202
Pyridostigmine, 190; *see also* Anticholinergic effects/syndrome

Rabbit syndrome, 186
Rape, 65, 242, 244, 261, 271–283, 309, 311, 325, 386–387, 407, 413; *see also* Crisis; Situational crises
    protocols, 277–282
    trauma syndrome, 273–276, 387
Rapid neuroleptization, *see* Haloperidol; Neuroleptization
Reality-testing, 16, 21, 197, 210, 214–215, 237
Recoil phase, 262, 265, 275; *see also* Crisis, phases
Regression, 80, 103, 211
Rehabilitation, 138, 146, 384, 388
Reorganization phase, 261–262, 275–276; *see also* Crisis, phases
Repeaters, 14–15, 76, 78, 229
Resource poor areas, *see* Rural communities
Restraint, 330, 355, 356, 381, 403; *see also* Physical restraint
Retirement, 244, 353
Right to refuse treatment, 50–53, 57

Right to treatment, 49–50, 57
Rigidity, 166, 185, 186; *see also* Parkinson's syndrome
Risk-rescue rating, 111, 119, 120; *see also* Suicide
Rogers vs. Commissioner, 41, 51
Rogers vs. Okin, 42, 43, 44, 57
Rum fits, 134, 136–137; *see also* Alcohol; Seizures
Runaway, 299, 303, 304, 310, 311, 316, 322, 337–340
Rural communities, 393–399
 resource poor areas—tables, 394, 395

Samaritans, 407, 409; *see also* Telephone
Scales, suicide rating
 hopelessness, 115
 ideation, 112
 intent, 116
 Los Angeles, 122
 risk-rescue, 119
 Tuckman–Youngman, 121
Schizoaffective disorder, 87, 205, 221, 228
Schizophrenia, 25, 26, 63, 83, 85, 87, 92, 94, 100, 157, 163, 168, 188, 189, 203–204, 221, 228, 233, 327, 329, 356, 367; *see also* Psychoses
School phobia, *see* Phobias; School refusal
School refusal, 240, 303, 304, 311, 340–346
Secobarbital, 148; *see also* Barbiturates
Secondary prevention programs, 385, 387–388
Sedative-hypnotics, *see* specific agents
Seizures, 64, 86, 92, 136–137, 138, 148, 149, 152, 153, 156, 166, 167, 190, 251, 256, 277, 329, 330, 361; *see also* Rum fits; specific drugs; Temporal lobe epilepsy
Self-neglect, 21, 219, 222
Sexual abuse, *see* Child abuse; Child neglect; Rape
Short-term psychotherapy, 5, 11, 16, 94; *see also* Counseling; Crisis intervention; Emergency psychotherapy
Simple phobia, 240, 241–242; *see also* Phobias
Situational crises, 9–10, 65, 91, 104, 261–262, 386–387, 401; *see also* Disasters; Rape
Sleep disturbances, *see* Depression; Hypersomnia; Insomnia; Nightmares
Social phobia, 240, 241–242; *see also* Phobias
Social supports, *see* Support network
Sodium amytal interview, 238
Somatization disorder, 236, 239
Standards of care, 53–54
Stealing, 316, 334, 336
Stimulants, *see* specific agents
"STP," 27, 162; *see also* Hallucinogens

Stress response, 221
Subdural hematoma, 361
Substance abuse, 86, 122, 141–179, 290, 361, 374, 429; *see also* specific agents
Suicide, 219, 220, 222, 228, 229, 237, 287, 289, 303, 304, 306, 311, 312, 363, 365–366, 374, 375, 380, 382, 395, 404, 412, 420, 427, 428; *see also* Overdose
 attempts, 32–33, 34, 98, 101, 104, 120–121, 150
 demographics—table, 99
 hopelessness scale, 111, 114, 115
 ideas, 98
 ideation scale, 111, 112, 114
 in children and adolescents, 314–325, 331, 336
 intent scale, 111, 114, 116–118
 legal issues, 54–56
 potential/treatment—table, 107
 prevention, 385, 407, 408
 rates—table, 121
 toxic drugs in suicide—table, 32
Support networks, 7, 9, 14, 78, 85, 102–103, 107, 111, 200, 221, 229, 267, 287, 291, 294, 324, 362, 365, 387, 396, 417, 418, 419, 420, 422, 425, 426
Sympathomimetics, *see* Amphetamine; Cocaine
Systems therapy, 5, 421, 385; *see also* Family, therapy

Tachycardia, 134, 138, 144, 152, 160, 172, 234, 240, 258
Tarasoff decision, 45
Tardive dyskinesia, 188–189
Telephone, 110, 293, 377, 379, 380, 385, 397, 403, 407–415, protocol, 412, 428; *see also* Hotlines
Temazepam, 68; *see also* Benzodiazepines
Temper tantrums, 328
Temporal lobe epilepsy, 25, 87, 207, 256–257, 329
Tertiary prevention programs, 388, 389
Tetany, 236
Tetracycline, 280
THC, *see* Marijuana
Therapeutic alliance, *see* Therapeutic relationship
Therapeutic communities, 146, 147, 174
Therapeutic relationship, 6, 10, 11, 16, 71–72, 75, 106, 107–108, 111, 195, 213–214, 224, 225, 297, 324, 339, 353–354, 363, 376, 381, 382, 402, 409, 421, 429, 432; *see also* Countertransference; Transference

Thiamine, 62, 133, 135, 207, 212, 360; *see also* Alcohol

Thioridazine, 33, 64, 183, 190, 359, 363; *see also* Antipsychotic agents; Phenothiazines

Thiothixene (Navane), 29, 64; *see also* Antipsychotic agents

Thioxanthenes, 64

Thought content, *see* Mental status examination

Thought disorder, *see* Delusions; Hallucinations; Psychoses; Schizophrenia

Thought flow, *see* Mental status examination

Tolerance, 149; *see also* specific agents

Toluene, *see* Inhalants

Toxic psychosis; *see also* Delirium; Organic disorders; Psychosis; specific agents
toxic drugs in suicide—table, 32
toxic states, management—table, 182

Toxic screen, 202, 235

Training, 389–390

Transference, 15, 16, 17, 72, 75, 76, 77, 78, 79, 109, 324, 374, 430, 432; *see also* Countertransference; Therapeutic relationship

Treatment alliance, *see* Therapeutic relationship; Transference

Treatment planning, 7, 12–14, 86, 107, 110, 214–217, 222; *see also* specific disorders

Tremor, 144, 150, 153, 155, 162, 181, 185

Triage, 8, 354–355, 385–386, 387, 425, 426

Trifluoperazine, 33, 64, 133, 212; *see also* Antipsychotic agents; Phenothiazines

Trihexyphenidyl, 65, 186, 187, 188; *see also* Antiparkinson agents

Truancy, 322, 328, 340, 341

Tyramine, 70

Uremia, 360

Vasopressors, 34

Venereal disease, 280

Violence, 22, 25, 29, 83–95, 145, 156, 165, 168, 197–198, 243, 285–292, 305, 306, 311, 325–332, 355, 363, 373–374, 375, 380, 381, 382, 395, 397, 403, 404; *see also* Battered women; Child abuse; Dangerousness; Domestic violence; Physical restraint
antisocial or aggressive behavior—table, 85
pharmacological treatment of violence—table, 92

Vital signs, 23, 63, 135, 137, 182, 190, 202, 221, 222, 234; *see also* Physical examination

Vomiting, *see* Nausea

Weight problems, 220, 221, 224, 225, 227, 311; *see also* Anorexia nervosa; Obesity

Wernicke's disease, 62, 132, 133, 137, 202, 203, 207, 209, 212, 226, 360; *see also* Alcohol

Withdrawal, *see* specific agents

Wrist slashing, 100, 229, 230; *see also* Depression; Suicide

Date Due

SEP 2 8 1986			
OCT 1 2 1998			
FEB 2 4 1989			
NOV 2 1 1991			
DEC 0 9 1986			
OCT 2 3 1998			
OCT 2 9 1997			
DEC 0 3 1997			
NOV 1 0 1997			